T0259568

Undiagnosed and Rare Diseases in Children

Editors

ROBERT M. KLIEGMAN
BRETT J. BORDINI

PEDIATRIC CLINICS
OF NORTH AMERICA

www.pediatric.theclinics.com

Consulting Editor
BONITA F. STANTON

February 2017 • Volume 64 • Number 1

ELSEVIER

1600 John F. Kennedy Boulevard • Suite 1800 • Philadelphia, Pennsylvania, 19103-2899

http://www.theclinics.com

THE PEDIATRIC CLINICS OF NORTH AMERICA Volume 64, Number 1
February 2017 ISSN 0031-3955, ISBN-13: 978-0-323-49671-1

Editor: Kerry Holland
Developmental Editor: Casey Potter

© **2017 Elsevier Inc. All rights reserved.**

This periodical and the individual contributions contained in it are protected under copyright by Elsevier, and the following terms and conditions apply to their use:

Photocopying

Single photocopies of single articles may be made for personal use as allowed by national copyright laws. Permission of the Publisher and payment of a fee is required for all other photocopying, including multiple or systematic copying, copying for advertising or promotional purposes, resale, and all forms of document delivery. Special rates are available for educational institutions that wish to make photocopies for non-profit educational classroom use. For information on how to seek permission visit www.elsevier.com/permissions or call: (+44) 1865 843830 (UK)/(+1) 215 239 3804 (USA).

Derivative Works

Subscribers may reproduce tables of contents or prepare lists of articles including abstracts for internal circulation within their institutions. Permission of the Publisher is required for resale or distribution outside the institution. Permission of the Publisher is required for all other derivative works, including compilations and translations (please consult www.elsevier.com/permissions).

Electronic Storage or Usage

Permission of the Publisher is required to store or use electronically any material contained in this periodical, including any article or part of an article (please consult www.elsevier.com/permissions). Except as outlined above, no part of this publication may be reproduced, stored in a retrieval system or transmitted in any form or by any means, electronic, mechanical, photocopying, recording or otherwise, without prior written permission of the Publisher.

Notice

No responsibility is assumed by the Publisher for any injury and/or damage to persons or property as a matter of products liability, negligence or otherwise, or from any use or operation of any methods, products, instructions or ideas contained in the material herein. Because of rapid advances in the medical sciences, in particular, independent verification of diagnoses and drug dosages should be made.

Although all advertising material is expected to conform to ethical (medical) standards, inclusion in this publication does not constitute a guarantee or endorsement of the quality or value of such product or of the claims made of it by its manufacturer.

The Pediatric Clinics of North America (ISSN 0031-3955) is published bimonthly by Elsevier Inc., 360 Park Avenue South, New York, New York 10010-1710. Months of issue are February, April, June, August, October, and December. Periodicals postage paid at New York, NY and additional mailing offices. Subscription prices are $208.00 per year (US individuals), $589.00 per year (US institutions), $281.00 per year (Canadian individuals), $784.00 per year (Canadian institutions), $338.00 per year (international individuals), $784.00 per year (international institutions), $100.00 per year (US students and residents), and $165.00 per year (international and Canadian residents and students). To receive students/resident rare, orders must be accompanied by name of affiliated institution, date of term, and the signature of program/residency coordinator on institution letterhead. Orders will be billed at individual rate until proof of status is received. Foreign air speed delivery is included in all Clinics subscription prices. All prices are subject to change without notice. **POSTMASTER:** Send address changes to The Pediatric Clinics of North America, Elsevier Health Sciences Division, Subscription Customer Service, 3251 Riverport Lane, Maryland Heights, MO 63043. **Customer Service: 1-800-654-2452 (US and Canada). From outside of the US and Canada: 1-314-447-8871. Fax: 1-314-447-8029. For print support, E-mail: JournalsCustomerService-usa@elsevier.com. For online support, E-mail: JournalsOnlineSupport-usa@elsevier.com.**

Reprints. For copies of 100 or more, of articles in this publication, please contact the Commercial Reprints Department, Elsevier Inc., 360 Park Avenue South, New York, NY 10010-1710. Tel.: 212-633-3874; Fax: 212-633-3820; E-mail: reprints@elsevier.com.

The Pediatric Clinics of North America is also published in Spanish by McGraw-Hill Inter-americana Editores S.A., Mexico City, Mexico; in Portuguese by Riechmann and Affonso Editores, Rua Comandante Coelho 1085, CEP 21250, Rio de Janeiro, Brazil; and in Greek by Althayia SA, Athens, Greece.

The Pediatric Clinics of North America is covered in MEDLINE/PubMed (Index Medicus), Excerpta Medica, Current Contents, Current Contents/Clinical Medicine, Science Citation Index, ASCA, ISI/BIOMED, and BIOSIS.

PROGRAM OBJECTIVE
The goal of the *Pediatric Clinics of North America* is to keep practicing physicians and residents up to date with current clinical practice in pediatrics by providing timely articles reviewing the state-of-the-art in patient care.

TARGET AUDIENCE
All practicing pediatricians, physicians and healthcare professionals who provide patient care to pediatric patients.

LEARNING OBJECTIVES
Upon completion of this activity, participants will be able to:
1. Review common errors in the diagnosis of rare childhood diseases.
2. Discuss the presentation and diagnosis of rare childhood diseases.
3. Recognize how family education, counselling, and a team-based approach can impact the diagnosis and management of rare childhood diseases.

ACCREDITATION
The Elsevier Office of Continuing Medical Education (EOCME) is accredited by the Accreditation Council for Continuing Medical Education (ACCME) to provide continuing medical education for physicians.

The EOCME designates this enduring material for a maximum of 15 *AMA PRA Category 1 Credit*(s)™. Physicians should claim only the credit commensurate with the extent of their participation in the activity.

All other health care professionals requesting continuing education credit for this enduring material will be issued a certificate of participation.

DISCLOSURE OF CONFLICTS OF INTEREST
The EOCME assesses conflict of interest with its instructors, faculty, planners, and other individuals who are in a position to control the content of CME activities. All relevant conflicts of interest that are identified are thoroughly vetted by EOCME for fair balance, scientific objectivity, and patient care recommendations. EOCME is committed to providing its learners with CME activities that promote improvements or quality in healthcare and not a specific proprietary business or a commercial interest.

The planning committee, staff, authors and editors listed below have identified no financial relationships or relationships to products or devices they or their spouse/life partner have with commercial interest related to the content of this CME activity:
Donald Basel, MBBCh, FACMG; Brett J. Bordini, MD; Shanmuganathan Chandrakasan, MD; Yvonne E. Chiu, MD; Michael J. Chusid, MD; Dominic O. Co, MD, PhD; Craig Erker, MD; Anjali Fortna; John B. Gordon, MD; Paul Harker-Murray, MD, PhD; Kerry Holland; Debra Jablonski, RN; Robert M. Kliegman, MD; Subra Kugathasan, MD; Indu Kumari; Molly Marquardt Smith, BA; Julie McCarrier, MS, CGC; Priya Monrad, MD; James J. Nocton, MD; Hillary W. Petska, MD, MPH; John M. Routes, MD; Barbara E. Ruggeri, MLIS; Lynn K. Sheets, MD; Mark D. Simms, MD, MPH; Bonita F. Stanton, MD; Megan Suermann; Julie-An Talano, MD; Suresh Venkateswaran, PhD; James W. Verbsky, MD, PhD; Molly J. Youssef, MD.

The planning committee, staff, authors and editors listed below have identified financial relationships or relationships to products or devices they or their spouse/life partner have with commercial interest related to the content of this CME activity:
Gisela Chelimsky, MD's spouse is a consultant/advisor for Lundbeck and Ironwood Pharmaceuticals, Inc.
Thomas Chelimsky, MD is a consultant/advisor for Lundbeck and Ironwood Pharmaceuticals, Inc.
David P. Dimmock, MD is a consultant/advisor for BioMarin; Audentes Therapeutics; and Complete Genomics Incorporated, and has research support from Demeter Therapeutics; Genzyme Corporation, a Sanofi Company; Shire, BioMarin; and Cytonet, acquired by Promethera Biosciences.
Christopher Inglese, MD is on the speakers' bureau for Lundbeck.
Michael W. Lawlor, MD, PhD is a consultant/advisor for Audentes Therapeutics and Guidepoint Global, LLC, and has research support from Audentes Therapeutics; Solid BioSciences; A Foundation Building Strength; and Demeter Therapeutics.
Arthur B. Meyers, MD receives royalties/patents from Elsevier.

UNAPPROVED/OFF-LABEL USE DISCLOSURE
The EOCME requires CME faculty to disclose to the participants:

1. When products or procedures being discussed are off-label, unlabelled, experimental, and/or investigational (not US Food and Drug Administration [FDA] approved); and
2. Any limitations on the information presented, such as data that are preliminary or that represent ongoing research, interim analyses, and/or unsupported opinions. Faculty may discuss information about pharmaceutical agents that is outside of FDA-approved labelling. This information is intended solely for CME and is not intended to promote off-label use of these medications. If you have any questions, contact the medical affairs department of the manufacturer for the most recent prescribing information.

TO ENROLL

To enroll in the *Pediatric Clinics of North America* Continuing Medical Education program, call customer service at 1-800-654-2452 or sign up online at http://www.theclinics.com/home/cme. The CME program is available to subscribers for an additional annual fee of USD 290.

METHOD OF PARTICIPATION

In order to claim credit, participants must complete the following:
1. Complete enrolment as indicated above.
2. Read the activity.
3. Complete the CME Test and Evaluation. Participants must achieve a score of 70% on the test. All CME Tests and Evaluations must be completed online.

CME INQUIRIES/SPECIAL NEEDS

For all CME inquiries or special needs, please contact elsevierCME@elsevier.com.

Contributors

CONSULTING EDITOR

BONITA F. STANTON, MD
Founding Dean, School of Medicine, Professor of Pediatrics, Seton Hall University, South Orange, New Jersey

EDITORS

ROBERT M. KLIEGMAN, MD
Professor and Chair Emeritus, Department of Pediatrics, Medical College of Wisconsin, Children's Hospital of Wisconsin, Milwaukee, Wisconsin

BRETT J. BORDINI, MD
Assistant Professor, Department of Pediatrics, Section of Hospital Medicine, Nelson Service for Undiagnosed and Rare Diseases, Children's Hospital of Wisconsin, Medical College of Wisconsin, Milwaukee, Wisconsin

AUTHORS

DONALD BASEL, MBBCh, FACMG
Associate Professor, Chief of Genetics, Department of Pediatrics, Medical College of Wisconsin, Children's Hospital of Wisconsin, Milwaukee, Wisconsin

BRETT J. BORDINI, MD
Assistant Professor, Department of Pediatrics, Section of Hospital Medicine, Nelson Service for Undiagnosed and Rare Diseases, Children's Hospital of Wisconsin, Medical College of Wisconsin, Milwaukee, Wisconsin

SHANMUGANATHAN CHANDRAKASAN, MD
Assistant Professor, Department of Pediatrics, Division of Hematology, Oncology and BMT, Emory University School of Medicine and Children's Healthcare of Atlanta, Atlanta, Georgia

GISELA CHELIMSKY, MD
Division of Pediatric Gastroenterology, Department of Pediatrics, Medical College of Wisconsin, Milwaukee, Wisconsin

THOMAS CHELIMSKY, MD
Department of Neurology, Medical College of Wisconsin, Milwaukee, Wisconsin

YVONNE E. CHIU, MD
Associate Professor, Section of Pediatric Dermatology, Department of Dermatology; Department of Pediatrics, Medical College of Wisconsin, Milwaukee, Wisconsin

MICHAEL J. CHUSID, MD
Professor, Infectious Diseases, Department of Pediatrics, Medical College of Wisconsin, Wauwatosa, Wisconsin

DOMINIC O. CO, MD, PhD
Assistant Professor, Section of Pediatric Rheumatology, Department of Pediatrics, Medical College of Wisconsin, Milwaukee, Wisconsin

DAVID P. DIMMOCK, MD
Associate Professor, Division of Genetics, Department of Pediatrics, Human Molecular Genetics Center, Medical College of Wisconsin, Milwaukee, Wisconsin

CRAIG ERKER, MD
Instructor, Division of Pediatric Hematology/Oncology/Blood and Marrow Transplant, Medical College of Wisconsin, Milwaukee, Wisconsin

JOHN B. GORDON, MD
Children's Hospital of Wisconsin, Professor, Medical College of Wisconsin, Milwaukee, Wisconsin

PAUL HARKER-MURRAY, MD, PhD
Assistant Professor, Division of Pediatric Hematology/Oncology/Blood and Marrow Transplant, Medical College of Wisconsin, Milwaukee, Wisconsin

CHRISTOPHER INGLESE, MD
Associate Professor, Section of Pediatric Neurology, Department of Neurology, Medical College of Wisconsin, Milwaukee, Wisconsin

DEBRA JABLONSKI, RN
Children's Hospital of Wisconsin, Milwaukee, Wisconsin

ROBERT M. KLIEGMAN, MD
Professor and Chair Emeritus, Department of Pediatrics, Medical College of Wisconsin, Children's Hospital of Wisconsin, Milwaukee, Wisconsin

SUBRA KUGATHASAN, MD
Professor of Pediatrics and Human Genetics, Department of Pediatrics, Division of Gastroenterology; Emory University School of Medicine and Children's Health Care of Atlanta, Atlanta, Georgia

MICHAEL W. LAWLOR, MD, PhD
Associate Professor, Division of Pediatric Pathology, Department of Pathology and Laboratory Medicine, Neuroscience Research Center, Medical College of Wisconsin, Milwaukee, Wisconsin

JULIE McCARRIER, MS, CGC
Medical College of Wisconsin, Children's Hospital of Wisconsin, Milwaukee, Wisconsin

ARTHUR B. MEYERS, MD
Associate Professor of Radiology, University of Central Florida College of Medicine, Orlando, Florida

PRIYA MONRAD, MD
Assistant Professor, Department of Child and Adolescent Neurology, Medical College of Wisconsin, Milwaukee, Wisconsin

JAMES J. NOCTON, MD
Professor, Department of Pediatrics, Medical College of Wisconsin, Pediatric Rheumatologist, Children's Hospital of Wisconsin, Milwaukee, Wisconsin

HILLARY W. PETSKA, MD, MPH
Children's Hospital of Wisconsin, Assistant Professor, Medical College of Wisconsin, Milwaukee, Wisconsin

JOHN M. ROUTES, MD
Professor, Department of Pediatrics, Children's Research Institute, Medical College of Wisconsin, Milwaukee, Wisconsin

BARBARA E. RUGGERI, MLIS
Clinical Services Librarian, Medical College of Wisconsin, Children's Hospital of Wisconsin, Milwaukee, Wisconsin

LYNN K. SHEETS, MD
Children's Hospital of Wisconsin, Professor, Medical College of Wisconsin, Milwaukee, Wisconsin

MARK D. SIMMS, MD, MPH
Professor and Chief, Section of Developmental Pediatrics, Department of Pediatrics, Medical College of Wisconsin; Medical Director, Child Development Center, Children's Hospital of Wisconsin, Milwaukee, Wisconsin

MOLLY MARQUARDT SMITH, BA
Department of Pediatrics, Medical College of Wisconsin; Access Center Supervisor, Children's Hospital of Wisconsin, Milwaukee, Wisconsin

JULIE-AN TALANO, MD
Associate Professor, Division of Pediatric Hematology/Oncology/Blood and Marrow Transplant, Medical College of Wisconsin, Milwaukee, Wisconsin

SURESH VENKATESWARAN, PhD
Research Associate, Department of Pediatrics, Division of Pediatric Gastroenterology; Emory University School of Medicine, Atlanta, Georgia

JAMES W. VERBSKY, MD, PhD
Associate Professor of Pediatrics and Microbiology/Molecular Genetics, Pediatric Rheumatology, Medical College of Wisconsin, Milwaukee, Wisconsin

MOLLY J. YOUSSEF, MD
Resident, Department of Dermatology, Medical College of Wisconsin, Milwaukee, Wisconsin

Contents

> The scientific process of analysis and deduction is frequently, often subconsciously, used by physicians to develop a differential diagnosis based on patients' symptoms. Common disorders are most frequently diagnosed in general practice. Rare diseases are uncommon and frequently remain undiagnosed for many years. Cognitive errors in clinical judgment delay definitive diagnosis. Whole-exome sequencing has helped identify the cause of undiagnosed or rare diseases in up to 40% of children. This article provides experiences with an undiagnosed or rare disease program, where detailed data accumulation and a multifaceted analytical approach assisted in diagnosing atypical presentations of common disorders.

> Patients with undiagnosed or rare diseases often remain without a diagnosis for many years. Many are misdiagnosed or treated symptomatically without having an identified underlying disease process. Health care providers in general practice and subspecialists are equipped to diagnose diseases commonly seen. Most practitioners are unlikely to be familiar with uncommon manifestations of a common disorder and have little or no experience with rare diseases. Multidisciplinary teams are effective in reviewing patients with undiagnosed and rare diseases and in developing a new diagnostic strategy for appropriate evaluation. A medical librarian and an access coordinating navigator are essential members of the team.

> Although primary immunodeficiencies typically present with recurrent, chronic, or severe infections, autoimmune manifestations frequently accompany these disorders and may be the initial clinical manifestations. The presence of 2 or more autoimmune disorders, unusual severe atopic disease, or a combination of these disorders should lead a clinician to consider primary immunodeficiency disorders.

Most neurodevelopmental disorders are defined by their clinical symptoms and many disorders share common features. Recently there has been an increase in the number of children diagnosed with autism spectrum disorder, although concerns have been raised about the accuracy of the reported prevalence rates. This article reviews the essential features of autism spectrum disorder and describes other conditions that may include similar symptoms that may be misdiagnosed as autism spectrum disorder (primary communication disorders, anxiety disorders, attachment disorders, intellectual disability, vision and hearing impairment, and normal variations). An approach to differential diagnosis is discussed with particular attention to evaluation of young children.

This article discusses non-classical forms of inflammatory bowel disease (IBD) mainly occurs in infants and very young children. Defects in every aspect of the immune system, such as neutrophils, T-cell and B-cell lymphocytes, and macrophages are associated with IBD in infants. Also, non lympho-hematopoietic defects with primary defects in enterocytes can also lead to IBD-like manifestations. Clinical vignettes are presented and the genetic origins and possible management strategies are outlined. Early evaluation of these patients is important because identification of underlying immune defects would facilitate the use of better-targeted therapy for the specific genetic defect.

Mitochondrial disease (MD) occurs when alteration of mitochondrial respiratory chain complex function caused by genetic mutation produces a detectable disease state. These mutations may be found in either the nuclear or mitochondrial genomes, and may only be present in a subset of cells or body tissues. Thus, the phenotype of MD is extremely variable and the definitive diagnosis of MD is complex. This article provides a brief description of a strategy used in the diagnosis of MD, by integrating data from clinical, imaging, pathologic, molecular, and enzymatic assessments. Additional information on characteristic findings seen in classic MD syndromes is also provided.

Structural autonomic disorders (producing structural damage to the autonomic nervous system or autonomic centers) are far less common than functional autonomic disorders (reflected in abnormal function of a fundamentally normal autonomic nervous system) in children and teenagers. This article focuses on this uncommon first group in the pediatric clinic. These disorders are grouped into 2 main categories: those characterized by hypoventilation and those that feature an autonomic neuropathy.

The idiopathic vasculitides are a group of inflammatory and immune-mediated conditions associated with inflammation of blood vessels. They affect multiple organ and body systems, and vary in their clinical manifestations, severity, prognosis, and pathology. They frequently present a diagnostic challenge for clinicians because of their complexity, overlapping features, and similar findings to other noninflammatory, genetic, or infectious conditions. This article summarizes some of the common pediatric vasculitides, emphasizing both the characteristic and unusual clinical manifestations of these diseases.

Childhood fever of unknown origin (FUO) is most often related to an underlying infection but can also be associated with a variety of neoplastic, rheumatologic, and inflammatory conditions. Repeated, focused reviews of patient history and physical examination are often helpful in suggesting a likely diagnosis. Diagnostic workup should be staged, usually leaving invasive testing for last. Advances in molecular genetic techniques have increased the importance of these assays in the diagnosis of FUO in children.

Differentiating Guillain-Barré syndrome (GBS) from inherited neuropathies and other acquired peripheral neuropathies requires understanding the atypical presentations of GBS and its variant forms, as well as historical and physical features suggestive of inherited neuropathies. GBS is typically characterized by the acute onset of ascending flaccid paralysis, areflexia, and dysesthesia secondary to peripheral nerve fiber demyelination. The disorder usually arises following a benign gastrointestinal or respiratory illness, is monophasic, reaches a nadir with several weeks, and responds to immunomodulatory therapy. Inherited neuropathies with onset before adulthood, whose presentation may mimic Guillain-Barré syndrome, are reviewed.

Children with medical complexity and victims of medical child abuse may have similar clinical presentations. Atypical or unexplained signs and symptoms due to rare diseases may lead providers to suspect medical child abuse when not present. Conversely, medical child abuse may be the cause of or coexist with medical complexity. Careful consideration of whether or not medical child abuse is present is essential when assessing a child with medical complexity since either diagnosis has significant consequences for children and families.

Genomic sequencing is the diagnostic test of choice for families with undiagnosed or rare diseases seeking an explanation for their child's complex medical concerns. The desire to find answers can easily bias interpretation of sequencing results, and thus the counseling process is designed to facilitate informed decision making and set realistic expectations for possible outcomes. The patient case examples serve to highlight the various challenges and complexities encountered with the clinical application of genomic sequencing and to reflect some of the data that has been accrued during the past 5 years of clinical experience.

PEDIATRIC CLINICS OF NORTH AMERICA

THE CLINICS ARE AVAILABLE ONLINE!
Access your subscription at:
www.theclinics.com

Foreword

Undiagnosed and Rare Childhood Diseases

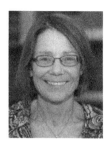

Bonita F. Stanton, MD
Consulting Editor

As medical students and residents, we quickly gain experience and begin to recognize common disorders in our patients, and gradually, unusual manifestations of common disorders. Over time, as maturing pediatricians, we learn about and recognize uncommon disorders among the children for whom we care.

And then one day, we come across a problem that we believe we have never before encountered—and are not sure we have even read about it. Or, we read about a disorder that we think we have never seen—and realize that we have seen it in one or more of our patients—but did not recognize it.

In this issue of *Pediatric Clinics of North America*, the authors present in a logical and clear fashion unusual forms of common disorders and uncommon conditions that may mimic more common diseases. All of these conditions are important to contemplate in our differential diagnoses, and the articles help us to organize our thinking in this regard.

I suspect that this issue will provide at least a few "ah-ha!" moments for each of us as we think about patients for whom we have cared over the years, especially those for whom no diagnosis seemed to fit quite right.

This issue will provide fascinating—and helpful—reading for every pediatrician.

Bonita F. Stanton, MD
School of Medicine
Seton Hall University
400 South Orange Avenue
South Orange, NJ 07079, USA

E-mail address:
bonita.stanton@shu.edu

Preface

Undiagnosed and Rare Diseases

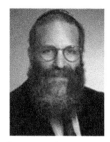
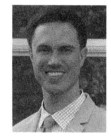

Robert M. Kliegman, MD   Brett J. Bordini, MD
Editors

The many and rapid advances in new disease discovery and advanced diagnostic testing in pediatric medicine have made it difficult for all practitioners to be kept current. In 1968, Gordon Avery described a highly lethal undifferentiated disorder, "intractable diarrhea of infancy"; in 2016, there are over 50 identifiable causes of an early onset and also potentially lethal inflammatory bowel disease-like syndrome.[1,2] Almost all practitioners have cared for children with chronic, progressive diseases that do not fit a common or definable diagnosis. Although symptoms are treated, the patients remain undiagnosed and often uncured. Unfortunately, symptomatic therapy for the wrong disease can lead to drug-related toxicities and the relentless progression of the undiagnosed disorder.

This issue of *Pediatric Clinics of North America* highlights the experience of a predominantly single center's program to help identify the disease cause of children whose parents have been on a diagnostic odyssey to discover the cause of their child's undiagnosed disease. Written from a clinical perspective, the authors have helped identify common cognitive diagnostic errors as well as suggestive diagnostic clues to help uncover the underlying disease process.

Because the Institute of Medicine has now highlighted the impact of diagnostic errors, we hope this issue will bring an informed awareness to clinicians by assisting them in avoiding diagnostic errors.[3] Furthermore, and of greater significance to our patients, we hope this issue also helps clinicians recognize unusual manifestations of common disorders as well as known features of rare diseases. These two categories represent the majority of undiagnosed diseases in children.

Robert M. Kliegman, MD
Department of Pediatrics
Medical College of Wisconsin
Children's Hospital of Wisconsin
Children's Corporate Center
999 North 92nd Street–Suite C450
Milwaukee, WI 53226, USA

Pediatr Clin N Am 64 (2017) xvii–xviii
http://dx.doi.org/10.1016/j.pcl.2016.10.002
0031-3955/17/© 2016 Published by Elsevier Inc.

pediatric.theclinics.com

Brett J. Bordini, MD
Department of Pediatrics
Medical College of Wisconsin
Children's Hospital of Wisconsin
Children's Corporate Center
999 North 92nd Street–Suite C560
Milwaukee, WI 53226, USA

E-mail addresses:
rkliegma@mcw.edu (R.M. Kliegman)
bbordini@mcw.edu (B.J. Bordini)

REFERENCES

1. Avery GB, Villavicencio O, Lilly JR, et al. Intractable diarrhea in early infancy. Pediatrics 1968;41(4):712–22.
2. Grossman AB, Baldassano RN. Inflammatory bowel disease. In: Kliegman RM, Stanton BF, St Geme JW III, et al, editors. Nelson textbook of pediatrics. 20th edition. Philadelphia: Elsevier; 2016. p. 1819–31.
3. Balogh EP, Miller BT, Ball JR, editors. Committee on Diagnostic Error in Health Care; Board on Health Care Services; Institute of Medicine; The National Academies of Sciences, Engineering, and Medicine: Improving Diagnosis in Health Care. 2015. Available at: http://www.nap.edu/21794. Accessed September 1, 2016.

How Doctors Think

Common Diagnostic Errors in Clinical Judgment—Lessons from an Undiagnosed and Rare Disease Program

Robert M. Kliegman, MD*, Brett J. Bordini, MD,
Donald Basel, MBBCh, James J. Nocton, MD

KEYWORDS

- Undiagnosed or rare diseases (URDs) • Whole-exome sequencing • Misdiagnosis

KEY POINTS

- Patients who have been misdiagnosed or who remain undiagnosed may experience continued suffering or a progression in their disease, leading to potential disabilities and even preventable life-threatening complications.
- Misdiagnosis or lack of a specific diagnosis leads to unnecessary diagnostic testing and invasive procedures, which, in addition to increasing patient suffering and risking complications, add major costs to the health care system.
- Whole-exome sequencing (WES) is the diagnostic test of choice for children with undiagnosed or rare diseases (URDs) after traditional laboratory and imaging studies have not yielded a diagnosis.

Medicine is a science of uncertainty and an art of probability.

—*William Osler[1]*

DEFINING RARE AND UNDIAGNOSED DISEASES

A rare disease is defined in the United States as one affecting fewer than 200,000 patients; however, there are more individual rare diseases than there are common diseases, cumulatively affecting more than 25 million people.[2,3] Nonetheless, health care providers are more likely to see patients within the narrower spectrum of highly prevalent common diseases than they are to encounter patients with a much less prevalent individual rare disease. Although some rare diseases, such as Huntington chorea, may have characteristic findings that facilitate diagnosis, the presenting

Department of Pediatrics, Medical College of Wisconsin, Children's Hospital of Wisconsin, 999 North 92nd Street, Suite C450, Milwaukee, WI 53226, USA
* Corresponding author. Children's Corporate Center, Children's Hospital of Wisconsin, 999 North 92nd Street, Suite C450, Milwaukee, WI 53226.
E-mail address: rkliegma@mcw.edu

Pediatr Clin N Am 64 (2017) 1–15
http://dx.doi.org/10.1016/j.pcl.2016.08.002
0031-3955/17/© 2016 Elsevier Inc. All rights reserved.

pediatric.theclinics.com

manifestations of rare diseases are often nonspecific, such as weight loss, weakness, fatigue, or fever. When signs and symptoms are nonspecific, initial diagnostic impressions may favor diseases seen commonly within the scope of a practice, leading many rare diseases to be initially misdiagnosed or to remain undiagnosed.

Many but not all patients with an undiagnosed disease have a rare disease. Both common and rare diseases may present atypically and remain undiagnosed for weeks to decades despite multiple subspecialist consultations and extensive laboratory and imaging studies. Given that both common and rare diseases may remain undiagnosed despite these evaluations, classifying a disease as "undiagnosed" is challenging. Time is an imperfect criterion, because symptoms may remain incomplete and static or may evolve over a prolonged period. Furthermore, nonspecific signs or symptoms of a rare disease may truncate the evaluation process if they leave a health care provider with the impression of a more common disease. The perpetuation of incomplete or inaccurate diagnostic labels may lead to an inability to alter the course of a diagnostic evaluation and to significant delays in appropriate diagnosis and therapy. Complexity is an imperfect criterion as well, because some undiagnosed diseases may be restricted to a single symptom or organ system, whereas others may have systemic manifestations necessitating evaluation and management by multiple specialties. Undiagnosed diseases may be analogous to the definition historically applied to patients with fever of unknown origin, which requires both the passage of a certain period of time as well as a progression from basic to more aggressive or even invasive diagnostic procedures. Some undiagnosed diseases may be as simple as an adolescent with 6 months of headache, eventually diagnosed with pseudotumor cerebri, or as complex as a child originally thought to have treatment-refractory chronic autoimmune demyelinating polyneuropathy, who was found 10 years after initial presentation to have a rare form of riboflavin transporter deficiency (**Table 1**).

THE CHALLENGES OF EVALUATING UNDIAGNOSED OR RARE DISEASES

Children with URDs have often been evaluated by individual subspecialists in medical centers across the country and have been on a diagnostic odyssey for many years or even decades. Delays in diagnosis are often multifactorial, although they may be categorized broadly as either inherent to the disease process or related to pitfalls in the diagnostic evaluation. Diagnostic pitfalls may be further classified as patient-specific, physician-specific, or related to limitations in various diagnostic modalities. In many ways, the structure of the health system promotes these diagnostic pitfalls, because individual expertise and practice are promoted. The cognitive process of an experienced clinician often relies on experience and gut instincts or on disease pattern recognition to formulate a diagnosis. Thus, despite adherence to a rigid scientific methodology of data collection, analysis, and deductive inference, the prioritization and interpretation of data ultimately rely on that individual expert opinion and are subject to individual bias or error. The development of a URD program, in which a core of experienced clinicians collaborate with relevant subspecialists, mitigates many of these individual biases and ensures a more rigorous application of the scientific method when analyzing available data.

Disease-specific Factors

One reason for delayed diagnosis is the all-too-true aphorism, "diseases do not read the textbook." For example, patients with endocarditis rarely have all or any of the classic physical findings associated with this disease.[4] Some patients with periodic fever syndromes or other autoinflammatory diseases may not have fever, individuals

Table 1
Examples of undiagnosed diseases

Initial Diagnosis/Manifestation	Final Diagnosis
Neurologic	
Cardiomyopathy delayed myopathy	Myofibrillar myopathy
Late-onset autistic regression	Kleefstra syndrome
Autoimmune polyneuropathy	Riboflavin transporter deficiency
Laryngitis	Miller Fisher variant Guillain-Barré syndrome with vocal cord paralysis
Hypotonia	Nemeline myopathy
Siblings with neurodegenerative disorder	*NDUF10A* (mitochondrial complex 1)
Microcephaly, absent speech	*NDUFV3* mutation
Hypotonia	*LAMA* dystroglycanopathy
Seizures	*SCN2B* mutation
Inflammatory, immune, infectious, infiltrative	
IBD	XIAP
IBD	IPEX
Obstructive hydrocephalus	fHLH
Congenital infection	fHLH
Nonimmune hydrops	fHLH
Nonimmune hydrops	Congenital neuroblastoma
CRMO	LCH
Orbital cellulitis	LCH
Neonate with urticaria	NOMID
Rule out sepsis	Dengue fever
Rule out sepsis	Rat-bite fever
Pneumonia with effusion	Lymphoma
Recurrent lymphadenitis	ALPS
Evans syndrome	ALPS
Viral meningitis	Tuberculous meningitis
Pulmonary alveolar proteinosis	CD40 ligand deficiency
Arthritis	Hyper-IgD syndrome
Central nervous system vasculitis	ADA-2 deficiency
Interstitial lung disease	CGD
CVID	CTLA4 deficiency
Neutropenia	*GATA2* deficiency
Other	
Chronic fatigue syndrome	Addison disease
Hepatic failure	Citrin deficiency
Intestinal pseudo-obstruction	Intestinal leiomyositis
Anorexia nervosa	Celiac disease
Growing pains	Scurvy
Lymphedema, microphthalmia	Oculo-facial-digital syndrome
Cardiomyopathy	Semialdehyde dehydrogenase deficiency
Atypical HUS	*DGKE* mutation

(continued on next page)

Table 1 (*continued*)	
Initial Diagnosis/Manifestation	**Final Diagnosis**
Failure to thrive, increased respiratory effort	Marshall-Smith syndrome (*NFIX*)
SCID	*HDAC8*-associated Cornelia de Lange
Microphthalmia, high myopia, pigmentary choroidopathy	*EFTUD2* mutation
Intrauterine fetal demise	Coffin-Siris syndrome (*ARID1B*)
Hypermobility EDS	Noonan syndrome (*KRAS*)
Scoliosis, renal disease	Coffin-Siris syndrome (*ARID1B*)
Myopathy, hypotonia	Arterial toruosity syndrome

Abbreviations: ADA, adenosine deaminase; ALPS, autoimmune lymphoproliferative syndrome; CGD, chronic granulomatous disease; CRMO, chronic recurrent multifocal osteomyelitis; CVID, common variable immunodeficiency disease; EDS, Ehlers-Danlos syndrome; HUS, hemolytic uremic syndrome; IBD, inflammatory bowel disease; LCH, Langerhan cell histiocytosis; NOMID, neonatal-onset multisystem inflammatory disease; SCID, severe combined immunodeficiency disease; XIAP, X-linked inhibition of apoptosis.

with hyper–immunoglobulin D (IgD) syndrome may have normal levels of IgD, and hyperkalemia may be present in the classic hypokalemic form of Bartter syndrome. The great masqueraders of the past century—lupus, tuberculosis, and syphilis—still exist but have been joined by others, including hemophagocytic syndromes, periodic fever/autoinflammatory syndromes, neuroimmunologic diseases, and other autoimmune and immunodeficiency syndromes. In addition to having patients whose disease evolution and diagnostic evaluation have persisted for a prolonged time period, most large pediatric hospitals have cared for patients with URDs who have evaded a specific diagnosis in the early phase of their disease and who present acutely with a serious or catastrophic illness. In the authors' experience, these acutely ill patients represent approximately 15% to 20% of patients; they require immediate consultation as well as aggressive and rapid diagnostic evaluation.

Patient-specific Factors

Families of children with URD may be viewed with certain negative biases. They are often anxious from the persistence of their child's chronic undiagnosed medical illness. These families have often shared the diagnostic odyssey with multiple physicians and have reached a point where they are over-reporting the minutest details in hopes of discovering the clue or clues that will lead to a diagnosis. This may result in a diagnostician presented with an overwhelming amount of information, all of it seemingly equally important to the family, making it difficult to form an accurate representation of the child's signs and symptoms. There may be some suspicion on the part of health care providers that the information is even factitious and an effort to force further diagnostic testing. Parents and families may be perceived as doctor-shopping as part of their effort to find answers to their questions. In addition, because of unsatisfactory previous interactions with the health care system, these families may not always speak well of their past experiences. An attribution error from this negative stereotype may lead to an inappropriate diagnosis of Munchausen syndrome by proxy (also known as medical child abuse or factitious disorder by proxy). Although it is essential to be aware of this possibility, the diagnosis of Munchausen syndrome by proxy in a child with a URD should be considered and made in a manner identical to all other diagnoses considered: after careful review of all available information; consideration of the specific pattern and details of the signs, symptoms, laboratory, imaging, and other data; and deliberate and thoughtful conversations with the patient, family members, and all involved health care providers. This diagnosis should not be made prematurely or simply because nothing else fits.

Physician-specific Factors: Issues in Clinical Judgment

Two important maxims in the evaluation of children with URDs are to expect the unexpected and to never say never. During the evaluation of many patients, well-intended and often senior experts in their field have made statements like, "I have never seen this symptom in the proposed disease," "It cannot be this," and, even mistakenly, "It must be this." This appeal to authority often results in avoidable diagnostic errors. Despite evidence of convincing geographic clustering and the development of a preceding unusual rash in a majority of patients, the originally described patients with Lyme arthritis were most frequently misdiagnosed as having juvenile rheumatoid arthritis.[5] Statements like, "In my experience" or "We see this," are more authoritative than evidence based and eventually lead to a diagnostic momentum that excludes consideration of other disorders. Once a diagnosis is fixed in a medical record, in particularly a multiyear record, it is most often perpetuated, assumed to be correct, and difficult to question or rethink.

Appeals to authority can increase the tendency toward confirmation bias, in which the clinician seeks out only information that affirms a diagnosis and excludes facts that contradict the initial diagnosis. Atypical or new clinical findings may be a clue to the real diagnosis and should not be ignored. Overcoming confirmation bias is particularly problematic if a physician advocating for a particular diagnosis is a senior subspecialist recognized as an expert in the field, because it often prevents the entire team from considering other possible diseases. Even independent of appeals to authority, confirmation bias is detrimental to the diagnostic process because many URDs are atypical or uncommon manifestations of a common disease or are unrecognized manifestations of a rare disease. Always maintain a broad differential diagnosis and do not eliminate disorders from consideration solely because they initially do not seem to fit. On a busy hospital service or in a clinic setting, there may be a tendency to rule out a diagnosis too quickly. Once a diagnosis is incorrectly considered ruled out, it is difficult to rethink that diagnosis even in spite of evidence suggesting the excluded disease. Published clinical descriptions of diseases — in particular newly described diseases — tend to be biased in favor of the most commonly recognized manifestations and should be interpreted with caution. The true breadth of clinical manifestations of a specific disease may be much more extensive than suggested by descriptions in textbooks or in the literature. Recently, genomic testing has provided molecular evidence that many disorders exhibit greater clinical heterogeneity than previously appreciated. Always ask, "Do any of the features match what we know regarding a specific disease?" and "Could this be a condition I have seen before, but with a new or different clinical pattern?"

An attribution error in URDs occurs when minimizing signs, symptoms, or laboratory data. This is typified by the use of slight or slightly before describing an abnormality. Classically used by medical students who are unsure whether they hear a cardiac murmur or see a rash, when used by more experienced health care workers, the term, *slight*, may deemphasize an actual critical finding. Slight tachycardia should be stated as tachycardia if the heart rate is elevated above a normal range; the same is true for abnormal laboratory data. A sodium level of 150 mEq/L is elevated and abnormal; it may suggest a specific condition. These types of findings should not be overlooked in the child with an undiagnosed disease. Every symptom, every finding on the physical examination, and every discovery on laboratory testing and imaging should be considered potentially important clues that lead to a correct diagnosis.

Some children with URDs may appear seemingly healthy. Because many of the complaints of URDs may be vague or vexing, and because there is frequently considerable family anxiety regarding the lack of a diagnosis, the significance of the illness may not be appreciated or the parents may be thought of as over-reacting. This type of benign thinking is a type of affective error, where emotions may interfere with diagnostic judgment. "This child looks too well" or "Hoping for the good" or expecting that "Nothing really bad could be wrong with this child" clouds diagnostic decision making. Because most practitioners see common disorders on a day-to-day basis, they may miss the zebra among the horses. Because common diseases are common, a neutropenia may be assumed the result of viral suppression or drug induced, when a patient in fact has leukemia; a child presenting with tachypnea and fever initially diagnosed with pneumonia may have salicylate toxicity; or an athlete with prolonged knee pain initially diagnosed as a sprain may have osteogenic sarcoma. Conversely, significant family anxiety may lead to malignant thinking, another affective error in which a health care provider favors potential diagnoses with higher acuity or an increased risk for morbidity or mortality, simply as a function of that anxiety. Diagnosticians need to be self-aware of the tendency for these types of errors and to maintain the same impartial and broad differential diagnosis for a given set of signs and symptoms, even when a child appears generally well or in the context of significant family anxiety.

Perpetuating a diagnosis over time, whether due to appeals to authority, confirmation bias, attribution errors, benign thinking, or other affective errors, should be a cause to go back to the beginning of the illness and review all information available. Adolescent-onset behavioral and neurologic regression in a child originally diagnosed with autism may actually be a metabolic or neurodegenerative disorder. Recurrent episodes of swelling initially thought to be allergic reactions may eventually be diagnosed as episodes of hereditary angioedema or as nephrotic syndrome if the swelling is predominantly periorbital. Abdominal pain attributed to constipation but persisting despite evidence of normal stool output may in fact be porphyria, familial Mediterranean fever, lupus, or even malrotation with intermittent volvulus. Skin lesions that may appear eczematous or psoriasiform, when present in an unusual distribution restricted over the small joints of the hands, may be correctly diagnosed as associated with dermatomyositis.

Limitations in Diagnostic Testing

When evaluating children with URDs, it is important to recognize the limitations of diagnostic testing. Rarely is a diagnostic test 100% sensitive or specific, and as such, the positive and negative predictive values are often not ideal. Test results should not be considered dichotomously as ruling a particular condition either "in" or "out" but rather as increasing or decreasing the post-test probability of that condition in accordance with the positive or negative predictive value of that test as well as any other findings or results from laboratory or imaging studies. Laboratory error should be considered as well. There may be a tendency to believe the hard data of a particular test result more than believing eyes, ears, and hands and to trust that test results are more accurate and definitive than information gathered from history and physical examination. Finally, the absence of a positive laboratory test does not always disprove a diagnosis. For example, most but not all patients with lupus have a positive antinuclear antibody test; fewer have positive anti–double-stranded DNA titers.[6] Only 80% to 90% of patients with endocarditis have positive blood cultures.[4] The long QT syndrome (LQTS) has traditionally been diagnosed based on an age-specific length of the QT interval.[7–9] There are more than 1000 genetic variants that account for approximately 80% of patients with LQTS. Nonetheless, 30% of patients with a gene mutation and resultant risk for arrhythmias do not demonstrate an abnormal QT interval on standard ECG testing.

THE APPROACH TO DIAGNOSING UNDIAGNOSED OR RARE DISEASES

Recurrent themes from the evaluation of patients with URD who have been successfully diagnosed include the critical steps of maintaining a complete and fluid differential diagnosis and considering disease mimics and disease chameleons. Mimics are diseases whose signs and symptoms overlap with other diseases despite being distinct disorders. Central nervous system demyelinating disorders, such as acute disseminated encephalomyelitis, multiple sclerosis, neuromyelitis optica, and various leukoencephalopathies, frequently mimic each other. Chameleons are disorders that present with incomplete, atypical, disguised, or poorly recognized manifestations. For example, lupus may present with chorea, congenital syphilis may present solely with hepatitis, congenital neuroblastoma may present as nonimmune hydrops, and a periodic fever syndrome may present without fever. Potential diagnoses may be inappropriately excluded from consideration if expert opinion or medical literature does not acknowledge the less common symptom or sign as a manifestation of that disorder.

The evaluation of patients with URD should always involve considering the following 3 questions: Could this be an unusual presentation of a common disease? Could this be a rare disease? Could my patient have more than one disease? It has been stated, "Where you hear hoof beats, think horses not zebras." This was meant to say that common diseases occur commonly and that zebras—rare diseases—are uncommon. Nonetheless, when approaching patients with URDs, unusual, atypical, or previously unknown manifestations of a common disease must be considered ("Where you do not hear hoof beats, horses might still be present") as well as those rare and unrecognized zebras. Physicians specializing in the care of URD patients can be designated zebra hunters, but they might also be hunting horses in zebra coats, common diseases presenting in an uncommon fashion. Furthermore, the combination of detailed phenotyping and genomic sequencing has revealed clear evidence of multiple disease states in individuals; hoof beats may represent a herd of both horses and zebras. In addition to unusual manifestations of common diseases or poorly recognized manifestations of rare diseases, another category deserves mention: the unicorn. As the ability to correlate phenotypes and functional bioassays with molecular genetic findings improves, new diseases not currently in the diagnostic catalogs will be identified. Once discovered, the elusive unicorn will become recognized as a new but rare disease.

Data Gathering

When evaluating a child with a URD, it is critical to obtain and comprehensively review the entirety of the medical record, inclusive of any institutions that have evaluated the patient previously. The review should be conducted objectively and in a manner that consciously avoids potential sources of bias that may perpetuate inaccurate diagnostic labels. It is of paramount importance to obtain actual imaging studies or pathology material and not just written interpretations. One of the authors' patients underwent heart transplantation for restrictive cardiomyopathy at another institution 10 years prior to presenting with recent-onset muscle wasting and weakness.

Obtaining tissue of the diseased heart from the original medical center helped confirm the diagnosis of a myofibrillar myopathy. In another situation, a child with chronic headaches was reported to have normal CT of the head and treated for headaches with medication and biofeedback at a different institution. Two years later, the patient was discovered to have a brain tumor that was present on the original CT scan but not appreciated by the original radiologists. Avoid making assumptions without the actual data. It is too easy to assume that a radiologist's interpretation is correct or that a pathologist performed all the appropriate analyses on a tissue sample. Re-reviewing this clinical information with another set of eyes sometimes leads to detection of previously overlooked critical findings.

Data Analysis and Hypothesis Generation

It is important to distill a patient's history and results of previous diagnostic testing into a clearly defined phenotype of the disease because arriving at a correct diagnosis is contingent on generating a hypothesis based on an accurate phenotype. When defining the phenotype, it is critical to consider which findings are likely to represent primary pathology, which represent morbidity secondary to that pathology, which may be true although unrelated to the underlying disease, and which may be consequences of therapy or otherwise iatrogenic in nature. For example, recurrent pneumonias may be a direct manifestation of primary ciliary dyskinesia or may be secondary to restrictive lung disease from neuromuscular weakness. The clinician should be aware, however, that phenotypic heterogeneity can confound this analysis. Molecular heterogeneity underlies some degree of phenotypic variability, because there is growing evidence that certain individual clinical entities can be caused by mutations in multiple genes. Conversely, mutations in a single gene may be associated with multiple and vastly different phenotypes, depending on whether the changes induce an increase or a decrease in gene expression or which active region of the gene product is impacted, resulting in altered functional interactions with other proteins. For example, separate mutations in SCN5A have been associated with Brugada syndrome, LQTS-3, dilated cardiomyopathy, familial atrial fibrillation, and congenital sick sinus syndrome.[7] Thus, finding a pathogenic variant in a gene may not always be diagnostic of a specific disease, particularly if that variant is associated with a phenotype markedly distinct from that of the patient. In those circumstances, pairing specific variants with a specific phenotype helps diagnose the disease.

With the phenotype characterized, data should be analyzed systematically, with an approach that uses abductive, deductive, and inductive methods as appropriate. The generation of a differential diagnosis based on objective data is an example of abductive reasoning, in which specific observations, such as physical examination findings or laboratory results, are synthesized in an attempt to work forward and arrive at a unifying diagnosis. Abductive approaches lend themselves to probabilistic analyses, in which the positive and negative predictive values of various diagnostic assays are used to determine if a particular diagnosis is more likely or less likely based on the results. Using this approach, a diagnosis can be iteratively arrived at by using sensitive and specific tests to either confirm or reject hypotheses regarding the ultimate diagnosis. When symptoms are vague or incomplete, the differential diagnosis may be too broad to allow for a directed testing strategy. In these circumstances, it may be more useful to adopt an inductive approach. Inductive reasoning takes specific observations and works backward in an attempt to derive general principles about underlying pathophysiology. A straightforward example of an inductive approach is failure to thrive in infants, working backward from a specific observation (ie, insufficient weight gain) to propose potential underlying mechanisms, such as insufficient caloric intake, malabsorption, or increased caloric demands. With this differential pathophysiology generated, a testing strategy can then be developed, aimed at confirming or rejecting these hypotheses. An inductive approach can be helpful when manifestations are vague or when the differential diagnosis includes disease mimics or chameleons. When there are insufficient objective measures by which suspicion for a particular disease process in a probabilistic fashion could be increased or decreased, the use of deductive reasoning may be useful. Deductive approaches begin with general principles and attempt to align a patient's presentation with those general principles. The use of disease-based criteria is an example of a deductive approach and has proved invaluable in diseases for which definitive testing strategies may not exist, although these criteria are not without limitations.[10]

Over-reliance on disease-based criteria

When a disease does not have a definitive diagnostic manifestation or an appropriately sensitive and specific laboratory test, experts in the field often develop criteria to help facilitate the diagnosis. These criteria are often based on limited clinical information and are developed by consensus opinion. Criteria may subsequently be modified as the understanding of the disease evolves, such as the recent revisions of the Jones criteria used to diagnose rheumatic fever that are believed to miss fewer patients who may have rheumatic fever.[11]

Although it is tempting to adhere strictly to published criteria when considering a diagnosis, this approach has significant potential for error. The true sensitivity and specificity of such criteria are often unknown. The criteria are also often insufficiently detailed to allow for consideration of the clinical nuances or unique manifestations of certain diseases. For example, polyarthritis is one of the major criteria within the Jones criteria, but it is far more helpful to define the specific characteristics of the arthritis when rheumatic fever is a diagnostic consideration. If the arthritis is migratory, transient, and disproportionately painful, these are more characteristic of rheumatic fever than if these characteristics were not present. Over-reliance on criteria may truncate exploration for alternate diagnoses or prevent consideration of the disease in question because a patient does or does not meet criteria. Furthermore, these criteria are often based on the known, typical manifestations of disease and fail to account for incomplete, atypical, or unusual clinical findings.

Kawasaki disease is an excellent example of the potential for error when relying strictly on published clinical criteria to make a diagnosis, particularly when a disease can present with atypical or incomplete findings. The criteria for Kawasaki disease have been established for many years, but recent experience has demonstrated a high incidence of incomplete or atypical cases that do not meet the classic case definition.[12] Patients have developed the primary serious sequela of Kawasaki disease, coronary artery aneurysms, without ever developing a sufficient number of clinical manifestations that satisfy the published criteria. Infants with Kawasaki disease are particularly less likely to develop clinical criteria that satisfy the published case criteria. There are also multiple reports of Kawasaki disease in children presenting solely with fever and lymphadenopathy.[13,14] Strict reliance on the classic criteria may result in failure to diagnose patients at risk for coronary artery aneurysms.

For many criteria-based diagnoses, the abnormalities are present simultaneously, such as in rheumatic fever or Kawasaki disease. Other diseases, however, for which diagnostic criteria have been developed, may have symptoms or laboratory abnormalities that are separated over time. In these instances, the diagnosis is more challenging, and premature exclusion for not meeting criteria potentially prevents an accurate diagnosis from eventually being made. Children labeled as having idiopathic immune thrombocytopenia have over time developed other disorders, such as lupus or autoimmune lymphoproliferative syndrome. The authors have watched the progression of familial hemophagocytic lymphohistiocytosis (fHLH) from a fever of unknown origin with unremarkable serum ferritin levels to full expression of clinical and laboratory criteria over a 4-week to 8-week time course. Consistently remaining open-minded to the evolution of disease over time, reviewing the complete history and physical examination periodically, and repeating laboratory tests all aid diagnostic evaluation and help prevent diagnostic errors or oversights.

Clinical criteria may also prove insufficient when genetic heterogeneity results in wide phenotypic variation. The potentially lethal disorder Marfan syndrome has specific clinical criteria to aid in diagnosis.[15–17] These clinical criteria are age related and have variable phenotypic expression. Mutations in the FBN1 gene are thought responsible for the Marfan fibrillinopathy. There are more than 300 unique mutations in this gene, which may also produce sporadic thoracic aortic aneurysm/dissection syndrome and various skeletal dysplasias. When criteria-based diagnosis is compared with the presence of a mutation in FBN1, 12% of suspected patients who do not meet clinical diagnostic criteria have the mutation, whereas in those who meet clinical criteria only 66% have a FBN1 mutation.[17]

Hypothesis Testing

After all relevant clinical data have been gathered and analyzed and hypotheses regarding the underlying pathophysiology of the URD have been generated, a testing strategy that maximizes the yield while minimizing the burden on the patient and family should be developed. If noninvasive diagnostic measures yield accurate and reliable results, they should be favored, but invasive measures should not be shied away from if they are going to prove critical in establishing the diagnosis. In all situations, particularly in situations in which invasive diagnostic procedures are to be used, tissue should always be obtained from the most affected yet most conveniently accessed site. If physical examination reveals proximal muscle weakness and a mitochondrial disorder is suspected, performing quantitative and qualitative analyses on mitochondria derived from the impacted muscle tissue should be favored over performing such assays on mitochondria derived from peripheral blood samples. In situations where patient symptoms are progressing rapidly or patients are critically ill, functional bioassays, such as perforin granzyme testing for hemophagocytic lymphohistiocytosis, should be considered over molecular genetic techniques if they offer sufficient sensitivity and specificity, because they may allow for more rapid diagnosis and institution of therapy while awaiting molecular genetic confirmation. Ultimately, genetic testing may be required to arrive at a diagnosis.

With increasing recognition and publication of genotype-phenotype correlations, it may be tempting to restrict testing to specific candidate genes. Reliance on specific single-gene testing, however, may result in missing the diagnosis of a suspected disease. Clinicians are often pleased when a gene becomes associated with a clinical syndrome. Unfortunately, the new diagnostic gene may be responsible for only some but not all cases of the disease. FOXP3 mutations are associated with the immune dysregulation, polyendocrinopathy, enteropathy, X-linked (IPEX) syndrome. Not all patients presenting with features of IPEX, however, have mutations in FOXP3. To date, 4 other genes (CD25, STAT5b, ITCH, and STAT1) that produce an IPEX-like syndrome have been identified, and more are likely to be discovered.[18,19] Testing for FOXP3 mutations alone misses patients with mutations in other genes.

fHLH is another genetic disorder originally thought due solely to mutations in the perforin gene. The understanding of the fHLH phenotype has evolved and now includes 5 clinical subtypes and 4 known genes: *PRF1* (FHL2), *UNC13D* (FHL3), *STX11* (FHL4), and *STXBP2* (FHL5), with more likely to be discovered.[20] Reliance on single-gene testing does not identify all patients with fHLH. Other examples of multiple genes causing a known disease include tuberous sclerosis (*TSC1* and *TSC2*) and Noonan syndrome (*RAF1, NF1, NRAS, PTPN11, SOS1, SOS2, KRAS, BRAF, SOC2, LZTR1,* and *RIT1*).

Value and limitations of genetic testing and sequencing

Genetic testing can be approached in many ways. Targeted single-gene analysis is used less often in current clinical practice because many disorders are associated with more than 1 gene. For this reason, gene panels using next-generation, or high-throughput, sequencing techniques have been developed. Disorders whose significant clinical findings overlap are often included on the same gene panel. An example of this is the Thoracic Aortic Aneurysm and Dissection gene panel that screens for the genes associated with several disorders, including Marfan syndrome, Loeys-Dietz syndrome, and vascular Ehlers-Danlos, among others, all of which are associated with dilation of the ascending aortic root. The technology used to sequence and analyze multiple candidate genes for related disorders is also used at the genomic level: whole exome sequencing (WES), in which the coding portion of the genome is sequenced, and whole-genome sequencing (WGS), in which the entire genomic content is sequenced. WES interrogates approximately 24,000 genes, which equates to approximately 1% of the entire genome. The quality of the sequencing depends on the quality of the original DNA sample, the depth of sequencing, and bioinformatic support for the analysis. Run as a single test on an affected individual, it can identify the underlying genetic cause in as many as 25% of individuals. The power of this analysis increases if the biological parents are analyzed as a trio, which increases diagnostic yield to as high as 40%. Many of the identified pathogenic variants (mutations) are autosomal dominant, whereas a smaller percentage is autosomal recessive.[21–25]

Given the enormity of data that such technology can generate, principles for categorizing variants (mutations) have been established; the results of such a test are not always in the traditional positive or negative format. Variants that have been well defined as disease causing are clearly pathogenic and are categorized as such; however, variants in a gene, whether or not known to be disease causing, may be categorized as "likely pathogenic," "variants of unknown significance," "likely benign," or "single nucleotide variants (SNVs)" that are common in the general population. The American Board of Medical Genetics and Genomics has recommended a series of guidelines to standardize how laboratories define variants in these categories, but ultimately the classification is performed by a testing laboratory service. It is thus important to know the general practices of a reference sequencing laboratory so that the data provided can be appropriately interpreted.

WES is an invaluable tool in the evaluation of URD. Once viewed as a research tool, WES is now permanently established as the standard test for patients of all ages with URDs. It is important to realize that WES in itself is limited by the analysis; more importantly, it is critical to recognize that this analysis is empowered by the clinical data that define a patient's phenotype. It is ultimately the description of a patient's phenotype, aided by objective physical, laboratory, and imaging findings and derived from the extensive evaluation process that most patients with URDs undergo, that allows the raw data of WES to inform a final diagnosis. The experiences from multiple medical centers have demonstrated the effectiveness of WES in ending the diagnostic odyssey for 25% to 40% of patients, depending on the underlying disease manifestations. The authors' experience has been that individuals with clearly defined phenotypes tend to have the highest yield; in the pediatric literature, developmental delay and seizures are more likely to yield an answer.[21–25] In addition, by providing a definitive diagnosis, WES results in lower medical costs by reducing the number of unnecessary investigations and improves management by providing disease-specific treatments or even cures.[25–27] WES is also used as a tool to aid in the identification of novel disease genes as well as expanding the phenotype of known diseases.

Definitive results from WES are a humbling experience for physicians who have been considered outstanding diagnosticians. In some patients, WES may confirm a

Table 2
Potential limitations of whole exome sequencing

Limitation	Comments
VUS	WES may reveal >20,000 VUSs. Computerized and manual review needed to narrow down number Sanger sequencing to confirm variant presence or bioassay to assess significance Annual review to determine if VUS now reported as disease causing Collaborate with disease-specific research group to further evaluate VUS.
CNV	Sequencing unable to detect deletions or duplications Large deletions may create loss of heterozygosity, but currently SNV density not be sufficient to emulate CNV evaluation of a microarray. WGS anticipated to resolve this limitation.
Complex genetic mechanisms	Uniparental disomy, epigenetic influences cannot be detected through exome sequencing.
Tandem repeat sequences	Long runs of tandem repeats are not well sequenced in general and require additional assays to be evaluated. For example, triple-repeat associated with Huntington disease is not detected with WES.
Deep intronic sequences, 5' regulatory sequences, microRNA	Require WGS; examples include insulators, enhancers, promotors, operon silencers; for example, Pierre Robin sequence and *SOX9* enhancer.
mtDNA	WES may detect nuclear mitochondrial genes. WGS may improve detection of mtDNA mutations.
Gaps in sequencing	Not all regions of the genes are equally covered; some regions are GC rich (more common in the first exon of a gene). Not all regions covered to sufficient depth for reliable variant calling. WES platforms do not uniformly read all gene sequences at the same depth. Certain genes, which have repeated sequences, for example, collagens, prove too complex to align on the reference sequence and thus risk inaccurate variant calling.
Presence of pseudogene	Alignment of next-generation sequencing fragments is difficult and thus variant calling in these genes is unreliable. Using targeted primers for Sanger sequencing eliminates these concerns.
Structural genomic variants (aneuploidy, large copy number variants, inversions)	Require chromosome analysis, microarray or more complex molecular techniques to resolve.

Abbreviations: CNV, copy number variation; GC, guanine cytosine; mtDNA, mitochondrial DNA mutations; VUS, variants of unknown significance; WES, whole exome sequencing; WGS, whole genome sequencing.

suspicion about a rare disease, but in others the unexpected diagnosis emphasizes the limits of a traditional linear approach to making a diagnosis. Although the linear process of taking a history, doing a physical examination, and ordering laboratory tests based on an abductively derived differential diagnosis often reveals a final diagnosis for common disorders, this approach has less utility in patients with URDs.

Despite the remarkable utility of WES in evaluating children with URDs, the technology is not without limitations. Awareness of these limitations may provide further direction for evaluation if WES does not result in a definitive diagnosis (**Table 2**). It is most important to appreciate that although all of the genes are sequenced, not all regions of the gene are equally covered and thus there may be gaps in the sequencing that are not readily apparent. For this reason, WES is not an ideal catch-all and it is better to order a targeted genetic test when a specific mongeneic disorder is suspected. Finally, WES does not detect deletions, duplications, and certain complex genomic mechanisms. Such alterations are better detected via microarray or other analysis.

WGS is currently not used as frequently as WES, but, in time, it is expected to replace WES as the standard of care for patients with URDs. The major restriction of WGS is the cost of analysis, which is 3-fold more than WES. A decade ago, WES cost approximately $100,000, whereas the current average cost approximates $4500. The rate of technological advancement is rapidly reducing these costs and it will not be long before the $1000 genome. The power of WGS is that it captures all regulatory sequences and all SNVs; thus, with a single test, large copy number variations will be able to analyzed, eliminating the need for microarray analysis, while providing for the analysis of any known gene.[28] The biggest limitation to the amount of data WGS generates is the ability to interpret and apply the results clinically. Other potential limitations to WES are noted in **Table 2**. These limitations should in no way underestimate the great value of WES in ending the diagnostic odyssey of 25% to 35% of patients with aURDs. The authors anticipate an even higher success rate with WGS.

SUMMARY

Diagnostic errors create significant burdens for both patients and the health care system.[29–31] Patients who have been misdiagnosed or who remain undiagnosed may experience continued suffering or a progression in their disease, leading to potential disabilities and even preventable life-threatening complications. Misdiagnosis or lack of a specific diagnosis leads to unnecessary diagnostic testing and invasive procedures, which, in addition to increasing patient suffering and risking complications, add major costs to the health care system.

The cognitive clinical judgment concerns outlined in this article hopefully will help create an awareness of past errors and inform clinicians of improved ways to approach patients with URDs. The use of WES has greatly expanded the ability to diagnose misdiagnosed or URD patients; WES/WGS is no longer experimental and should be covered by all insurance providers in patients with URDs when an appropriate evaluation has not yielded a diagnosis. Both awareness of cognitive errors and utilization of WES/WGS will save patients from continued suffering and the health care system from unnecessary and excessive health care costs.

REFERENCES

1. Bean RB, Bean WB. Sir William Osler: aphorisms from his bedside teachings and writings. New York: H. Schuman; 1950. p. 129.

2. Gahl WA, Adams DR, Markello TC, et al. Genetic approaches to rare and undiagnosed diseases. In: Kliegman R, editor. Nelson textbook of pediatrics. 20th edition. Philadelphia: Elsevier; 2016. p. 629–33. Chapter 83.
3. Tifft CJ, Adams DR. The National Institutes of Health undiagnosed diseases program. Curr Opin Pediatr 2014;26:626–33.
4. Baddour LM, Wilson WR, Bayer AS, et al. Infective endocarditis in adults: diagnosis, antimicrobial therapy, and management of complications. Circulation 2015;132:1435–86.
5. Steere AC, Malawista SE, Snydman DR, et al. An epidemic of oligoarticular arthritis in children and adults in three Connecticut communities. Arthritis Rheum 1977;20:7–17.
6. Petri M, Orbai AM, Alarcón GS, et al. Derivation and validation of the systemic lupus international collaborating clinics classification criteria for systemic lupus erythematosus. Arthritis Rheum 2012;64(8):2677–86.
7. Campuzano O, Sarquella-Brugada G, Cesar S, et al. Genetics of inherited arrhythmias in pediatrics. Curr Opin Pediatr 2015;27:665–74.
8. Tester DJ, Ackerman MJ. Genetics of long QT syndrome. Methodist Debakey Cardiovasc J 2014;10(1):29–33.
9. Behere SP, Shubkin CD, Weindling SN. Recent advances in the understanding and management of long QT syndrome. Curr Opin Pediatr 2014;26:727–33.
10. Osimani B. "Modus Tollens" probabilized: deductive and inductive methods in medical diagnosis. MEDIC, Methodology and Education for clinical Innovation 2009;17(1-2):43–9.
11. Gewitz MH, Baltimore RS, Tani LY, et al. Revision of the Jones criteria for the diagnosis of acute rheumatic fever in the era of doppler echocardiography. Circulation 2015;131(20):1806–18.
12. Newberger JW, Takahashi M, Gerber MA, et al. Diagnosis, treatment, and long-term management of Kawasaki disease: a statement for health professionals from the committee on rheumatic fever, endocarditis, and Kawasaki disease, council on cardiovascular disease in the young, American Heart Association. Pediatrics 2004;114(6):1708–33.
13. Kanegaye JT, Van Cott E, Tremoulet AH, et al. Lymph-node-first presentation of Kawasaki disease compared with bacterial cervical adenitis and typical Kawasaki disease. J Pediatr 2013;162:1259–63.
14. Nomura Y, Arata M, Koriyama C, et al. A severe form of Kawasaki disease presenting with only fever and cervical lymphadenopathy at admission. J Pediatr 2010;156:786–91.
15. Bolar N, Van Laer L, Loeys BL. Marfan syndrome: from gene to therapy. Curr Opin Pediatr 2012;24:498–504.
16. Robinson PN, Booms P, Katzke S, et al. Mutations of FBN1 and genotype-phenotype correlations in Marfan syndrome and related fibrillinopathies. Hum Mutat 2002;20:153–61.
17. Loeys B, Nuytinck L, Delvaux I, et al. Genotype and phenotype analysis of 171 patients referred for molecular study of the fibrillin-1 gene FBN1 because of suspected Marfan syndrome. Arch Intern Med 2001;161:2447–54.
18. Verbsky JW, Chatila TA. Immune dysregulation, polyendocrinipathy, enteropathy, X-linked (IPEX) and IPEX-related disorders: an evolving web of heritable autoimmune diseases. Curr Opin Pediatr 2013;25:708–14.
19. Uhlig HH. Monogenic diseases associated with intestinal inflammation: implications for the understanding of inflammatory bowel disease. Gut 2013;62:1795–805.
20. Janka GE, Lehmberg K. Hemophagocytic syndromes – an update. Blood Rev 2014;28:135–42.

21. Yang Y, Muzny DM, Xia F, et al. Molecular findings among patients referred for clinical whole-exome sequencing. JAMA 2014;312(18):1870–9.
22. Lee H, Deignan JL, Dorrani N, et al. Clinical exome sequencing for genetic identification of rare Mendelian disorders. JAMA 2014;312(18):1880–7.
23. Iglesias A, Anyane-Yeboa K, Wynn J, et al. The usefulness of whole-exome sequencing in routine clinical practice. Genet Med 2014;16(12):922–31.
24. Soden SE, Saunders CJ, Willig LK, et al. Effectiveness of exome and genome sequencing guided by acuity of illness for diagnosis of neurodevelopmental disorders. Sci Transl Med 2014;6(265):265ra168.
25. Taylor RW, Pyle A, Griffin H, et al. Use of whole-exome sequencing to determine the genetic basis of multiple mitochondrial respiratory chain complex deficiencies. JAMA 2014;312(1):68–77.
26. Worthey EA, Mayer AN, Syverson GD, et al. Making a definitive diagnosis: successful clinical application of whole exome sequencing in a child with intractable inflammatory bowel disease. Genet Med 2011;13(3):255–62.
27. Dauber A, Stoler J, Hechter E, et al. Whole exome sequencing reveals a novel mutation in CUL7 in a patient with an undiagnosed growth disorder. J Pediatr 2013;162:202–4.
28. Scacheri CA, Scacheri PC. Mutations in the noncoding genome. Curr Opin Pediatr 2015;27:659–64.
29. Khullar D, Jha AK, Jena AB. Reducing diagnostic errors – why now? N Engl J Med 2015;373:2491–5.
30. Singh H, Graber ML. Improving diagnosis in health care – the next imperative for patient safety. N Engl J Med 2015;373:2493–5.
31. Institute of Medicine. Improving diagnosis in health care. Washington, DC: National Academies of Sciences, Engineering, and Medicine; 2015. Available at: http://iom.nationalacademies.org/Reports/2015/Improving-Diagnosis-in-Healthcare.aspx.

FURTHER READINGS

Berman JJ. Rare diseases and orphan drugs: keys to understanding and treating the common diseases. San Diego (CA): Academic Press/Elsevier; 2014.
Groopman J. How doctors think. Boston: Houghton Mifflin; 2007.
Kliegman RM, Stanton BF, St. Geme JW III, et al. Nelson textbook of pediatrics. 20th edition. Philadelphia: Elsevier; 2016.
Montgomery K. How doctors think: clinical judgment and the practice of medicine. Oxford (United Kingdom): Oxford University Press; 2013.
Mukherjee S. The laws of medicine: Field notes from an uncertain science. TED Books. New York: Simon & Schuster; 2015.

The Team-Based Approach to Undiagnosed and Rare Diseases

Robert M. Kliegman, MD*, Barbara E. Ruggeri, MLIS,
Molly Marquardt Smith, BA

KEYWORDS

- Undiagnosed or rare diseases • Team approach • Multidisciplinary

KEY POINTS

- Patients with undiagnosed and rare diseases (URDs) are often misdiagnosed.
- A team approach to the appropriate diagnosis of patients with URDs has been successful.
- Parents appreciate the team approach and ability to have the evaluation at one institution.

None of us is as smart as all of us.

—*Ancient Japanese Proverb*

Patients with URDs may be on a diagnostic odyssey for years or even decades. (See Robert M. Kliegman and colleagues' article, "How Doctors Think Common Diagnostic Errors in Clinical Judgment—Lessons from an Undiagnosed and Rare Disease Program," in this issue.) Many have complex symptoms that do not suggest an obvious diagnosis, whereas a significant number have been misdiagnosed and inappropriately treated for a disease they do not have. The process of diagnosing and appropriately managing URDs is fraught with challenges. Most patients begin the diagnostic odyssey for their complex medical condition under the care of a single physician but eventually seek further evaluation via referrals to multiple individual subspecialists. These referrals may lead to fragmenting of the medical record across various health care systems or even misalignment of diagnostic impressions and evaluation strategies within the same health care system. An additional challenge in pediatrics is that disease progression or developmentally related changes in the patient's physiology, such as the onset of puberty, may alter a patient's phenotype over time. Furthermore, most children, independent of their underlying pathophysiology, undergo developmental changes in their ability to communicate their symptoms, leading to a dynamically evolving understanding of their phenotype. Finally, patients who remain undiagnosed or misdiagnosed for many

---

Department of Pediatrics, Medical College of Wisconsin, Children's Hospital of Wisconsin, 999 North 92nd Street, Suite C450, Milwaukee, WI 53226, USA
* Corresponding author. Children's Corporate Center, Children's Hospital of Wisconsin, 999 North 92nd Street, Suite C450, Milwaukee, WI 53226
E-mail address: rkliegma@mcw.edu

Pediatr Clin N Am 64 (2017) 17–26
http://dx.doi.org/10.1016/j.pcl.2016.08.003
0031-3955/17/© 2016 Elsevier Inc. All rights reserved.

years often develop adverse behavioral or psychological reactions to their chronic medical condition or may acquire unintended or unrecognized side effects of inappropriate treatments that complicate the diagnostic evaluation.

Common medical disorders comprise most patient encounters in both general and subspeciality practices. The traditional diagnostic approach of an individual physician taking a history, conducting a physical examination, generating a differential diagnosis, and obtaining any indicated laboratory and imaging studies frequently yields a diagnosis for most patients presenting with common ailments. Undiagnosed diseases may represent atypical or poorly recognized manifestations of a common disease or, as often noted in pediatric patients, the presentation of a rare and often genetic disorder. (See Robert M. Kliegman and colleagues' article, "How Doctors Think Common Diagnostic Errors in Clinical Judgment—Lessons from an Undiagnosed and Rare Disease Program," in this issue.) For the physician who cares for patient after patient with the more common disorders in general practice, the usual response to a patient's complaint is to consider that complaint within the scope of their practice. Uncomplicated disorders, such as the common cold, headaches, asthma, abdominal pain, or constipation, are readily recognized and diagnosed by a single physician familiar with both the patient and the management of common ailments. When a diagnosis fails to fit the usual pattern of disease, however, because of duration, the unanticipated involvement of other organ systems, abnormal responses to therapy, or additional atypical features, the patient may be referred to a specialist. This specialty referral may result in an appropriate diagnosis but may also be subject to the cognitive biases inherent within that medical specialty. Within each specialty, there is often a comfort zone in managing that specialty's organ-specific symptoms; there may be less familiarity when symptoms do not fit. Each practice has an experiential proficiency with the diseases that are highly prevalent within their specialty. In contrast, individual rare disorders have a very low prevalence, and many practitioners may not have ever cared for or even read about patients with rare disorders. (See Robert M. Kliegman and colleagues' article, "How Doctors Think Common Diagnostic Errors in Clinical Judgment—Lessons from an Undiagnosed and Rare Disease Program," in this issue.) Cumulatively, there are too many individual rare disorders for any single practitioner to be aware of, let alone be able to diagnose, without the help of a team. When the traditional approach to medical diagnosis leaves patients undiagnosed, they require a team-based approach exemplified by the Japanese proverb, "None of us is as smart as all of us."

TEAM DYNAMICS

The authors' URD team includes providers from most pediatric subspecialties, including hospitalists, geneticists, radiologists, and pathologists. Other essential health professionals on the team include a medical librarian and an access-coordinating specialist. Each subspecialist brings to the evaluation experience and expertise as both a pediatrician and a subspecialty physician and is instrumental in providing insights into the nuances associated with particular symptoms or the disease processes considered in the differential diagnosis. For example, although arthritis is a criterion in the recently modified Jones criteria for rheumatic fever,[1] the observation that the arthritis is migratory, polyarticular, and exquisitely tender may not be discussed in published articles or textbooks or even in the criteria themselves. Such subtleties are frequently observed, however, in patients with URD, and awareness of these clinical pearls improves the diagnostic process.

The composition of a team is aided in great part by the incorporation of established members whose regular participation in multiple patient case team reviews over time has led to the development of a group thought process. The authors make a conscious effort to recognize common cognitive errors and are highly suspicious of authoritative statements, such as, "It cannot be this disease," "In my experience I have never seen this," "We have already ruled out this disease," or "It must be this disease." In addition to recognizing errors or biases in the diagnostic process by working together to review many complex URD patients, the team has developed the ability to collectively recognize unusual or rare patterns of disease manifestations. Most general physicians use pattern recognition to diagnose common disorders, such as swollen edematous eyes, thought to represent an ocular allergy. But sometimes these swollen eyes are a manifestation of nephrotic syndrome (**Table 1**). Members of the URD team have developed sensitivity to uncommon manifestations of common or even rare diseases, such as neurologic symptoms associated with familial hemophagocytic lymphohistiocytosis, Langerhans cell histiocytosis, autoimmune encephalitis, lupus, neurosarcoidosis, Wilson disease, or other inborn errors of metabolism.[2]

After careful review of all the available medical records and team-based discussions, the authors are able to identify misdiagnosed patients who have been treated inappropriately for many years; for example, the misdiagnosis of chronic Lyme disease instead of Addison disease or anorexia nervosa instead of celiac disease (see **Table 1**).

Although common things do happen commonly, and when you hear hoof beats you should initially think of horses, the patients the authors see with URDs are often zebras (uncommon manifestations of a common disease or a poorly recognized manifestation of a rare disease). Team members may be considered "zebra hunters."

INITIATING THE TEAM PROCESS—REFERRAL

Patients are referred to the URD team from within the Wisconsin-based health care system and from throughout the United States. Those from outside of Wisconsin are usually self-referred, although a growing number are new referrals from the physician who cared for the original self-referred patient. A majority of these patients have involvement of more than 1 organ system and have complex and chronic unresolved or progressive disorders that have lasted many years. In contrast, approximately 15% to 20% of the referrals are acutely and critically ill children admitted to the authors' hospital with complex symptomatology but without an immediately obvious diagnosis. (See Robert M. Kliegman and colleagues' article, "How Doctors Think Common Diagnostic Errors in Clinical Judgment—Lessons from an Undiagnosed and Rare Disease Program," in this issue.)

Out-of-state referrals go through the hospital's access center, whereas those within the health care system request a consultation through the internal referral system, which is available 24 hours a day, 7 days a week. A member of the team contacts out-of-town families, discusses their concerns, explains the URD program process, and asks if they would like to be reviewed by the team.

DATA GATHERING AND SYNTHESIS

If the family wishes to pursue evaluation with the URD team, the access center registers the patient in the electronic health record and works with the family to request all medical records from every institution, clinic, and hospital that has cared for the patient and to request copies of all of the actual imaging studies and slides of all tissue samples obtained by biopsy or tissue resection. Having the team obtain and then review all imaging and pathology studies is essential for many reasons. Imaging abnormalities may be missed in the original report or may be subject to a more informed interpretation when new symptoms develop or the disease progresses. A child with headaches, who had a report of a "normal" CT scan and who was treated with

Table 1
Diagnostic errors in general practice

Presentation	Initial Diagnosis	Final Diagnosis
Weakness and fatigue	Chronic Lyme disease	Addison disease
Periorbital edema	Allergy	Nephrotic syndrome
Cervical lymphadenopathy	Bacterial adenitis	Kawasaki disease Cat-scratch disease Branchial cleft cyst
Weight loss	Anorexia nervosa	IBD Celiac disease
Thrombocytopenia	ITP	SLE ALL ALPS
Red urine	Nephritis	Autoimmune hemolytic anemia Rhabdomyolysis
Extremity pain	Sprain	Osteomyelitis Osteosarcoma
Joint or bone pain	JIA	ALL Lymphoma Neuroblastoma Scurvy
Aseptic meningitis	Viral meningitis	ADEM Autoimmune encephalitis Parameningeal infection Tuberculosis
Tachypnea	Pneumonia	DKA Salicylate toxicity Pulmonary embolism
Pallor, fatigue, microcytosis	Iron deficiency anemia	Crohn disease
Facial swelling	Cellulitis	Cold panniculitis Mosquito hypersensitivity Tooth abscess Poison ivy
Drop attacks	Seizures	Dysrhythmia Narcolepsy
Emesis	Gastroenteritis	Increased ICP Pancreatitis UTI Poisoning
Recurrent emesis	Gastroenteritis	Inborn errors of metabolism Malrotation
Jaundice	Hepatitis	Autoimmune hemolytic anemia HUS
Abdominal pain	Constipation	UTI HSP IBD Lower lobe pneumonia Testicular/ovarian torsion Pancreatitis Hepatitis

(continued on next page)

Table 1 *(continued)*		
Presentation	Initial Diagnosis	Final Diagnosis
Dysuria	UTI	Peritonitis (ruptured appendix)
Pharyngitis	Group A streptococcus	Mononucleosis Lemierre disease

Abbreviations: ADEM, acute disseminated encephalomyelitis; ALL, acute lymphoblastic leukemia; ALPS, autoimmune lymphoproliferative syndrome; DKA, diabetic ketoacidosis; HSP, Henoch-Schön-lein purpura; HUS, hemolytic uremic syndrome; IBD, inflammatory bowel disease; ICP, intracranial pressure; ITP, immune (idiopathic) thrombocytopenia; JIA, juvenile idiopathic arthritis; SLE, systemic lupus erythematosus; UTI, urinary tract infection.

medication and biofeedback later developed abnormal pubertal development and worsening headaches and was found to have a craniopharyngioma. When the original CT scan was reviewed, there was evidence of the tumor at that time. Conversely, because of the exquisite sensitivity of MRI, many patients have lesions detected on brain MRI scans. Most of these lesions are not pathologic and may be considered "incidentalomas" or "unidentified bright objects."[3,4] Unfortunately these nonpathologic MRI findings often are misinterpreted and may lead to a mistaken diagnosis if not interpreted within the context of a team-based evaluative approach.

When all of the paper and electronic medical records are available, all of the data (notes, laboratory results, and reports) are reviewed by at least 2 members of the team and are summarized. One common phenomenon noted in these multiyear, multiconsultation medical records is the perpetuation of errors copied from one note to another, which then often influences clinical judgment. A child treated for asthma with prolonged corticosteroids was initially labeled as having drug-induced adrenal suppression but was eventually inappropriately labeled as adrenally insufficient and then as having Addison disease. Another child who underwent whole-exome sequencing was found to have 1 copy of a potentially disease-causing gene; however, it was a variant of unknown significance (VUS). This VUS was never reported to be disease-causing; in addition, the child had only 1 potentially abnormal variant allele in a recessive disorder. Furthermore, an unaffected parent also had one copy of the VUS. Nonetheless, the genetic disorder appeared repeatedly over time as the patient's diagnosis.

THE TEAM MEETING

After reviewing and summarizing a patient's history, a whole-team meeting is scheduled. Although all team members are invited (51 current members), the meeting is planned based on the availability of the subspecialists considered essential for the discussion. For a child with seizures, pancytopenia, fever, splenomegaly, and high ferritin levels, for example, neurology, radiology, hematology, immunology, rheumatology, and genetic specialists are required in addition to the core members of the team, which include experienced diagnosticians who were the founding members of the URD team. Prior to the meeting, all team members review the case summary and have access to the medical records downloaded in the electronic medical record system. Questions about symptoms and possible symptom-based etiologies that help inform the team discussion are given to the medical librarian to research.

The team discussion lasts 1.5 to 2 hours and has always uncovered new aspects to the patient's issues. It has been impressive and a universal observation that when many different clinicians review a medical record, they come away with different and often important insights not thought of or identified previously. Thus, the proverb, "None of us is smarter than all of us," is fulfilled.

THE DIAGNOSTIC EVALUATION

After a discussion of the differential diagnosis, a diagnostic strategy is developed with the goal of involving team members in that evaluation during a planned visit to the authors' institution. If a subspecialist (eg, movement disorders) is not a member of the team, communication is arranged with that faculty member and an appointment arranged when a visit (usually 2–3 days) to the campus is planned. When indicated (and it is often), new imaging modalities are involved, such as interventional radiology, or tissue-specific biopsies of skin are ordered for dermatosis, liver for hepatic dysfunction, muscle for histology, special stain and mitochondrial studies, bone marrow for cytopenias, and bone for unexplained skeletal imaging findings.

The access center then works with the family and required consultants to coordinate the visit, get interim medical records, and obtain preapproval for the visit from the insurance companies. During the visit, the family is shepherded through the campus by access center staff and the consultants are informed of one another's findings. The last consultant visit usually includes a wrap-up session with any results, conclusions, follow-up plans, or change in treatments discussed with the family. Further follow-up with the family is continued by phone, the electronic health record, or e-mail; reports are sent to a patient's primary care physician and suggestions for local consultation, testing, or treatment that can be performed when the patient returns home are discussed with the primary care provider or local subspecialist.

There are some exceptions to this idealized team process. In some circumstances, after discussion with the family and reviewing the medical records, the pattern of symptoms suggests a specific need to see a consultant with experience with the patient's issues. A child with "chronic fatigue syndrome" who has salt craving, hyperpigmentation, and orthostatic dizziness should be seen immediately by an endocrinologist to be evaluated for Addison disease. If this is confirmed, the diagnostic odyssey ends with the endocrinologist. If it is not confirmed, a whole-team meeting is held, this time with more familiarity with the patient and the laboratory or other findings.

Another exception is an acutely and critically ill patient who despite immediate and preliminary testing remains undiagnosed in the hospital. In such cases, a URD service consultation is obtained and is answered by 1 of the 4 clinical diagnosticians who were founding members of the URD program. The consultant reviews all past and present medical records, meets with the family, examines the patient, and begins initial conversations with the treating team. Additional subspecialty consultations are often necessary and are usually requested from the appropriate URD team subspecialist if available. In addition, all imaging or pathology studies are reviewed side-by-side with a URD team radiologist or pathologist, to go over findings, expand the differential diagnosis, and suggest further testing. The URD team consultant remains involved and each day reviews the medical record, visits the patient and family, and rounds with the primary team to maintain a constant dialogue. If a patient's diagnosis does not become obvious after the initial diagnostic strategy, a team meeting is urgently arranged.

ROLE OF MEDICAL LIBRARIAN AND LITERATURE REVIEW

Rapid advances in the biomedical sciences over the past decade have created an information overload for clinicians that have made it extremely difficult to be fully aware of newly discovered diseases, diagnostic tests, and therapies, let alone review articles meant to be a basis for continuing medical education. When faced with a patient with a URD, busy clinicians have little time to search the bound journal volumes on the library shelves or the electronic cloud containing vast resources available to help develop a differential diagnosis.

In its recent Institute of Medicine report, *Improving Diagnosis in Health Care*, the Committee on Diagnostic Error in Health Care recognized that clinicians may be ill equipped to navigate diagnostic dilemmas alone in a landscape of rapid growth of biomedical discoveries as well as diagnostic tests and treatments. As part of the solution to reducing diagnostic error, the committee states that a "diagnostic process ideally involves collaboration among multiple health care professionals, the patient, and the patient's family."[5] A clinical medical librarian must be included in the diagnostic team; this person provides skilled information retrieval that assists the team approach to diagnostic decision making.

A systematic review of information-seeking behavior of clinicians suggested that more than half of the clinical questions a clinician needs for diagnosing or treating a patient may go unanswered.[6] Clinicians tend to look for answers to clinical questions that are quick and easy to locate. The challenging questions in patients with URD often take too much time to investigate. The librarianship program embeds the librarian where the actual information needs occur and improves information retrieval by locating answers to challenging clinical questions. The librarian attends rounds and team meetings to hear the case history as well as the team discussion. When the issues are identified that require more information, the medical librarian can attempt to find answers on the spot to help in real time or conduct a more thorough literature search shortly after the meeting. Having the opportunity to hear the issues and needed information in the actual clinical context enables a medical librarian to select search terms and filter articles that have more relevance to the patient. With years of involvement attending teaching rounds and team meetings, the medical librarian may perceive information needs from listening to the discussion and provide articles on those topics without being asked. For example, a search on the etiology of urticaria in neonates and infants produced references that included neonatal-onset multisystem inflammatory disease (NOMID) in the differential diagnosis. This approach to the patient was supported by the faculty and subsequently the patient was diagnosed with NOMID.

The clinical medical librarian is invaluable in the diagnostic process and is involved before, during, and after the diagnostic team meeting. Before the case conference, the medical librarian may perform a broad scope review of the literature initiated by first impressions that may guide the diagnostic strategy. The search usually relates to unusual presentations of known disease or the implications of a patient's current diagnosis with new symptoms. A literature search may often identify mimics of a disease, such as the mimics of cerebral palsy (metabolic or neurodegenerative disorders).[7] Search strategies often need to look for a unifying disease among a constellation of symptoms—What diseases are associated with peripheral neuropathy and optic atrophy? Many of these questions retrieve a large set of search results. To help locate review articles on mimics, differential diagnosis, and case reports of unusual presentations, the librarian creates a list of synonyms for look-alikes and mimics, MeSH headings, and key words that have proved helpful in yielding unusual case reports and have helped identify useful information for the team (**Box 1**).

During the team meeting, the medical librarian listens for additional needed information; the medical librarian then attempts to find answers during the team discussion or performs a more informed and detailed literature search based on the team conclusions after the meeting. During one discussion, the medical librarian identified case reports that supported imaging of the spine to look for a cause of communicating

Box 1
Suggested MeSH[a] Headings and key words and phrases to find rare or unusual presentations of known diseases, condition mimics, differential diagnosis, diagnostic errors

(MeSH) Diagnosis, differential	Novel presentation	Misdiagnosis	Simulant
(MeSH) Diagnostic errors	Unusual presentation	Resemble	Chameleon
(MeSH) Delayed diagnosis	Uncommon presentation	Mistaken	Mislead
Atypical	Like	Masquerade	Mimic

[a] MeSH is the National Library of Medicine controlled vocabulary list of medical subject headings used to describe each journal article in MEDLINE.

hydrocephalus. Later, the medical librarian provided a short summary of the etiologies of communicating hydrocephalus found in the literature. At another team meeting, a geneticist mentioned a condition that seemed similar to the patient's except that the patient did not have sensorineural hearing loss. The librarian found an article on a similar syndrome without the hearing loss. This article on Fazio-Londe syndrome, which involves bulbar palsy and peripheral neuropathy due to riboflavin transporter deficiency, was similar to the patient's eventual diagnosis.[8]

CASE REVIEW

The team does not always have the answer at first and that holds true for the medical librarian. One of the most valuable sessions is a team meeting that discusses the outcomes of all cases reviewed during the year. One particular case had perplexed everyone for months. As the authors reviewed the correct diagnosis (determined by exome sequencing) that was originally missed, the librarian reviewed the previous literature search. Based on the wrap-up discussion, the librarian used new search terms and found a case report that would have helped the team earlier. The librarian reviewed the MeSH terms and discovered additional key words that could have uncovered this report. By attending outcome meetings, this valuable feedback gives the librarian an opportunity to learn what was useful and what could be improved in performing a literature search for a patient with URD.

ROLE OF THE ACCESS CENTER

Children's Hospital of Wisconsin uses an access center that facilitates local and more often distant patients to negotiate and coordinate multiday multispecialty consultation and diagnostic testing. The goal of the access center is to maximize the efficiency and yield of the diagnostic evaluation. The highly trained access navigators serve as liaisons with all clinical areas (inpatient, outpatient, laboratory, and imaging). They help gather medical records and register and schedule children for appointments. They also assist with insurance approval and nearby lodging. Since 2013, the access center has worked with more than 500 patient families from out-of-state locations to be seen at specialty clinics across several different areas of clinical expertise.

When a family inquires about the Undiagnosed and Rare Disease Program, their first contact is usually with a navigator in the access center. The navigator takes all the information from the parent or guardian and enters it into the electronic health system. This includes patient demographics, insurance, preferred method of contact, and main health concern. Families use the navigator as a single point of contact because their visit often is complex.

After the first call or general request, the navigator directly notifies the URD team leader with basic information along with a parent's or guardian's main concern. While the team leader reviews the information, the navigator works with the family to collect medical records, which is often from multiple unrelated medical facilities.

When a patient's family inquires about a URD consultation, they can be assured that many different specialists from all areas of the hospital review their previous medical history. The navigators also help with this area to ensure that everyone receives the appropriate medical records.

The navigator attends the team meeting and is attentive to the diagnostic plan the team develops. Thereafter, the navigator obtains any additional records, including actual imaging studies or biopsy tissue and coordinates the multispecialty and diagnostic visit to the institution.

Feedback from parents has been uniformly positive. Parents appreciate the coordinated diagnostic evaluation at a single institution and the collaboration between multiple subspecialists as well as the ongoing communication with the family.

SUMMARY

Diagnostic errors create significant burdens for both patients and the health care system. Patients who have been misdiagnosed or who remain undiagnosed may experience ongoing or progressive suffering secondary to their disease, leading to potential disabilities and even preventable life-threatening complications. Misdiagnosis or lack of a specific diagnosis leads to unnecessary diagnostic testing and invasive procedures, which, in addition to increasing patient suffering and risking complications, add major costs to the health care system.

The Institute of Medicine report suggests that a diagnostic team have the following[5]:

- Shared goals
- Clear roles
- Mutual trust
- Effective communication
- Measurable outcome

These characteristics are even more essential for the evaluation of children with URDs. In addition to team members' specialty-based experience, skills, and knowledge, their participation in team case reviews helps them recognize past diagnostic errors that may lead to misdiagnosis and inappropriate treatment. Having an insight and constant awareness of the common cognitive errors, biases, and short-cuts that clinicians unknowingly commit improves the team-based evaluation and redirects the diagnostic strategy to finding a resolution to the diagnostic odyssey of the child with URD.

REFERENCES

1. Gewitz MH, Baltimore RS, Tani LY, et al. Revision of the Jones criteria for the diagnosis of acute rheumatic fever in the era of Doppler echocardiography. Circulation 2015;131(20):1806–18.
2. Janka GE, Lehmberg KL. Hemophagocytic syndromes – an update. Blood Rev 2014;28:135–42.
3. Hitzeman N, Cotton E. Incidentalomas: Initial management. Am Fam Physician 2014;90:784–9.
4. Lee HY, Kim JC, Chang DS, et al. Unidentified bright objects on brain magnetic resonance imaging affect vestibular neuritis. Clin Exp Otorhinolaryngol 2015; 8(4):364–9.
5. Committee on Diagnostic Error in Health Care, Board health Care Services, Institute of Medicine, et al. Improving diagnosis in health care. Washington, DC: Nat

Acad Sci; 2015. p. 31–80, 145–6. Available at: http://www.nap.edu/catalog/21794/improving-diagnosis-in-health-care. Accessed January 30, 2016.

6. Del Fiol G, Workman TE, Gorman PN. Clinical questions raised by clinicians at the point of care: a systematic review. JAMA Intern Med 2014;174(5):710–8.

7. Leach EL, Shevell M, Bowden K, et al. Treatable inborn errors of metabolism presenting as cerebral palsy mimics: systematic literature review. Orphanet J Rare Dis 2014;9:197.

8. Bosch AM, Stroek K, Abeling NG, et al. The brown-vialetto-van laere and fazio londe syndrome revisited: natural history, genetics, treatment and future perspectives. Orphanet J Rare Dis 2012;7:83.

Immunodeficiency Presenting as an Undiagnosed Disease

John M. Routes, MD[a],*, James W. Verbsky, MD, PhD[b]

KEYWORDS

- Primary immunodeficiencies • Common variable immunodeficiency • Autoimmunity
- Granulomatous and lymphocytic interstitial lung disease • IPEX
- Immune dysregulation, polyendocrinopathy, enteropathy, X-linked

KEY POINTS

- Autoimmunity is frequent in primary immunodeficiencies and may be the presenting clinical manifestation.
- Common variable immunodeficiency (CVID) is the most common primary immunodeficiency and is characterized by a low serum immunoglobulin G (IgG) and either a low IgA or IgM and exclusion of secondary causes of hypogammaglobulinemia.
- With the use of high-dose gamma globulin replacement, noninfectious complications of CVID are the most common cause of death.
- Hypomorphic mutations of forkhead box P3 (FOX P3) may reduce the severity and delay the clinical manifestations of immune dysregulation, polyendocrinopathy, enteropathy, X-linked.

INTRODUCTION

Primary immunodeficiencies (PIDs) are a diverse set of immunologic disorders that are intrinsic to the immune system. With the widespread use of high-throughput DNA sequencing, the number of monogenic causes of PIDs has increased dramatically and currently is more than 250 individual genes. Despite these advances in identifying the genetic cause of increasing numbers of PIDs, common variable immunodeficiency (CVID) is by far the most common PID; but the molecular nature of the disorder remains to be defined. Regardless of the cause of a PID, the clinical phenotype is extremely diverse in many cases and may present with autoimmunity or other unusual

[a] Department of Pediatrics, Children's Research Institute, Medical College of Wisconsin, Children's Clinics Building, Suite B440, 9000 West Wisconsin Avenue, Milwaukee, WI 53226-4874, USA; [b] Department of Pediatrics, Children's Corporate Center, Children's Research Institute, Medical College of Wisconsin, Suite C465, 9000 West Wisconsin Avenue, Milwaukee, WI 53226-4874, USA
* Corresponding author.
E-mail address: jroutes@mcw.edu

Pediatr Clin N Am 64 (2017) 27–37
http://dx.doi.org/10.1016/j.pcl.2016.08.007
0031-3955/17/© 2016 Elsevier Inc. All rights reserved.

but serious disorders rather than recurrent infections. In this article, the authors highlight 2 cases of PID that presented with unusual clinical manifestations that led to a delay in diagnosis.

CASE 1: AUTOIMMUNE CYTOPENIAS AND LUNG DISEASE

A 17-year-old girl presented to her primary care provider with a 2- to 3-week history of shortness of breath and bruising without known trauma. Her medical history is significant for only allergic rhinitis, which she thinks is worsening, with increased nasal congestion and 3 episodes of sinusitis over the last year. Her only medication is loratadine for symptoms of allergic rhinitis. The remainder of the personal history and family history are unremarkable. Physical examination is remarkable for bruises on the left thigh, left forearm, and right shoulder. Pertinent laboratory findings include the following: hemoglobin (Hgb) 8.1 g/dL, platelets 15,140/μL, and a positive direct Coombs (immunoglobulin G [IgG]). The patient was diagnosed with Evan syndrome and treated with prednisone with a normalization of the platelet count and Hgb.

One year after discontinuing prednisone, the patient again presented with bruising. Hgb was 8.5 g/dL and the platelet count was 11,000/μL. The physical examination was notable for bruising and an enlarged spleen 4 cm below the left midclavicular line. Bone marrow examination revealed large megakaryocytes but no evidence of malignancy. A computed tomography (CT) scan of the abdomen demonstrated splenomegaly, scattered adenopathy, and nodular and ground-glass abnormalities in the lower lungs zones. Based on these findings, a high-resolution CT (HRCT) of the chest was performed that revealed large nodules with ground-glass abnormalities in the lower lung zones and mediastinal adenopathy. PET-CT imaging revealed hypermetabolic lymph nodes in the mediastinum, abdomen, and right inguinal region, with increased uptake in the nodular lesions of the lower lung zones. Biopsy of the right inguinal lymph node revealed noncaseating granulomas but was negative for malignancy. Cultures were negative for routine pathogens, fungi, and mycobacteria. Pulmonary medicine performed a transbronchial biopsy that demonstrated noncaseating granulomas, and a presumptive diagnosis of sarcoidosis was made. The patient was treated with prednisone with resolution of the anemia and thrombocytopenia. However, following 4 months of corticosteroids, there was only a small decrease in the radiographic abnormalities on HRCT of the chest and no changes in the mild restrictive lung disease as determined by complete pulmonary function tests. Corticosteroids were slowly tapered, and other therapeutic options were entertained.

Over the next 2 months the patient had 2 episodes of sinusitis. Clinical immunology was consulted for evaluation of possible immunodeficiency. Quantitative immunoglobulins demonstrated a low IgG (250 mg/dL), absent IgA (<10 mg/dL), and low IgM (12 mg/dL). Postimmunization titers to diphtheria, tetanus, and pneumococcal vaccine polyvalent were nonprotective; the diagnosis of CVID was made. Video-assisted thoracoscopic lung biopsy was performed and demonstrated granulomatous and lymphocytic interstitial lung disease (GLILD). The patient underwent treatment with azathioprine and rituximab, and an HRCT scan of the chest 6 months after beginning immunosuppressive therapy showed marked improvement of the parenchymal abnormalities and pulmonary function.

COMMON VARIABLE IMMUNODEFICIENCY

CVID is the most common PID to be followed by a clinical immunologist and requires regular therapy.[1] Recent data from the European Society for Immunodeficiencies (ESID) registry and the United States Immunodeficiency Network registry showed that CVID accounted for 20% to 30% of all reported PIDs.[2] The estimated prevalence of CVID has been estimated at between 1:10,000 and 1:100,000 of the population.[3] The wide variation in the prevalence of the disease is likely multifactorial, but underdiagnosis likely contributes to these discrepancies. The diagnosis of CVID is frequently delayed with studies reporting a median of 5 to 9 years from the onset of symptoms to the diagnosis of CVID.[4–6]

DEFINITION AND LABORATORY TEST RESULTS' ABNORMALITIES

The diagnostic criteria for CVID based on a recent international consensus document are summarized in **Box 1**.[1] The current guidelines to diagnosis CVID do not require the typical clinical manifestations (eg, recurrent infections, autoimmunity) to be present in a patient at the time of the diagnosis, a feature that is not present in alternative diagnostic criteria.[7] The enumeration of lymphocyte subsets in patients with CVID reveals several abnormalities. In contrast to congenital agammaglobulinemias, B cells are typically present in peripheral blood. However, in approximately 10% of patients, B cells are profoundly reduced or absent, which may portend a poorer prognosis.[8] B-cell subset analysis is useful in identifying patients at risk to develop complications of the disorder. For example, low numbers of isotype class switched B cells (CD27$^+$, IgM$^-$, IgD$^-$) in peripheral blood correlates with an increased risk of multisystemic granulomatous disease and splenomegaly.[9] T-cell abnormalities are common and may include T-cell lymphopenia, anergy, and poor response to mitogens. A subset of patients with CVID may have profoundly reduced numbers of CD4 T cells (<200 cells per microliter).[10] These patients are much more likely to have noninfectious and infectious complications of CVID and are at risk for increased mortality.

CAUSE

CVID is a clinical syndrome with a common laboratory phenotype. The protean clinical manifestations of CVID likely represent the many heretofore-unidentified causes of the disorder. Many reserve the diagnosis of CVID to those PIDs that meet the international criteria (see **Box 1**) and for which no monogenic cause has been found.[1] Depending on the ethnicity of a population, CVID is familial in approximately 5% to 25% of the

---

Box 1
Diagnostic criteria for common variable immunodeficiency

- Decreased serum IgG at least 2 SD less than the mean adjusted for age
- Decreased IgA and/or IgM
- Age of onset more than 2 years of age
- Poor specific antibody response to vaccinations
- Exclusion of other causes of hypogammaglobulinemia
  - Drugs (eg, corticosteroids, rituximab)
  - Single-gene defects (eg, congenital agammaglobulinemias, hyper-IgM syndromes)
  - Malignancy (eg, B-cell lymphomas, chronic lymphocytic leukemia, Good syndrome)
  - Protein-losing states (eg, nephrotic syndrome, protein-losing enteropathy)
  - Other (eg, chromosomal abnormalities, HIV-1 infection, bone marrow failure)

Adapted from Bonilla FA, Barlan I, Chapel H, et al. International consensus document (ICON): common variable immunodeficiency disorders. J Allergy Clin Immunol Pract 2016;4:38–59.

cases.[11] Heterozygous mutations in the transmembrane activator and calcium-modulator and cyclophilin-ligand interactor (TACI) gene are found in 5% to 10% of patients and are associated with a dramatically increased risk to develop CVID, whereas homozygous mutations of TACI invariably lead to a CVID-like disorder.[12–14] Interestingly, in contrast to patients with CVID and heterozygous mutations in TACI, patients with homozygous mutations do not have autoimmune complications typically found in CVID.[14] With the increasing use of high-throughput DNA sequencing, there are several monogenic disorders that share many of the features of CVID (eg, CD19 deficiency, CTLA4 deficiency, Inducible T cell costimulator deficiency).[1] Consequently, many clinical immunologists perform either targeted gene sequencing or whole-exome sequencing in patients with CVID with an unusual clinical phenotype (eg, severe clinical phenotype, early age of onset).

CLINICAL MANIFESTATIONS

The onset of the clinical manifestations of CVID is highly variable. In the United States, the mean age for the diagnosis of CVID is the third decade of life.[6] In contrast, data from the ESID registry found that more than 30% of patients with CVID had an onset of disease at less than 10 years of age, with 38% of males diagnosed before 10 years of age.[5] Regardless of these differences, CVID should be considered in any person with unusually severe, frequent, or chronic infections who is greater than 2 years of age.

Recurrent upper and/or lower respiratory tract infections (RTIs) (bronchitis, sinusitis, otitis media, and pneumonia) are a hallmark of CVID occurring in greater than 90% of such patients. Encapsulated bacteria (*Haemophilus influenzae, Streptococcus pneumoniae*) and atypical bacteria (*Mycoplasma or Ureaplasma* spp) are common pathogens.[15,16] As most clinical laboratories do not culture for *Mycoplasma sp* and serology cannot be used to reliably diagnose infection in antibody-deficient patients, antimicrobial therapy for RTIs should include coverage for atypical pathogens. Opportunistic infections are uncommon in patients with CVID unless T-cell counts are profoundly reduced.[17] Gastrointestinal (GI) tract infections with bacteria pathogens similar to those in immunocompetent hosts are common. Infections with *Giardia lamblia* may be particularly severe and difficult to treat and often require a longer duration of therapy than in an immunocompetent host. Recently, chronic norovirus infection has been implicated in the enteropathy that occurs in CVID.[18]

There has been a marked decline in mortality due to infection with the use of high-dose antibody replacement therapy.[19] In contrast, morbidity and mortality due to noninfectious complications has appreciably increased. Noninfectious complications are extremely common and occur in more than 60% of patients with CVID and include chronic lung disease, GI tract disease, liver disease, autoimmune disease, and cancer.[8] Autoimmune cytopenias are especially common and complicate 29% of patients with CVID. Autoimmune thrombocytopenia is the most common, but Coombs-positive autoimmune hemolytic anemia and autoimmune neutropenia occur as well. GI complications include chronic enteropathy and inflammatory bowel disease. The risk to develop B-cell lymphomas is increased in CVID and similar to individuals infected with human immunodeficiency virus type 1 (HIV-1). These lymphomas are due to EBV in only a minority of cases. Increased risk of early mortality in CVID is found in patients with functional or structural lung disease, GI tract disease, liver disease, and B-cell lymphomas.[8]

The pulmonary complications of CVID are diverse and a major cause of morbidity and mortality.[20–22] With the use of HRCT scans of the chest as a mandatory screen for pulmonary disease, clinically significant pulmonary disease was found to be present in more than one-third of patients.[20] Bronchiectasis is the most common and may be present in as many as 60% of patients as determined by HRCT of the chest. Gamma globulin replacement therapy markedly reduces pyogenic lung infections.[19] However, gamma globulin only contains IgG; some studies suggest that antibody replacement will not fully prevent the development of bronchiectasis.[19] Therapy for bronchiectasis is similar to those patients with bronchiectasis without immunodeficiency and emphasizes the mobilization of secretions. Based on studies of patients with bronchiectasis without immunodeficiency that showed decreased infectious exacerbations, chronic azithromycin prophylaxis is frequently used in patients with CVID and bronchiectasis.[23,24]

Diffuse interstitial lung disease (ILD) occurs in 20% to 30% of patients with CVID and includes GLILD, cryptogenic organizing pneumonia (COP), and B-cell lymphomas, which include bronchus-associated lymphoid tissue lymphomas or higher-grade B-cell lymphomas.[20,21] Apart from COP, which seems to respond to corticosteroid therapy,[25] other forms of diffuse ILD are resistant to corticosteroid therapy and do not respond to gamma globulin replacement therapy.

Granulomatous disease, which can occur in virtually any organ but most commonly in the lung, spleen, liver, bone marrow, and/or GI tract, is reported to occur in approximately 10% to 25% of patients with CVID. As standard screening tests for granulomatous disease are infrequently performed, the diagnosis may be significantly delayed or missed altogether. GLILD is the pulmonary manifestation of a multisystemic granulomatous disease.[20,21] The diagnosis of GLILD is based on the constellation of histopathologic findings that typically occur in the same biopsy and include non-necrotizing granulomas, lymphocytic interstitial pneumonitis (LIP), and follicular bronchiolitis.[21,26] GLILD is not specific to CVID and has been reported in other PIDs, including CTLA4 haploinsufficiency,[27] lipopolysaccharide responsive beigelike anchor protein (LRBA) deficiency,[28] and hypomorphic mutations of the recombinase activating 1 (RAG1) gene.[29] The natural history of GLILD in CVID is not clearly defined, and some think that progressive pulmonary disease may not occur. In contrast, the authors reported that GLILD leads to progressive impairment and early mortality with moderate to severe pulmonary fibrosis in nearly 50%.[21,26]

The constellation of findings of non-necrotizing granulomas and mediastinal adenopathy led to the belief that GLILD was a form of sarcoidosis in patients with CVID. It is now established that the two disorders are distinct disorders with unique pathologic, radiographic, and clinical findings.[30] GLILD is a macronodular disease with a lower lung zone predominance, whereas sarcoidosis is typically micronodular with an upper lung zone predominance. Follicular bronchiolitis and LIP are much more predominant in GLILD compared with sarcoidosis. Other features characteristic of GLILD include a high prevalence of autoimmune cytopenias, frequent presence of hepatosplenomegaly, lack of spontaneous remission of lung disease, and failure to respond to corticosteroid therapy.[30]

The cause of GLILD is unknown, but the occurrence in other PIDs characterized by autoimmunity suggests that this may be a common response of the lung to immune dysregulation. It has been reported that the overproduction of tumor necrosis factor-α (TNF-α) may lead to the granulomatous disease in CVID.[31] TNF-α antagonists have been reported to successfully treat patients with GLILD, lending further support to this hypothesis.[32] In a retrospective study of 7 patients, rituximab/azathioprine therapy was found to markedly improve the radiographic abnormalities on HRCT of the chest and pulmonary function of patients with CVID and GLILD.[33] This approach needs to be validated in a properly controlled, placebo-controlled, prospective study.

Replacement gamma globulin, administered either subcutaneously or by vein, is the treatment of choice for all patients with CVID.[34,35] A typical starting dosage of gamma globulin is 400 mg/kg to 600 mg/dL per month. Although measurement of serum IgG is useful, the doses of gamma globulin are increased to prevent serious infections. Patients with granulomatous disease, bronchiectasis, or marked splenomegaly require a higher dose of gamma globulin to prevent infection compared with patients without these complications.[34]

CASE 2: ATOPY AND ENTEROPATHY

A 6-year-old Caucasian boy with a strong history of atopic diseases was referred for consultation for possible immune problems with high IgE (1228 KU/mL) and low albumin (1.8 mg/dL). The patient had a long-standing history of moderate to severe atopic dermatitis (starting at 10 months of age) that was recalcitrant to standard therapy, eosinophilic esophagitis (treated with oral budesonide), multiple food allergies, and moderate persistent asthma. Apart from the atopic disease, the patient had a 6-month history of intermittent diarrhea (4–5 loose stools per day, 2–3 days per week). The patient was small (projected height 65 in) but on a normal growth curve, although markedly smaller than the older sibling (projected height of 78 in). No past history of unusual, frequent, or chronic infections. Family history was initially noncontributory. Physical examination was notable for poorly controlled atopic dermatitis. Laboratory evaluation showed an elevated IgE (1228 KU/mL), numerous IgE-specific positive skin tests to foods, low serum IgG 334 (mg/dL) with a normal IgA and IgM, complete blood count with moderate eosinophilia (1876 cells per microliter), low albumin (1.8 mg/d/), normal total protein, normal urine analysis, and normal stool alpha-1 antitrypsin. Upper endoscopy and colonoscopy were normal. Flow cytometry was normal, including a normal number of regulatory T cells.

The initial therapeutic plan focused on optimal treatment of atopic diseases and eosinophilic esophagitis with a planned capsule endoscopy to definitively identify the source of the protein loss. On the subsequent visit, a repeat family history was obtained and was notable for a maternal cousin with 2 boys, one who died after a liver transplant and the other with an undefined "problem with the immune system." Based on this history, the FOX P3 gene was sequenced on the authors' patient and a damaging mutation was found. The patient underwent hematopoietic stem cell transplant (HSCT) with resolution of the severe atopic diseases and enteropathy. It was subsequently determined the deceased boy and sibling carried the diagnosis of immunodeficiency, polyendocrinopathy, enteropathy, X-linked (IPEX).

INTRODUCTION: IMMUNODEFICIENCY, POLYENDOCRINOPATHY, ENTEROPATHY, X-LINKED

There are 2 predominant mechanisms whereby autoreactive T cells are prevented from causing autoimmunity/immunodysregulation.[36] As T cells mature in the thymus, autoreactive T cells are deleted in a process known as negative selection. However, negative selection is not a perfect process; rare autoreactive T cells escape the thymus into the periphery and are a potential cause of autoimmune disease. Through a process known as peripheral tolerance, autoreactive T cells in the periphery are suppressed by a special type of T cell known as regulatory T cells (T_R).[37] There are 2 types of T_R, those that are produced in the thymus and constitutively express the lineage-specific transcription factor FOX P3 known as natural T_R ($_nT_R$) and inducible T_R ($_iT_R$) that are induced in the periphery from FOX P3 negative CD4 lymphocytes. Both $_nT_R$ and $_iT_R$ (referred from this point on as T_R) are essential in the maintenance of peripheral tolerance. Damaging mutations in the FOX P3 gene resulting in either defective function or decreased/absent numbers of T_R allow for the unchecked proliferation of activated T cells leading to autoimmunity and lymphoproliferation and the disease IPEX.[38]

CLINICAL MANIFESTATIONS AND DIAGNOSIS

The classic presentation of IPEX is the clinical triad of enteropathy, endocrinopathy, and severe dermatitis (**Box 2**) with the usual onset in early infancy.[38,39] Patients with enteropathy have frequent watery stools, but bloody diarrhea may be present. Food allergies frequently complicate the enteropathy and lead to worsening diarrhea in addition to the more usual forms of food allergy, such as urticaria or anaphylaxis.[40] The patients may develop a protein-losing enteropathy with concomitant failure to thrive. The small bowel is most commonly involved in the enteropathy, although colonic involvement is also seen. Biopsy of the small bowel reveals a predominantly lymphocytic infiltrate with blunted villi, crypt hyperplasia, and/or abscesses, which are not pathognomic for the disorder. Autoimmune hepatitis is frequently present in patients with enteropathy and may be severe.[40]

The endocrinopathies most commonly associated with IPEX are type 1 diabetes mellitus and autoimmune thyroiditis, although other endocrinopathies have been reported (see **Box 2**). The clinical manifestations of type 1 diabetes mellitus typically occur early in infancy and neonatal hyperglycemia may be present. The disease is progressive with a lymphocytic infiltrate of the islet cells with or without anti-islet cell antibodies.[41] Autoimmune thyroiditis is also common, and antithyroid antibodies are frequently present.

The eczematous rash found in patients with IPEX is similar to that described in patients with atopic dermatitis and may be severe.[42] Similar to patients with atopic dermatitis, the serum IgE correlates with the extent of disease and food allergies may worsen the extent of disease.

Other common complications of IPEX include autoimmune cytopenias and autoimmune nephritis. Autoimmune cytopenias, which are present in approximately 50% of patients, include Coombs positive hemolytic anemia, immune neutropenia, and immune thrombocytopenia.[43] Autoimmune nephritis, most commonly lymphocytic interstitial nephritis, occurs in one third of patients and may worsen with the use of calcineurin inhibitors.

Serious infections (eg, meningitis, pneumonia, sepsis) occur in approximately 50% of patients with IPEX, although the cause for this can be explained by the loss of barrier

---

Box 2
Common clinical features of immune dysregulation, polyendocrinopathy, enteropathy, X-linked

Endocrinopathies (type I diabetes mellitus, autoimmune thyroiditis, autoimmune adrenal disease/adrenal failure, hypopituitarism)

Atopic disease (eczema, asthma, food allergies, eosinophilic esophagitis)

Autoimmune enteropathy

Inflammatory bowel disease

Autoimmune renal disease

Autoimmune liver disease

Autoimmune cytopenias

function (GI tract, skin), autoimmune neutropenia, protein-losing enteropathy resulting in hypogammaglobulinemia, and immunosuppressive medications. Infections of any severity can worsen the autoimmune and allergic manifestations of IPEX and should be treated promptly. Common pathogens include cytomegalovirus, *Staphylococcus* sp, *Enterococcus* sp, and *Candida* sp.[44,45]

The diagnosis of IPEX requires the demonstration of a damaging mutation of the FOX P3 gene. Flow cytometry enumerating the number of T_R cells (CD4+, CD25+, FOX P3+ T cells) is a useful screen for IPEX. Null mutations of FOX P3 (complete loss of gene function) leads to the classic presentation of IPEX with an absence of FOX P3 T_R cells by flow cytometry. In contrast, hypomorphic mutations of FOX P3 (partial loss of gene function) may lead to a delayed onset of disease without the classic IPEX triad.

Patients with IPEX initially require intense immunosuppression to manage the auto-inflammatory complications of the disorder. Dietary avoidance of food allergens may be difficult because of several foods involved and may require the use of amino acid–based formulas. In nearly all patients, IPEX is fatal unless definitive HSCT is performed.

SUMMARY

CVID is the most common serious PID, and delays in the diagnosis are frequent. The case of CVID illustrated an uncommon clinical presentation of this disorder: recurrent autoimmune cytopenias and diffuse parenchymal lung disease that was initially diagnosed as sarcoidosis. Approximately 5% to 10% of patients with Evan syndrome (autoimmune cytopenia involving at least 2 blood elements) have or develop CVID. Additionally, the presence of autoimmune cytopenias is further increased in patients with GLILD and CVID and is not uncommonly a presenting clinical manifestation. The authors' patient also had increasing numbers of sinus infections, a problem originally attributed to allergies. Therefore, the differential diagnosis of patients with Evan syndrome, in particular those with diffuse ILD or recurrent or chronic RTIs, should include CVID. Similarly, CVID should be considered in patients with sarcoidosis with unusual complications, such as autoimmune cytopenias, marked splenomegaly, and recurrent or chronic RTIs.

The difficulty of making an early diagnosis of PIDs caused by single-gene defects is magnified by variations in the penetrance of the disease (the proportion of people expressing the characteristic phenotype) and variable expressivity (phenotype of the disease varies among different people). The second case of IPEX illustrates these points. This patient initially presented with severe atopic disease that was somewhat resistant to the usual therapy. The patient subsequently developed a protein-losing enteropathy with the typical laboratory findings of low albumin, normal total protein, low IgG, and normal IgA and IgM. Obtaining a family history of immunodeficiencies in boys on the maternal side of the family was critical. Hypomorphic mutation of FOX P3 may have a delayed presentation or lack the classic features of the disorder. IPEX should be considered in any boy with early onset enteropathy. In this case, the combination of severe atopic disease and late-onset, relatively mild protein-losing enteropathy was suspicious for IPEX even in the absence of endocrinopathy. An increasing number of PIDs (eg, signal transducer and activator of transcription [STAT]1 gain of function, STAT5B deficiency, CD25 deficiency, CTLA4 haploinsufficiency, LRBA deficiency) can also present with similar clinical manifestations and would need to be excluded if no mutation of FOX P3 was found.

In summary, PIDs can present with diverse clinical manifestations apart from infection. Clinicians need to consider PID in any patient with a combination of unusual clinical manifestations, in particular in combination with autoimmunity.

ACKNOWLEDGMENTS

The authors acknowledge Amy Vega for her excellence in editing the article.

REFERENCES

1. Bonilla FA, Barlan I, Chapel H, et al. International consensus document (ICON): common variable immunodeficiency disorders. J Allergy Clin Immunol Pract 2016;4(1):38–59.
2. Gathmann B, Binder N, Ehl S, et al. The European internet-based patient and research database for primary immunodeficiencies: update 2011. Clin Exp Immunol 2012;167(3):479–91.
3. Chapel H, Cunningham-Rundles C. Update in understanding common variable immunodeficiency disorders (CVIDs) and the management of patients with these conditions. Br J Haematol 2009;145:709–27.
4. Quinti I, Soresina A, Spadaro G, et al. Long-term follow-up and outcome of a large cohort of patients with common variable immunodeficiency. J Clin Immunol 2007;27:308–16.
5. Gathmann B, Mahlaoui N, CEREDIH, et al. Clinical picture and treatment of 2212 patients with common variable immunodeficiency. J Allergy Clin Immunol 2014; 134:116–26.e11.
6. Cunningham-Rundles C, Bodian C. Common variable immunodeficiency: clinical and immunological features of 248 patients. Clin Immunol 1999;92:34–48.
7. Ameratunga R, Woon ST, Gillis D, et al. New diagnostic criteria for CVID. Expert Rev Clin Immunol 2014;10:183–6.
8. Resnick ES, Moshier EL, Godbold JH, et al. Morbidity and mortality in common variable immune deficiency over 4 decades. Blood 2012;119(7):1650–7.
9. Wehr C, Kivioja T, Schmitt C, et al. The EUROclass trial: defining subgroups in common variable immunodeficiency. Blood 2008;111(1):77–85.
10. Malphettes M, Gérard L, Carmagnat M, et al. Late-onset combined immune deficiency: a subset of common variable immunodeficiency with severe T cell defect. Clin Infect Dis 2009;49:1329–38.
11. Vorechovsky I, Zetterquist H, Paganelli R, et al. Family and linkage study of selective IgA deficiency and common variable immunodeficiency. Clin Immunol Immunopathol 1995;77(2):185–92.
12. Salzer U, Chapel HM, Webster AD, et al. Mutations in TNFRSF13B encoding TACI are associated with common variable immunodeficiency in humans. Nat Genet 2005;37:820–8.
13. Castigli E, Wilson SA, Garibyan L, et al. TACI is mutant in common variable immunodeficiency and IgA deficiency. Nat Genet 2005;37:829–34.
14. Salzer U, Bacchelli C, Buckridge S, et al. Relevance of biallelic versus monoallelic TNFRSF13B mutations in distinguishing disease-causing from risk-increasing TNFRSF13B variants in antibody deficiency syndromes. Blood 2009;113(9): 1967–76.
15. Oksenhendler E, Gérard L, Fieschi C, et al. Infections in 252 patients with common variable immunodeficiency. Clin Infect Dis 2008;46:1547–54.
16. Gelfand EW. Unique susceptibility of patients with antibody deficiency to mycoplasma infection. Clin Infect Dis 1993;17(Suppl 1):S250–3.
17. Lucas M, Lee M, Lortan J, et al. Infection outcomes in patients with common variable immunodeficiency disorders: relationship to immunoglobulin therapy over 22 years. J Allergy Clin Immunol 2010;125:1354–60.e4.

18. Woodward JM, Gkrania-Klotsas E, Cordero-Ng AY, et al. The role of chronic norovirus infection in the enteropathy associated with common variable immunodeficiency. Am J Gastroenterol 2015;110:320–7.
19. Busse PJ, Razvi S, Cunningham-Rundles C. Efficacy of intravenous immunoglobulin in the prevention of pneumonia in patients with common variable immunodeficiency. J Allergy Clin Immunol 2002;109:1001–4.
20. Maarschalk-Ellerbroek LJ, de Jong PA, van Montfrans JM, et al. CT screening for pulmonary pathology in common variable immunodeficiency disorders and the correlation with clinical and immunological parameters. J Clin Immunol 2014; 34:642–54.
21. Bates CA, Ellison MC, Lynch DA, et al. Granulomatous-lymphocytic lung disease shortens survival in common variable immunodeficiency. J Allergy Clin Immunol 2004;114:415–21.
22. Verma N, Grimbacher B, Hurst JR. Lung disease in primary antibody deficiency. Lancet Respir Med 2015;3(8):651–60.
23. Wong C, Jayaram L, Karalus N, et al. Azithromycin for prevention of exacerbations in non-cystic fibrosis bronchiectasis (EMBRACE): a randomised, double-blind, placebo-controlled trial. Lancet 2012;380:660–7.
24. Altenburg J, de Graaff CS, Stienstra Y, et al. Effect of azithromycin maintenance treatment on infectious exacerbations among patients with non-cystic fibrosis bronchiectasis: the BAT randomized controlled trial. JAMA 2013;309:1251–9.
25. Dibbern DA Jr, Claman HN, Dreskin SC. Dyspnea and pulmonary infiltrates in a 53-year-old woman with common variable immunodeficiency. Ann Allergy Asthma Immunol 2001;87:18–21.
26. Rao N, Mackinnon AC, Routes JM. Granulomatous and lymphocytic interstitial lung disease: a spectrum of pulmonary histopathologic lesions in common variable immunodeficiency-histologic and immunohistochemical analyses of 16 cases. Hum Pathol 2015;46(9):1306–14.
27. Schubert D, Bode C, Kenefeck R, et al. Autosomal dominant immune dysregulation syndrome in humans with CTLA4 mutations. Nat Med 2014;20:1410–6.
28. Alkhairy OK, Abolhassani H, Rezaei N, et al. Spectrum of phenotypes associated with mutations in LRBA. J Clin Immunol 2016;36(1):33–45.
29. Buchbinder D, Baker R, Lee YN, et al. Identification of patients with RAG mutations previously diagnosed with common variable immunodeficiency disorders. J Clin Immunol 2015;35:119–24.
30. Verbsky JW, Routes JM. Sarcoidosis and common variable immunodeficiency: similarities and differences. Semin Respir Crit Care Med 2014;35:330–5.
31. Mullighan CG, Fanning GC, Chapel HM, et al. TNF and lymphotoxin-alpha polymorphisms associated with common variable immunodeficiency: role in the pathogenesis of granulomatous disease. J Immunol 1997;159:6236–41.
32. Franxman TJ, Howe LE, Baker JR Jr. Infliximab for treatment of granulomatous disease in patients with common variable immunodeficiency. J Clin Immunol 2014;34:820–7.
33. Chase NM, Verbsky JW, Hintermeyer MK, et al. Use of combination chemotherapy for treatment of granulomatous and lymphocytic interstitial lung disease (GLILD) in patients with common variable immunodeficiency (CVID). J Clin Immunol 2013;33(1):30–9.
34. Gouilleux-Gruart V, Chapel H, Chevret S, et al. Efficiency of immunoglobulin G replacement therapy in common variable immunodeficiency: correlations with clinical phenotype and polymorphism of the neonatal Fc receptor. Clin Exp Immunol 2013;171:186–94.

35. Orange JS, Grossman WJ, Navickis RJ, et al. Impact of trough IgG on pneumonia incidence in primary immunodeficiency: a meta-analysis of clinical studies. Clin Immunol 2010;137:21–30.

36. Bluestone JA, Bour-Jordan H, Cheng M, et al. T cells in the control of organ-specific autoimmunity. J Clin Invest 2015;125(6):2250–60.

37. Ohkura N, Kitagawa Y, Sakaguchi S. Development and maintenance of regulatory T cells. Immunity 2013;38(3):414–23.

38. Verbsky JW, Chatila TA. Immune dysregulation, polyendocrinopathy, enteropathy, X-linked (IPEX) and IPEX-related disorders: an evolving web of heritable autoimmune diseases. Curr Opin Pediatr 2013;25:708–14.

39. Carneiro-Sampaio M, Coutinho A. Early-onset autoimmune disease as a manifestation of primary immunodeficiency. Front Immunol 2015;6:185.

40. Torgerson TR, Linane A, Moes N, et al. Severe food allergy as a variant of IPEX syndrome caused by a deletion in a noncoding region of the FOXP3 gene. Gastroenterology 2007;132:1705–17.

41. Wildin RS, Smyk-Pearson S, Filipovich AH. Clinical and molecular features of the immunodysregulation, polyendocrinopathy, enteropathy, X linked (IPEX) syndrome. J Med Genet 2002;39(8):537–45.

42. Halabi-Tawil M, Ruemmele FM, Fraitag S, et al. Cutaneous manifestations of immune dysregulation, polyendocrinopathy, enteropathy, X-linked (IPEX) syndrome. Br J Dermatol 2009;160(3):645–51.

43. Torgerson TR, Ochs HD. Immune dysregulation, polyendocrinopathy, enteropathy, X-linked: forkhead box protein 3 mutations and lack of regulatory T cells. J Allergy Clin Immunol 2007;120:744–50 [quiz: 751–2].

44. Gambineri E, Torgerson TR, Ochs HD. Immune dysregulation, polyendocrinopathy, enteropathy, and X-linked inheritance (IPEX), a syndrome of systemic autoimmunity caused by mutations of FOXP3, a critical regulator of T-cell homeostasis. Curr Opin Rheumatol 2003;15(4):430–5.

45. Williams KW, Ware J, Abiodun A, et al. Hypereosinophilia in children and adults: a retrospective comparison. J Allergy Clin Immunol Pract 2016;4(5):941–7.e1.

Eczema and Urticaria as Manifestations of Undiagnosed and Rare Diseases

 CrossMark

Molly J. Youssef, MD[a], Yvonne E. Chiu, MD[b,c],*

KEYWORDS

- Eczema • Urticaria • Nutritional deficiencies • Immunodeficiency syndromes
- Autoinflammatory syndromes • Mycosis fungoides

KEY POINTS

- Autoinflammatory syndromes should be suspected in a child with recurrent bouts of urticaria associated with other symptoms of inflammation (fever, arthritis, serositis, hepatosplenomegaly, ocular, and/or neurologic involvement).
- Immunodeficiency syndromes often present with a neonatal eczematous eruption along with recurrent infections, chronic lymphadenopathy, and/or failure to thrive.
- In a child with a chronic dermatitis that is unresponsive to treatment, biopsy may be warranted to rule out mycosis fungoides (MF).
- Nutritional deficiencies are important to consider in children presenting with recalcitrant dermatitis, often with characteristic locations and/or other clinical features.

INTRODUCTION

Eczema and urticaria are common cutaneous eruptions seen in children. In the vast majority of cases, they are skin-limited disorders that run a benign course. In rare instances, they may signify a more serious underlying disease such as an immunodeficiency or an autoinflammatory syndrome. This review highlights the signs and symptoms that should alert the clinician to suspect something more concerning.

ECZEMA

Eczematous eruptions are characterized by scaly pink papules and plaques, often with associated pruritus. The most common eczematous eruption of childhood is

Disclosure Statement: The authors have no conflicts of interest to disclose.
[a] Department of Dermatology, Medical College of Wisconsin, 9200 West Wisconsin Avenue, Milwaukee, WI 53226, USA; [b] Section of Pediatric Dermatology, Department of Dermatology, Medical College of Wisconsin, 9200 West Wisconsin Avenue, Milwaukee, WI 53226, USA; [c] Department of Pediatrics, Medical College of Wisconsin, Milwaukee, WI, USA
* Corresponding author. Department of Dermatology, Medical College of Wisconsin, 9200 West Wisconsin Avenue, Milwaukee, WI 53226.
E-mail address: ychiu@mcw.edu

atopic dermatitis, which affects nearly 13% of children in the United States.[1] Nearly two-thirds of children with atopic dermatitis have onset of skin manifestations before 1 year of age but typically after 2 months of age.[2] Atopic dermatitis has a predilection for the face, scalp, and extensor extremities in infants and young children, whereas flexural sites are more common in older children and adults. A personal or family history of atopy is also a clue for the diagnosis. Although eczema is often equated with atopic dermatitis, there are several other eczematous eruptions of the skin.

Because atopic dermatitis is such a common condition in childhood, it is important to recognize unusual clinical presentations that may indicate the need for further investigation. Many of the childhood diseases associated with eczematous eruptions benefit tremendously from early diagnosis. Some unusual, but very important, causes of eczema in childhood include:

- Primary immunodeficiencies:
  - Autosomal-dominant hyper-IgE syndrome (AD-HIES),
  - Dedicator of cytokinesis 8 gene (DOCK8) deficiency,
  - Phosphoglucomutase 3 (PGM3) deficiency,
  - Wiskott–Aldrich syndrome (WAS),
  - Severe combined immunodeficiency (SCID),
  - IPEX syndrome (immune dysregulation, polyendocrinopathy, enteropathy, X-linked syndrome), and
  - Netherton syndrome (NS).
- MF.
- Nutritional deficiencies:
  - Pellagra,
  - Kwashiorkor,
  - Zinc deficiency, and
  - Biotin deficiency.

Primary Immunodeficiencies

Eczematous dermatitis is a significant clinical feature of many primary immunodeficiency disorders. When severe and widespread eczema develops at birth or in the early neonatal period and is associated with recurrent or severe infections, chronic lymphadenopathy, significantly increased IgE levels, persistent eosinophilia, recalcitrant oral thrush, or failure to thrive, an evaluation for an underlying immunodeficiency may be warranted.[3] The specific clinical manifestations of primary immunodeficiencies with associated eczematous dermatitis are listed in **Table 1**. For many of these conditions, hematopoietic stem cell transplantation is the treatment of choice, although gene therapy and enzyme replacement are novel treatments under development for some immunodeficiency disorders.

Autosomal-dominant hyperimmunoglobulin E syndrome

AD-HIES is an immunodeficiency syndrome caused by dominant negative mutations in the signal transducer and activator of transcription 3 (STAT3) gene. STAT3 regulates processes involving cell growth and inflammation, with mutations in STAT3 leading to failure of T helper 17 cell differentiation and reduced IL-17 production.[4,5] AD-HIES is characterized by eczematous eruptions, skin abscesses, recurrent sinopulmonary infections, mucocutaneous candidiasis, and malignancies. The rash commonly presents within the first few weeks of life, which is earlier onset than is typical for atopic dermatitis. The eruption tends to start on the face and scalp. It may be papulopustular at onset but within the first year of life, an eczematous dermatitis develops

Table 1
Features of primary immunodeficiencies associated with eczematous dermatitis

Disease	Gene	Inheritance	Clinical Features	Lab Abnormalities
AD-HIES	*STAT3*	AD, less commonly sporadic	• Cold abscesses • Recurrent sinopulmonary infections • Mucocutaneous candidiasis • Coarse facies • Minimal trauma fractures • Scoliosis • Joint hyperextensibility • Retained primary teeth • Coronary artery tortuosity or dilation • Lymphoma	• High IgE (>2000 IU/µL) • Eosinophilia
DOCK8 deficiency	*DOCK8*	AR	• Severe mucocutaneous viral infections • Mucocutaneous candidiasis • Atopic features (asthma, allergies) • Squamous cell carcinoma • Lymphoma	• High IgE • Eosinophilia • With or without decreased IgM
PGM3 deficiency	*PGM3*	AR	• Neurologic abnormalities • Leukocytoclastic vasculitis • Atopic features (asthma, allergies) • Sinopulmonary infections • Mucocutaneous viral infections	• High IgE • Eosinophilia
WAS	*WASP*	XLR	• Hepatosplenomegaly • Lymphadenopathy • Atopic diathesis • Autoimmune conditions (especially hemolytic anemia) • Lymphoreticular malignancies	• Thrombocytopenia (<80,000/uL) • Low mean platelet volume • Eosinophilia is common • Lymphopenia • Low IgM, variable IgG

(continued on next page)

Table 1
(continued)

Disease	Gene	Inheritance	Clinical Features	Lab Abnormalities
SCID	Variable, depends on type	XLR and AR most common	• Recurrent, severe infections • Failure to thrive • Persistent diarrhea • Recalcitrant oral candidiasis • Omenn: lymphadenopathy, hepatospleno-megaly, erythroderma	• Lymphopenia common • Variable patterns of reduced lymphocyte subsets (T, B, natural killer cells) • Omenn: high lymphocytes, eosinophilia, high IgE
IPEX	FOXP3	XLR	• Severe diarrhea (autoimmune enteropathy) • Various autoimmune endocrinopathies (especially diabetes mellitus, thyroiditis) • Food allergies	• High IgE • Eosinophilia • Various autoantibodies
Netherton syndrome	SPINK5	AR	• Hair shaft abnormalities • Erythroderma • Ichthyosis linearis circumflexa • Food allergies • Recurrent gastroenteritis • Neonatal hypernatremic dehydration • Upper and lower respiratory infections	• High IgE • Eosinophilia

Abbreviations: AD, autosomal dominant; AD-HIES, autosomal-dominant hyper-IgE syndrome; AR, autosomal recessive; DOCK8, dedicator of cytokinesis 8 gene; Ig, immunoglobulin; IPEX, immune dysregulation, polyendocrinopathy, enteropathy, X-linked syndrome; PGM3, phosphoglucomutase 3; SCID, severe combined immunodeficiency; WAS, Wiskott–Aldrich syndrome.

with varying severity (**Fig. 1**). The presence of *Staphylococcus aureus* seems to be a provoking factor and cutaneous infections are common.[6–8] These patients may suffer from recurrent cold abscesses, most often secondary to *S aureus* and lacking typical features of warmth and erythema. All patients with AD-HIES have elevated serum IgE, usually with peak levels of greater than 2000 IU/μL, and eosinophilia is almost always present.[8] Children with severe atopic dermatitis may have greatly increased IgE levels and eosinophilia, so this feature alone is not diagnostic of AD-HIES. Craniofacial, musculoskeletal, dental, and vascular abnormalities can be extremely useful for diagnosing AD-HIES.[9,10] AD-HIES is also associated with an increased risk of malignancy, most commonly non-Hodgkin lymphoma.[7]

Dedicator of cytokinesis 8 gene deficiency

Mutations in the DOCK8 gene were discovered to be responsible for an autosomal-recessive form of hyper-IgE syndrome.[11] DOCK8 deficiency shares many similar clinical features with AD-HIES, including elevated serum IgE levels, eosinophilia, eczematous dermatitis, staphylococcal skin and sinopulmonary infections, and risk of lymphoma. However, unlike the neonatal pustular eruption that often occurs in AD-HIES, patients with DOCK8 deficiency tend to develop an eczematous rash in the classic atopic dermatitis areas. The eruption may begin beyond the neonatal period. In a study by Chu and colleagues,[12] the incidence of newborn rash was 24% in the DOCK8-deficient cohort, in contrast with 81% of patients with AD-HIES, although the DOCK8-deficient cohort had more severe dermatitis. Other distinguishing features of DOCK8 deficiency include the presence of multiple food and environmental allergies, asthma, and an increased risk of squamous cell carcinoma. Furthermore, nearly all patients with DOCK8 deficiency develop extensive, recurrent and treatment-resistant cutaneous viral infections owing to herpes simplex virus, varicella zoster virus, human papilloma virus, and/or molluscum contagiosum. DOCK8 deficiency has been shown to impair the development and survival of mature natural killer (NK) cells, which would contribute to the host susceptibility to viral infections.[13]

Phosphoglucomutase 3 deficiency

PGM3 deficiency is another autosomal-recessive form of hyper-IgE syndrome owing to a mutation in the PGM3 gene that results in dysfunction of the glycosylation pathway. This condition shares similar features with both AD-HIES and DOCK8 deficiency, including the development of eczematous dermatitis of variable severity. Neurologic impairment and leukocytoclastic vasculitis are unique features of PGM3 deficiency.[14]

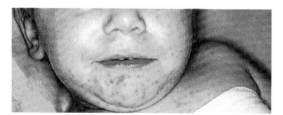

Fig. 1. Early papulopustular rash on the face of an infant with hyper-IgE syndrome. (*From* Olaiwan A, Marie-Oliveria C, Fraitag S, et al. Cutaneous findings in sporadic and familial autosomal dominant hyper-IgE syndrome: a retrospective, single-center study of 21 patients diagnosed using molecular analysis. J Am Acad Dermatol 2011;65:1169; with permission.)

Wiskott–Aldrich syndrome

WAS is an X-linked recessive condition characterized by thrombocytopenia and small dysfunctional platelets, recalcitrant eczematous dermatitis, and recurrent bacterial infections. It almost exclusively occurs in males with few reports of females affected.[15] WAS is secondary to loss-of-function mutations in the WAS protein (WASP) gene, which plays a role in lymphoid development and thereby affects both B and T lymphocyte function.[16] Owing to thrombocytopenia and platelet dysfunction from birth, patients often present initially with spontaneous bleeding, such as epistaxis or bloody stools. The dermatitis usually begins within the first few months of life and is indistinguishable from atopic dermatitis, but may be more generalized and/or severe. The face, scalp, and flexural areas are typically affected and secondary bacterial infections are common. Owing to the bleeding diathesis, excoriated areas are more likely to demonstrate serosanguinous crust, petechiae, and purpura. Recurrent bacterial infections, especially with encapsulated organisms, begin in infancy as maternal antibodies wane. Most children with WAS also develop autoimmune or inflammatory disease over time. Hemolytic anemia is the most common, but other conditions reported in patients with WAS include autoimmune neutropenia, painful cutaneous small vessel vasculitis, arthritis, cerebral vasculitis, inflammatory bowel disease, and renal disease.[17] In 1 study, nearly 25% of WAS patients developed malignancies including lymphoma and myelodysplasia.[18]

Severe combined immunodeficiency

SCID describes a group of disorders that arise from a variety of genetic defects and result in absent lymphocyte development and function. The most common types of SCID include an X-linked recessive form involving IL2RG mutations with loss of T and NK cell development, and an autosomal-recessive form involving RAG1 or RAG2 mutations with resultant loss of T-cell and B-cell development. Adenosine deaminase–SCID accounts for approximately 15% of cases, with deficiency of intracellular enzyme adenosine deaminase leading to the accumulation of metabolic precursors that are toxic to lymphocytes.[19] Infants tend to present between 3 and 6 months of life as maternal antibodies wane, although screening for SCID as part of the newborn panel has been more recently implemented in many states and leads to earlier diagnosis.[20] Typical features of SCID include recurrent and/or severe infections, persistent diarrhea, failure to thrive, and recalcitrant oral candidiasis. Infants may also develop a generalized dermatitis, which may be seborrheic or exfoliative. Omenn syndrome is a variant of SCID caused by deficiency of RAG protein, and nearly all infants with Omenn syndrome present with extensive skin inflammation or erythroderma (**Fig. 2**). Other common features of Omenn syndrome include hepatosplenomegaly, lymphadenopathy, alopecia, eosinophilia, and elevated IgE levels.[7,19]

Immune dysregulation, polyendocrinopathy, enteropathy, X-linked syndrome

IPEX syndrome is an X-linked recessive disorder owing to a mutation in the FOXP3 transcription factor resulting in abnormal development of T-regulatory cells.[21,22] Affected males typically present during the first months of life with severe watery diarrhea owing to autoimmune enteropathy, various autoimmune endocrinopathies (eg, early onset diabetes mellitus, thyroiditis), and chronic dermatitis. The dermatitis in infancy tends to be eczematous and is usually widespread affecting the trunk, lower extremities, and face. It is often recalcitrant to standard treatments and may be complicated by frequent staphylococcal superinfections and sepsis. Other reported cutaneous manifestations of IPEX syndrome include psoriasiform dermatitis, erythroderma, urticaria, alopecia, onychodystrophy, and cheilitis.[23,24] The majority

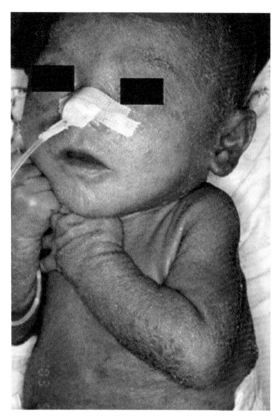

Fig. 2. Generalized exfoliative dermatitis in a 2-month-old boy with Omenn syndrome. (*From* Hsu C, Lee JY, Chao S. Omenn syndrome: a case report and review of literature. Dermatologica Sinca 2009;29:51; with permission.)

of patients with IPEX have markedly elevated IgE and eosinophils, and a variety of autoantibodies.[25]

Netherton syndrome

NS is an autosomal-recessive condition with a triad of ichthyosis, atopic diathesis, and hair shaft deformities. It is caused by mutations in the SPINK5 gene, which encodes a serine protease inhibitor and mutations ultimately leads to reduced desmosomal proteins.[26,27] NS typically presents in the neonatal or early infantile period with generalized ichthyosiform erythroderma. The scaly erythroderma tends to improve with age, but the majority of patients with NS will develop ichthyosis linearis circumflexa starting in toddler or early childhood years and appearing as migratory, serpiginous, and polycyclic scaly lesions with a characteristic peripheral double-edged scale.[28] Infants may also develop recurrent acute gastroenteritis, failure to thrive, and hypernatremic dehydration. NS has a classic hair shaft abnormality called trichorrhexis invaginata, resulting in easily broken hairs that appear as "bamboo hair" or "ball and socket" abnormalities under magnification. A recent study identified many immunologic abnormalities in patients with NS, including reduced memory B cells, skewed Th1 phenotype, impaired antibody amplification and class-switching, decreased NK cell cytotoxicity, and elevated proinflammatory cytokine levels.[29] These findings have led some to suggest that NS should be considered a primary immunodeficiency and helps to explain why patients with NS are susceptible to staphylococcal skin infections, respiratory infections, and sepsis. The majority of patients with NS also demonstrate an atopic diathesis with pruritic atopic dermatitis, food allergies, rhinitis, and/or asthma.[29]

Malignancy

Mycosis fungoides

MF is a type of primary cutaneous T-cell lymphoma and is predominantly a disease of older adults, with pediatric MF accounting for less than 5% of all MF cases. The clinical presentation of MF in children is quite variable and may occur at any age, even as early as infancy.[30] Hypopigmented MF is a variant that occurs most commonly in children, especially those with darker skin types. Children with hypopigmented MF present with hypopigmented macules and patches, which are often round and may have slight overlying scale. The lesions are usually asymptomatic and occur in sun-protected areas. Hypopigmented MF can easily be mistaken for postinflammatory hypopigmentation secondary to atopic dermatitis or other inflammatory conditions. MF in children may also present as erythematous, scaly papules and plaques, which can be pruritic and very closely mimic atopic dermatitis. There may be subtle clues of MF, such as poikilodermatous changes, atrophy, and telangiectasia. Frequently, it is the chronicity and recalcitrance to therapy that prompts skin biopsy and leads to the diagnosis of MF, often years after the lesions developed. Fortunately, most cases of pediatric MF represent very early stage disease without involvement of lymph nodes, viscera, or blood. It tends to follow an indolent course and progression to advanced-stage MF during childhood is rare.[30–32] Common treatment options for MF in children include phototherapy and topical steroids.

Nutritional Deficiencies

Nutritional deficiencies are important to consider in children presenting with recalcitrant dermatitis. Even children with adequate access to food can develop nutritional deficiencies secondary to chronic medical conditions, parental nutritional ignorance, food allergen avoidance, or restrictive diets. Identification of nutritional deficiencies is life saving for some children, and the conditions are often easily treatable.

Pellagra

Pellagra is a disorder resulting from a severe cellular deficiency of niacin, owing to inadequate dietary nicotinic acid or its precursor essential amino acid, tryptophan. Pellagra now rarely occurs in developed countries owing to dietary availability of niacin, but those with malabsorptive states, restrictive eating behaviors, and poor social circumstances (eg, homelessness) remain at particular risk. This condition is characterized by the classic triad of dermatitis, diarrhea, and dementia. The dermatitis begins as a well-demarcated scaling erythema, with similar appearance to a sunburn, on areas exposed to sunlight, heat, friction, or pressure. The face, neck, dorsal hands and arms, feet, and inguinal area are commonly affected; in infants, the diaper area is often involved. There may be associated burning sensation, pruritus, and/or tenderness. "Casal's necklace" is a term used for a characteristic red eruption with well-defined borders on the lower neck. Vesicles and bullae may be present. Over time, the erythema transitions to a dusky brown-red color, and later stages may demonstrate hyperkeratosis, scaling, fissuring, and shellaclike shiny appearance. Oral involvement, such as glossitis, cheilitis, aphthous ulcers, and fissuring, occurs in one-third of patients. Gastrointestinal manifestations may include diarrhea, poor appetite, nausea, vomiting, and abdominal pain. Neuropsychiatric disturbances can range broadly—from headache and irritability to confusion and psychosis. Measurement of urinary metabolites of niacin (N_1-methylnicotinamine and/or pyridine) can aid in the diagnosis of pellagra.[33,34]

Secondary pellagra occurs when adequate amounts of niacin are consumed in the diet, but other conditions interfere with its absorption or processing. Hartnup disease is a rare autosomal-recessive disorder caused by a mutation in the SLC6A19 gene, which encodes a transporter of neutral amino acids.[35] Loss of function of this transporter leads to inability to resorb tryptophan and other amino acids by the small intestine and renal tubules. Hartnup disease is often diagnosed in children between the ages of 3 and 9 years and manifests as a pellagralike cutaneous eruption and neurologic abnormalities (predominantly cerebellar ataxia). Diagnosis can be achieved by analysis of urine amino acids, and treatment consists of prolonged high doses of oral nicotinic acid.[36]

Kwashiorkor

Severe protein deficiency is most often seen in children of developing countries secondary to poverty and limited access to protein-containing foods. In higher income countries, protein deficiency is more commonly owing to food allergen avoidance and other restrictive diets, nutritional ignorance, and malabsorptive conditions.[37] The substitution of rice milk as a dietary staple for infants has become a common cause of protein deficiency in the United States.[38] The presence of protein deficiency without significant total caloric deficit results in a condition called kwashiorkor, with typical features including edema, hypoalbuminemia, and rash. The eruption appears as an erythematous, crusted, erosive, and desquamative dermatitis. The dermatitis tends to have an overlying reddish-brown scale with sharply marginated, raised edges that may seem to be "pasted-on" or similar to "flaky paint." The flexures, face, perioral area, and diaper area are most frequently affected, which differs from the rash on sun-exposed sites seen in pellagra. The edema seen in kwashiorkor tends to be prominent on the face, feet, and abdomen. Affected children often demonstrate mental status changes such as irritability or apathy. Treatment of children with kwashiorkor involves gradual introduction of a high-protein diet with careful attention to electrolyte imbalances and hydration status.[37]

Zinc deficiency

Zinc deficiency often manifests with an eczematous dermatitis but in characteristic locations that help to establish the diagnosis. Acrodermatitis enteropathica is an autosomal-recessive inherited disorder with mutations in SLC39A, which results in dysfunction of an intestinal zinc transporter, with subsequent severe zinc deficiency. Breastfeeding-related zinc deficiency can occur secondary to maternal mutations resulting in poor secretion of zinc into breastmilk, or in premature infants exclusively breastfed without zinc supplementation. In addition, there is a risk of zinc deficiency in patients with malabsorption as seen in inflammatory bowel disease and cystic fibrosis, as well as children receiving parenteral nutrition without zinc additive.[39,40] Whether zinc deficiency is congenital or acquired, it may present with a triad of diarrhea, acral and periorificial dermatitis, and alopecia. The dermatitis consists of eczematous pink scaly plaques, which can become vesicular, bullous, pustular, or desquamative. The lesions develop over the anogenital and periorificial areas, extensor extremities, scalp, fingers, and toes (**Fig. 3**). Secondary infection with *Candida albicans* is common on the face and may also lead to paronychia of the digits. Infants with zinc deficiency may demonstrate growth delay, poor feeding, apathy, and/or irritability.

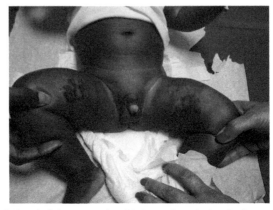

Fig. 3. The rash of zinc deficiency on the thighs and genitals of a breastfed infant.

Diagnosis is based on clinical suspicion and low serum zinc levels. Both acrodermatitis enteropathica and acquired forms of zinc deficiency are treated with zinc supplementation, and infants often show dramatic improvement of their symptoms within days.[40,41] Findings resembling acrodermatitis enteopathica have also been described in patients with biotin deficiency and certain organic acid disorders.

URTICARIA

Urticaria is owing to localized edema in the superficial dermis, leading to the characteristic pink or pale elevated swellings called wheals. Wheals may vary in size from a few millimeters to several centimeters. Urticarial lesions may assume an annular, polycyclic, or serpiginous pattern with clearing of the central region and coalescence of the wheals. Urticaria is classically pruritic and transient with individual wheals lasting less than 24 hours. Acute urticaria, defined as urticaria occurring for less than 6 weeks, is a common self-limited hypersensitivity response in children that is often secondary to infection, medications, or food allergies. However, chronic urticaria can be a manifestation of rare autoinflammatory syndromes and a clue to an underlying disorder.

Autoinflammatory syndromes are a rare category of inherited disorders characterized by recurrent fevers and episodic inflammation of multiple organ systems. Unlike autoimmune diseases, which exhibit autoreactive T lymphocytes or autoantibodies, the persistent inflammation in autoinflammatory syndromes is owing to aberrant regulation of the innate immune system where cytokine signaling pathways are activated in the absence of a recognizable infection.[42,43] Autoinflammatory syndromes should be suspected in a child with recurrent bouts of urticaria lasting months to years. The urticarial outbreaks are associated with other symptoms of inflammation such as fever, arthritis, serositis, hepatosplenomegaly, and ocular and/or neurologic involvement (**Table 2**). Infection or malignancy should be excluded through appropriate investigations.

Atypical urticaria are a common presenting feature in several autoinflammatory syndromes that present in childhood, including:

- Cryopyrin-associated periodic syndromes (CAPS)
  - Familial cold autoinflammatory syndrome
  - Muckle-Wells syndrome
  - Chronic infantile neurologic cutaneous articular syndrome/neonatal-onset multisystem inflammatory disease

Table 2
Febrile autoinflammatory diseases causing urticaria in children

Disease	Gene (Protein)	Inheritance	Attack Length	Timing of Onset	Cutaneous Features	Extracutaneous Clinical Features
FCAS	*NLRP3* (cryopyrin)	AD	Brief; Minutes–3 d	Neonatal or infantile	Cold-induced urticaria	• Arthralgia • Conjunctivitis • Headache
Muckle-Wells syndrome	*NLRP3* (cryopyrin)	AD	1–3 d	Neonatal, infantile, childhood (can be later)	Widespread urticaria	• Arthralgia/arthritis • Sensorineural hearing loss • Conjunctivitis/episcleritis • Headache • Amyloidosis
Chronic infantile neurologic cutaneous articular syndrome/neonatal-onset multisystem inflammatory disease	*NLRP3* (cryopyrin)	AD	Continuous flares	Neonatal or infantile	Widespread urticaria	• Deforming osteoarthropathy, epiphyseal overgrowth • Sensorineural hearing loss • Dysmorphic facies • Chronic aseptic meningitis, headaches, papilledema, seizures • Conjunctivitis/uveitis, optic atrophy • Growth retardation • Developmental delay • Amyloidosis
HIDS	*MVK* (mevalonate kinase)	AR	3–7 d	Infancy (<2 y)	• Intermittent morbilliform or urticarial rash • Aphthous mucosal ulcers • Erythema nodosum	• Arthralgia/arthritis • Cervical lymphadenopathy • Severe abdominal pain • Diarrhea/vomiting

(continued on next page)

Table 2
(continued)

Disease	Gene (Protein)	Inheritance	Attack Length	Timing of Onset	Cutaneous Features	Extracutaneous Clinical Features
						• Headache • Elevated IgD and IgA antibody levels • Elevated urine mevalonic acid during attacks
Tumor necrosis factor receptor-associated periodic syndrome	*TNFRSF1A* (TNFR1)	AD	>7 d	Childhood	• Intermittent migratory erythematous macules and edematous plaques overlying areas of myalgia, often on limbs • Periorbital edema	• Migratory myalgia • Conjunctivitis • Serositis • Amyloidosis
Systemic onset juvenile idiopathic arthritis	Polygenic	Varies	Daily (quotidian)	Peak onset at 1–6 y	• Nonfixed erythematous rash, may be urticarial • With or without Dermatographism • With or without Periorbital edema	• Polyarthritis • Myalgia • Hepatosplenomegaly • Lymphadenopathy • Serositis
PLAID	PLCG2	AD	N/A	Infancy	• Urticaria induced by evaporative cooling • Ulcers in cold-exposed areas	• Allergies • Autoimmune disease • Recurrent sinopulmonary infections • Elevated IgE antibody levels • Decreased IgA and IgM antibody levels • Often elevated antinuclear antibody titers

Abbreviations: AD, autosomal dominant; AR, autosomal recessive; Ig, immunoglobulin; PLAID, PLCγ2-associated antibody deficiency and immune dysregulation; SoJIA, systemic onset juvenile idiopathic arthritis.

- Hyperimmunoglobulinemia D with periodic fever syndrome (HIDS)
- Tumor necrosis factor receptor-associated periodic syndrome
- Systemic onset juvenile idiopathic arthritis
- PLCγ2-associated antibody deficiency and immune dysregulation (PLAID)

Cryopyrin-associated Periodic Syndromes

CAPS are a group of autoinflammatory syndromes caused by mutations in cryopyrin, also called NLRP3 (nucleotide-binding domain and leucine-rich repeat containing family, pyrin domain-containing 3).[44] When stimulated by various danger-associated molecular patterns and pathogen-associated molecular patterns, NLRP3 associates with other proteins to form the inflammasome, resulting in increased release of active IL-1β. Mutations in NLRP3 result in constitutive inflammasome activity and subsequent IL-1β secretion.

In the CAPS, a rash is usually the first notable symptom. The rash is typically migratory and resembling urticarica, but it is often nonpruritic and can be painful. The rash commonly has diurnal variation with minimal rash in the morning, gradual increase in severity throughout the day, and worst rash in the evening.[43] In familial cold autoinflammatory syndrome, the urticarial eruption is unique in that it occurs approximately 1 to 2 hours after exposure to cold temperature.[45,46] In addition to an urticarial eruption, all forms of CAPS are characterized by recurrent fevers and joint inflammation, usually presenting in infancy. The majority of individuals with Muckle-Wells syndrome suffer from a sensorineural hearing loss, whereas chronic infantile neurologic cutaneous articular syndrome/neonatal-onset multisystem inflammatory disease is the most severe of the cryopyrinopathies with neurologic abnormalities (including sensorineural hearing loss) and deforming osteoarthropathies. In addition, the development of secondary amyloidosis occurs in approximately 25% of patients with Muckle-Wells syndrome and chronic infantile neurologic cutaneous articular syndrome/neonatal-onset multisystem inflammatory disease. Amyloid deposition in the kidneys can lead to renal failure and is an important factor in overall prognosis.[42,46] Interestingly, the severity of clinical disease does not predict association with amyloidosis.[43] Treatment of CAPs is focused on decreasing IL-1β activity through the use of anakinra (IL-1 receptor antagonist), rilonacept (IL-1 trap), and canakinumab (IL-1β monoclonal antibody).[47–49]

Hyperimmunoglobulinemia D with Periodic Fever Syndrome

HIDS is an autosomal-recessive disease associated with mutations in the MVK gene. These mutations result in decreased activity of mevalonate kinase, resulting in decreased isoprenoid production and ultimately, increased IL-1β release.[50] Inflammatory symptoms begin within the first 1 to 2 years of life, often triggered by vaccinations. Cutaneous manifestations occur in two-thirds of patients with HIDS, and may include morbiliform and urticarial eruptions, as well as erythema nodosum (**Fig. 4**). Importantly, about one-half of patients develop aphthous ulcers in the mouth and/or genitals, which often leads to an incorrect diagnosis of Behçet disease.[51] Abdominal pain is also a common feature of HIDS.

Tumor Necrosis Factor Receptor-associated Periodic Syndrome

Caused by mutations in the TNFR1 gene, tumor necrosis factor receptor-associated periodic syndrome is unique in that febrile attacks are longer lasting, often 1 to 6 weeks.[52,53] Skin manifestations can resemble urticaria and include migratory erythematous macules or patches, edematous dermal plaques, serpiginous or annular

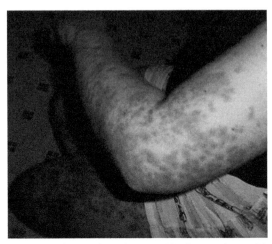

Fig. 4. Urticarial eruption on the trunk and extremities in a patient with hyperimmunoglobulinemia D with periodic fever syndrome. (*From* Brydges S, Athreya B, Kasther DL. Periodic fever syndromes in children. In: Cassidy JT, Petty RE, editors. Textbook of pediatric rheumatology. 5th edition. Philadelphia: Elsevier Saunders; 2005. p. 642–60; with permission.)

lesions, and periorbital edema.[42] Often there is a warm, tender erythematous swollen plaque that arises on the limbs near the trunk and migrates distally (**Fig. 5**). Skin lesions typically correlate with underlying myalgias.[45] Secondary amyloidosis may occur in 10% to 15% of patients.

Systemic-Onset Juvenile Idiopathic Arthritis

Systemic onset juvenile idiopathic arthritis is a polygenic autoinflammatory syndrome. Although it is officially classified as a subtype of juvenile idiopathic arthritis, it shares many similarities with the hereditary autoinflammatory syndromes.[54] The condition is characterized by daily high spiking fevers in association with an inflammatory arthritis lasting longer than 6 weeks.[55] In contrast with other forms of JIA, the diagnosis of systemic onset JIA requires an additional extraarticular finding, which may include hepatomegaly, splenomegaly, lymphadenopathy, serositis, or an evanescent rash. The rash typically consists of salmon pink or erythematous macules and urticarial plaques, with possible associated dermatographism, involving the trunk, neck, and extremities. The face, palms, and soles are almost always spared. The urticarial eruption with systemic onset juvenile idiopathic arthritis varies throughout the day; it tends to be worst in evening hours, correlating with fever spikes and arthritis flares.[42,44,46]

PLCγ2-associated Antibody Deficiency and Immune Dysregulation

PLAID is a recently described entity that may represent a distinct type of autoinflammatory syndrome with an associated immunodeficiency.[56] PLAID is an autosomal-dominant condition caused by a mutation in PLCG2, leading to the development of urticaria in early childhood.[57] The urticaria are typically induced by evaporative cooling; ulcers in cold-exposed areas are also seen. Patients with this condition also develop autoimmune disease and recurrent sinopulmonary infections. Some patients with PLAID have a more pronounced inflammatory syndrome with pneumonitis, colitis, eye inflammation, arthralgias, and blistering skin lesions.[58,59] Immunologic abnormalities include elevated IgE, decreased IgA and IgM, and decreased circulating B cells and NK cells.

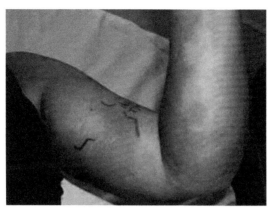

Fig. 5. Migrating erythematous plaques during an inflammatory attack in a patient with tumor necrosis factor receptor-associated periodic syndrome. (*From* van der Hilst JCH, van der Meer JWM, Drenth JPH. Autoinflammatory fever syndromes. In: Rich R, Fleisher T, Shearer E, et al, editors. Clinical immunology: principles and practice. 3rd edition. Philadelphia: Elsevier/Mosby; 2008. p. 899–908; with permission.)

SUMMARY

Eczema and urticaria may occasionally be the presenting complaint in a child with an underlying rare disease. Immunodeficiency syndromes should be suspected when eczema is associated with neonatal onset, recurrent infections, chronic lymphadenopathy, or failure to thrive. Nutritional deficiencies and MF are also in the differential diagnosis for a child with a recalcitrant eczematous eruption. Autoinflammatory syndromes should be suspected in a child with chronic urticaria, fever, and other systemic signs of inflammation. Even though these disorders are rare, early recognition of these disorders allows for appropriate treatment and decreased morbidity for the child.

REFERENCES

1. Silverberg JI, Simpson EL. Associations of childhood eczema severity: a US population based study. Dermatitis 2014;25:107–14.
2. Kay J, Gawkrodger DJ, Mortimer MJ, et al. The prevalence of childhood atopic eczema in a general population. J Am Acad Dermatol 1994;30:35–9.
3. Subbarayan A, Colarusso G, Hughes SM, et al. Clinical features that identify children with primary immunodeficiency diseases. Pediatrics 2011;127:810–6.
4. Holland SM, DeLeo FR, Elloumi HZ, et al. STAT3 mutations in the Hyper-IgE syndrome. N Engl J Med 2007;357:1608–19.
5. Ma CS, Chew GY, Simpson N, et al. Deficiency of Th17 cells in hyper IgE syndrome due to mutations in STAT3. J Exp Med 2008;205:1551–7.
6. Eberting CL, Davis J, Puck JM, et al. Dermatitis and the newborn rash in hyper-IgE syndrome. Arch Dermatol 2004;140:1119–25.
7. Pichard DC, Freeman AF, Cowen EW. Primary immunodeficiency update: part I. Syndromes associated with eczematous dermatitis. J Am Acad Dermatol 2015; 73:355–64.
8. Sowerwine K, Holland SM, Freeman AF. Hyper-IgE syndrome update. Ann N Y Acad Sci 2012;1250:25–32.
9. Freeman AF, Holland SM. Clinical manifestations of hyperIgE syndromes. Dis Markers 2010;29:123–30.

10. Freeman AF, Avila EM, Shaw PA, et al. Coronary artery abnormalities in hyper-IgE syndrome. J Clin Immunol 2011;31:338–45.
11. Zhang Q, Davis JC, Lamborn IT, et al. Combined immunodeficiency associated with DOCK8 mutations. N Engl J Med 2009;361:2046–55.
12. Chu EY, Freeman AF, Jing H, et al. Cutaneous manifestations of DOCK8 deficiency syndrome. Arch Dermatol 2012;148:79–84.
13. Crawford G, Enders A, Gileadi U, et al. DOCK8 is critical for the survival and function of NKT cells. Blood 2013;122:2015–61.
14. Zhang Y, Yu X, Ichikawa M, et al. Autosomal recessive PGM3 mutations link glycosylation defects to atopy, immune deficiency, autoimmunity, and neurocognitive impairment. J Allergy Clin Immunol 2014;133:1400–9.
15. Conley ME, Wang WC, Parolini O, et al. Atypical Wiskott-Aldrich syndrome in a girl. Blood 1992;80:1264–9.
16. Derry JM, Ochs HD, Francke U, et al. Isolation of a novel gene mutated in Wiskott-Aldrich syndrome. Cell 1994;78:635–44.
17. Dupuis-Girod S, Medioni J, Haddad E, et al. Autoimmunity in Wiskott-Aldrich syndrome: risk factors, clinical features, and outcome in a single-center cohort of 55 patients. Pediatrics 2003;111:e622–7.
18. Imai K, Morio T, Zhu Y, et al. Clinical course of patients with WASP gene mutations. Blood 2004;103:456–64.
19. Rivers L, Gaspar HB. Severe combined immunodeficiency: recent developments and guidance on clinical management. Arch Dis Child 2015;100:667–72.
20. Severe Combined Immunodeficiency (SCID). Centers for Disease Control and Prevention. Available at: http://www.cdc.gov/newbornscreening/scid.html. Accessed May 22, 2016.
21. Bennett CL, Christie J, Ramsdell F, et al. The immune dysregulation, polyendocrinopathy, enteropathy, X-lined syndrome (IPEX) is caused by mutations of FOXP3. Nat Genet 2001;27:20–1.
22. Sakaguchi S. The origin of FOXP3-expressing CD4+ regulatory T cells: thymus or periphery. J Clin Invest 2003;112:1310–2.
23. Nieves D, Phipps RP, Pollock SJ, et al. Dermatologic and immunologic findings in the immune dysregulation, polyendocrinopathy, enteropathy, x-linked syndrome. Arch Dermatol 2004;140:466–72.
24. Halabi-Tawil M, Ruemmele FM, Fraitag S, et al. Cutaneous manifestations of immune dysregulation, polyendocrinopathy, enteropathy, X-linked (IPEX) syndrome. Br J Dermatol 2009;160:645–51.
25. Barzaghi F, Passerini L, Bacchetta R. Immune dysregulation, polyendocrinopathy, enteropathy, X-linked syndrome: a paradigm of immunodeficiency with autoimmunity. Front Immunol 2012;3:1–25.
26. Chavanas S, Bodemer C, Rochat A, et al. Mutations in SPINK5, encoding a serine protease inhibitor, cause Netherton syndrome. Nat Genet 2000;25(2):141–2.
27. Descargues P, Deraison C, Bonnart C, et al. Spink5-deficient mice mimic Netherton syndrome through degradation of desmoglein 1 by epidermal protease hyperactivity. Nat Genet 2005;37:56–65.
28. Greene S, Muller S. Netherton's syndrome. J Am Acad Dermatol 1985;13(2):329–37.
29. Renner ED, Hartl D, Rylaarsdam S, et al. Comél-Netherton syndrome defined as primary immunodeficiency. J Allergy Clin Immunol 2009;124(3):536–43.
30. Zackheim HS, McCalmont TH, Deanovic FW, et al. Mycosis fungoides with onset before 20 years of age. J Am Acad Dermatol 1997;36(4):557–62.

31. Hodak E, Amitay-Laish I, Feinmesser M, et al. Juvenile mycosis fungoides: cutaneous T-cell lymphoma with frequent follicular involvement. J Am Acad Dermatol 2014;70(6):993–1001.
32. Yee KH, Koh MJ, Giam YC, et al. Pediatric mycosis fungoides in Singapore: a series of 46 children. Pediatr Dermatol 2014;31:477–82.
33. Hegyi J, Schwartz RA, Heygi V. Pellagra: dermatitis, dementia, and diarrhea. Int J Dermatol 2004;43:1–5.
34. Karthikeyan K, Thappa DM. Pellagra and skin. Int J Dermatol 2002;41:476–81.
35. Nozaki J, Dakeishi M, Ohura T, et al. Homozygosity mapping to chromosome 5 p 15 of a gene responsible for Hartnup Disorder. Biochem Biophys Res Commun 2001;284:255–60.
36. Patel AB, Prabhu AS. Hartnup disease. Indian J Dermatol 2008;53:31–2.
37. Liu T, Howard RM, Mancini AJ, et al. Kwashiorkor in the United States: fad diets, perceived and true milk allergy, and nutritional ignorance. Arch Dermatol 2001; 137:630–6.
38. Carvalho NF, Kenney RD, Carrington PH, et al. Severe nutritional deficiencies in toddlers resulting from health food milk alternatives. Pediatrics 2001;107:E46.
39. Cheng HC, Wang JD, Chen CH, et al. A young infant with periorficial and acral dermatitis. J Pediatr 2014;165:408.
40. Perafán-Riveros C, Franca LF, Alves AC, et al. Acrodermatitis enteropathica: case report and review of the literature. Pediatr Dermatol 2002;19:426–31.
41. Maverakis E, Fung MA, Lynch PJ, et al. Acrodermatitis enteropathica and an overview of zinc metabolism. J Am Acad Dermatol 2007;56:116–24.
42. Cush J. Autoinflammatory syndromes. Dermatol Clin 2013;31:471–80.
43. Shinkai K, McCalmont TH, Leslie KS. Cryopyrin-associated periodic syndromes and autoinflammation. Clin Exp Dermatol 2008;33:1–9.
44. Rigante D, Frediani B, Cantarini L. A comprehensive overview of the hereditary periodic fever syndromes. Clin Rev Allergy Immunol 2016. [Epub ahead of print].
45. Braun-Falco M, Ruzicka T. Skin manifestations in autoinflammatory syndromes. J Dtsch Dermatol Ges 2011;9:232–46.
46. Miyamae T. Cryopyrin-associated periodic syndromes: diagnosis and management. Paediatr Drugs 2012;14:109–17.
47. Hoffman HM, Rosengren S, Boyle DL, et al. Prevention of cold-associated acute inflammation in familial cold autoinflammatory syndrome by interleukin-1 receptor antagonist. Lancet 2004;364:1779–85.
48. Hoffman HM, Throne ML, Amar NJ, et al. Efficacy and safety of rilonacept (interleukin-1 Trap) in patients with cryopyrin-associated periodic syndromes: results from two sequential placebo-controlled studies. Arthritis Rheum 2008;58(8): 2443–52.
49. Lachmann HJ, Kone-Paut I, Kuemmerle-Deschner JB, et al. Use of canakinumab in the cryopyrin-associated periodic syndrome. N Engl J Med 2009;360(23):2416–25.
50. Mandey SH, Kuijk LM, Frenkel J, et al. A role for geranylgeranylation in interleukin-1β secretion. Arthritis Rheum 2006;54(11):3690–5.
51. van der Hilst JC, Bodar EJ, Barron KS, et al. Long-term follow-up, clinical features, and quality of life in a series of 103 patients with hyperimmunoglobulinemia D syndrome. Medicine (Baltimore) 2008;87(6):301–10.
52. McDermott MF, Aksentijevich I, Galon J, et al. Germline mutations in the extracellular domains of the 55 kDa TNF receptor, TNFR1, define a family of dominantly inherited autoinflammatory syndromes. Cell 1999;97(1):133–44.
53. Lachmann HJ, Papa R, Gerhold K, et al. The phenotype of TNF receptor-associated autoinflammatory syndrome (TRAPS) at presentation: a series of

158 cases from the Eurofever/EUROTRAPS international registry. Ann Rheum Dis 2014;73(12):2160–7.

54. Petty RE, Southwood TR, Manners P, et al. International League of Associations for Rheumatology classification of juvenile idiopathic arthritis: second revision. J Rheumatol 2004;31(2):390–2.

55. Behrens EM, Beukelman T, Gallo L, et al. Evaluation of the presentation of systemic onset juvenile rheumatoid arthritis: data from the Pennsylvania Systemic Onset Juvenile Arthritis Registry (PASOJAR). J Rheumatol 2008;35(2):343.

56. Gandhi C, Healy C, Wanderer AA, et al. Familial atypical cold urticaria: description of a new hereditary disease. J Allergy Clin Immunol 2009;124(6):1245–50.

57. Aderibigbe OM, Priel DL, Lee CC, et al. Distinct cutaneous manifestations and cold-induced leukocyte activation associated with PLCG2 mutations. JAMA Dermatol 2015;151(6):627–34.

58. Pichard D, Freeman A, Cowan E. Syndromes associated with mucocutaneous candidiasis and noninfectious cutaneous manifestations. J Am Acad Dermatol 2015;73(3):367–81.

59. Kanazawa N. Hereditary disorders presenting with urticaria. Immunol Allergy Clin N Am 2014;34(1):169–79.

Immune-Mediated Diseases of the Central Nervous System

A Specificity-Focused Diagnostic Paradigm

Dominic O. Co, MD, PhD[a],*, Brett J. Bordini, MD[b],
Arthur B. Meyers, MD[c], Christopher Inglese, MD[d]

KEYWORDS

- Central nervous system • Immune mediated • Neurologic dysfunction
- Immunopathology

KEY POINTS

- Immune-mediated diseases of the central nervous system show wide phenotypic and pathophysiologic heterogeneity.
- Precise definition of the phenotype of neurologic dysfunction and associated systemic findings focuses the diagnostic evaluation.
- Recognition of the clinical scenarios in which immune-mediated disease presents allows prompt diagnosis and management.

INTRODUCTION

Immune-mediated disease of the central nervous system (CNS) is as diverse in its phenotypes as it is in its pathogenesis. The challenge in approaching patients with immune-mediated disease of the CNS is to establish a sufficiently specific and timely diagnosis so as to allow for the presumptive treatment of a disease process for which specific biomarkers may be lacking, and for which physical findings and results from readily available diagnostic modalities may not be specific. Alternatively, specific biomarkers may exist to guide diagnosis, but the disease presentation may be protean and a clear diagnostic testing strategy may be elusive.[1–3] An additional challenge is that many of the

[a] Section of Pediatric Rheumatology, Department of Pediatrics, Medical College of Wisconsin, 8701 West Watertown Plank Road, Milwaukee, WI 53226, USA; [b] Section of Hospital Medicine, Department of Pediatrics, Medical College of Wisconsin, 8701 West Watertown Plank Road, Milwaukee, WI 53226, USA; [c] Department of Radiology, University of Central Florida College of Medicine, 6850 Lake Nona Blvd, Orlando, FL 32827, USA; [d] Section of Pediatric Neurology, Department of Neurology, Medical College of Wisconsin, 8701 West Watertown Plank Road, Milwaukee, WI 53226, USA
* Corresponding author.
E-mail address: dco@mcw.edu

Pediatr Clin N Am 64 (2017) 57–90
http://dx.doi.org/10.1016/j.pcl.2016.08.005
pediatric.theclinics.com
0031-3955/17/© 2016 Elsevier Inc. All rights reserved.

assays that lend specificity to the diagnosis have long turnaround times, and the acuity, severity, and progression of the underlying disease may mandate the initiation of treatment in the absence of confirmatory testing results. Given that the primary therapeutic modalities for most immune-mediated diseases of the CNS are designed to curb immunologic activity, it is of the utmost importance to exclude the possibility of an infectious process underlying the patient's symptoms, or to sufficiently establish that the patient's presentation is caused by an immunologic mechanism.[4,5]

Overcoming these challenges requires establishing the precise phenotype of the patient's neurologic dysfunction and delineating the involvement of other organ systems.[6] Defining the phenotype requires an appreciation of how pathologic changes in neurophysiology are expressed symptomatically and recognition of the wide phenotypic heterogeneity both within a disease category and a particular disorder. The process should encompass a multidisciplinary approach that incorporates the expertise of specialists in neurology, infectious diseases, neuroradiology, and (depending on individual patient circumstances) rheumatology, metabolic genetics, oncology, or pathology.[7] With a neuroanatomic and functional phenotype defined, a tiered diagnostic strategy should be used; one that can provide rapidly available and sensitive results to guide acute management via the exclusion of large categories of disease, as well as highly specific results to refine the diagnosis, although these assays may not return until later in the patient's course.[2] Furthermore, the diagnostic strategy should minimize unnecessary testing.[4] This process is aided by understanding which historical features, physical examination findings, and diagnostic assays are specific or even pathognomonic to the diagnosis, although clinicians should understand that certain immune-mediated diseases of the CNS lack sufficiently sensitive or specific testing modalities and require probabilistic diagnosis via the use of diagnostic criteria.[8] Clinicians should resist the temptation to have an unfocused diagnostic testing strategy, but should still recognize that historical and physical findings, or the results of rapidly available testing modalities, may not be able to narrow the differential diagnosis sufficiently to avoid extensive laboratory testing.[8]

FINDING SPECIFICITY IN A NONSPECIFIC DISEASE PROCESS

Immune-mediated diseases of the CNS show wide heterogeneity in both clinical presentations and underlying pathophysiology.[6] Aberrant immunologic activity leading to acute or subacute diffuse cerebral dysfunction can present with minimal manifestations or with severe or even life-threatening manifestations. Subtle subjective deficits in attention, information processing, and behavioral repertoires can develop on a spectrum with more overt signs of diffuse neuronal dysfunction, such as agitated delirium, catatonic mutism, or status epilepticus.[2,9,10] When evaluating a patient presenting with CNS dysfunction, the history, physical examination, and results of readily available diagnostic assays should allow the clinician to develop an initial differential diagnosis that restricts the patient's symptoms to broad categories of disease processes. Developing an evaluation and management strategy within these broad categories then becomes a matter of recognizing which particular signs, symptoms, and findings in that context suggest an immune-mediated mechanism, and which suggest alternative causes. Most presentations of immune-mediated CNS disease are in the following categories: (1) presentations in infants and toddlers, (2) presentations with the acute onset of focal neurologic deficits, (3) presentations characterized by encephalopathy or behavioral disturbances, (4) presentations characterized by seizures as the primary manifestation, and (5) presentations characterized by movement disorders as the primary manifestation.

PRESENTATIONS IN INFANTS AND TODDLERS

The differential diagnosis of acute or subacute-onset neurologic dysfunction in neonates and infants includes both congenital and acquired infection, metabolic or otherwise genetic encephalopathies, encephalopathic epilepsies, trauma, hypoxia, and other conditions that limit the effective delivery of oxygen and other substrates to, and removal of waste products from, the brain. Given that such diverse pathophysiologic mechanisms can result in similar phenotypic expressions of neurologic dysfunction, suspecting immune-mediated mechanisms as the cause of symptoms in infants and toddlers can be challenging. In the case of Aicardi-Goutières syndrome (AGS), which presents primarily as a mimic of TORCH (Toxoplasmosis, Other [syphilis, varicella-zoster, parvovirus B19], Rubella, Cytomegalovirus [CMV], and Herpes infections) or congenital human immunodeficiency virus (HIV) infection, the challenge is in recognizing which epidemiologic factors and findings differentiate the disorder from these infections. In the case of cerebral folate deficiency, the challenge is in recognizing the characteristic pattern of developmental regression, head growth deceleration, and associated findings to distinguish this disorder from other causes of developmental regression. Hemophagocytic lymphohistiocytosis (HLH) can present with a variety of neurologic symptoms, either in isolation or as part of a systemic inflammatory process that may mimic overwhelming infection or hematologic malignancy. Patients with opsoclonus-myoclonus-ataxia syndrome (OMAS) may present in early infancy, although this condition is discussed in further detail in the context of patients presenting with movement disorders.[11,12]

Aicardi-Goutières Syndrome

AGS is a genetic encephalopathy that often presents as a mimic of congenital infection. The disorder is mediated by mutations in genes related to the removal of infectious or endogenous nucleic acids.[13-15] The accumulation of nucleic acids is thought to mimic viral infection and trigger activation of Toll-like receptors of the innate immune system, in turn stimulating production of interferon-α (IFN-α) and leading to inflammatory cascades that result in neurologic signs and symptoms.[16] Although the understanding of the molecular and genetic basis of AGS is expanding considerably, the clinical presentation and progression can be divided into 2 main phenotypes: neonatal onset and later onset.[17]

The neonatal form presents with nonspecific features of encephalopathy, and affected neonates may show jitteriness, seizures, and poor feeding that may mimic neonatal sepsis. Findings include hepatosplenomegaly, anemia, thrombocytopenia, and increased transaminase levels. The head circumference, typically normal at birth, may progressively decrease relative to other normal trajectories of growth, although deceleration of head growth can begin in utero. Stagnation and even regression of motor and social milestones become apparent as the child's irritability persists. This neonatal presentation is reminiscent of TORCH infection or congenital infection with the HIV, although negative TORCH and HIV investigations, as well as the absence of microcephaly, retinopathy, hearing loss, or hydrocephalus, should direct attention to alternative diagnoses such as AGS. The localization of calcifications to the basal ganglia on neuroimaging (as opposed to a more diffuse pattern seen in TORCH infections), the intermittency of fever, and persistence of cerebrospinal fluid pleocytosis despite negative infectious studies are diagnostically important and distinguish AGS from other diseases.[13,17]

Children with later onset AGS present with subacute progressive encephalopathy as shown by irritability, loss of milestones, slowly progressive microcephaly or head growth deceleration, and episodic fever. On neurologic examination, pyramidal (spasticity) and extrapyramidal (dystonia) signs appear, because optic atrophy or pallor and ocular jerks are evidence of cortical blindness. Vascular necrotic cutaneous lesions (chilblains), hepatomegaly, increased transaminase levels, thrombocytopenia, glaucoma, hypothyroidism, diabetes mellitus, and antidiuretic hormone deficiency are non-neurologic features.[18] Thrombocytopenia, hypothyroidism, and diabetes deserve special mention because they are typically caused by immune thrombocytopenia purpura, autoimmune thyroiditis, and type I diabetes, respectively, and further show the central nature of autoimmunity in this disease.[19]

Diagnosis is supported by showing increased IFN-α and neopterin levels in the cerebrospinal fluid, or by showing an abnormal interferon expression signature on quantitative polymerase chain reaction analysis in peripheral blood mononuclear cells, although these tests are not widely available clinically.[19] Nonspecific cerebrospinal fluid lymphocytic pleocytosis should also be present, but the cerebrospinal fluid cell count and IFN-α signature can be normal, especially in the later stages of the disease after the active encephalopathic phase.[13] Neuroimaging studies may support diagnosis as well. The neuroimaging findings of AGS are typically characterized as having a triad of cerebral calcifications, white matter lesions, and cerebral atrophy. Head computed tomography (CT) scans provide the most sensitive evaluation for cerebral calcifications, which are typically seen within the basal ganglia, lobar white matter, and dentate nuclei.[20] Although cerebral calcifications are considered diagnostic of AGS, they may not be present on an initial CT scan. Head CT scans may also reveal cerebral atrophy and white matter lesions as decreased cerebral volume and hypoattenuating lesions in the white matter, respectively; however, MRI allows better characterization of these findings. The white matter lesions in AGS show increased signal intensity on T2-weighted and fluid-attenuated inversion recovery (FLAIR) MRI sequences. More severe lesions also show decreased signal intensity on T1-weighted images. White matter lesions show a lobar predominance with relative sparing of the periventricular, callosal, and capsular white matter and of the optic radiations.[20] The subcortical arcuate fibers are typically involved.[20] Two patterns of white matter involvement have been described: diffuse involvement of lobar white matter and an anteroposterior gradient with more intense involvement in the frontal lobes.[20] White matter disease can progress to cystic lesions, which has been described in the frontal and temporal white matter.[20]

Cerebral Folate Deficiency

Cerebral folate deficiency is characterized by decreased concentrations of 5-methyltetrahydrofolate in the cerebrospinal fluid, in the presence of normal blood folate concentrations. The 5-methyltetrahydrofolate deficiency is caused by inadequate transport of folate across the blood-brain barrier caused by decreased function of the folate receptor-alpha. This receptor dysfunction seems to be caused either by mutations in the FOLR1 gene,[21] which encodes the receptor, or by autoantibodies directed against the receptor.[22] If cerebral folate deficiency is promptly and appropriately diagnosed, supplementation with folinic acid can halt progression of symptoms.[21,23]

The disorder presents after normal pregnancies, deliveries, and neonatal periods with irritability, sleep disturbance, developmental stagnation or regression, and head growth deceleration. Hypotonia, spasticity, ataxia, and refractory seizures may ensue. Visual loss and later hearing loss occur, and some patients develop symptoms of autistic-type behaviors or psychosis.

Diagnosis in the setting of this presentation is supported by showing decreased 5-methyltetrahydrofolate concentrations in the cerebrospinal fluid (typically

<40 nmol/L) in the setting of normal blood folate concentrations.[23,24] If blood folate levels are reduced, dietary deficiencies and gastrointestinal absorption abnormalities should be excluded, as should systemic abnormalities in folate metabolism, such as methyltetrahydrofolate reductase (MTHFR) deficiency or dihydrofolate reductase deficiency. MTHFR deficiency is suggested by the presence of increased blood homocysteine and decreased blood methionine levels, whereas dihydrofolate reductase deficiency is suggested by megaloblastic anemia or pancytopenia. Specific assays for folate receptor-alpha antibodies are available, and analysis for *FOLR1* gene mutations, deletions, or duplications can be performed. Frontotemporal atrophy and periventricular and subcortical demyelination may be noted on neuroimaging, as well as nonspecific white matter lesions that show increased signal intensity of T2-weighted and FLAIR sequences.[21,22]

The differential diagnosis of cerebral folate deficiency includes methyltetrahydrofolate reductase deficiency, dihydrofolate reductase deficiency, Kearns-Sayre syndrome, Rett syndrome, AGS, 3-phosphoglycerate dehydrogenase deficiency, dihydropteridine reductase deficiency, mitochondrial complex 1 encephalomyopathy, and aromatic amino acid decarboxylase deficiency.

Hemophagocytic Lymphohistiocytosis and the Macrophage Activation Syndrome

HLH is a syndrome of uncontrolled immune activation that causes a picture of disseminated intravascular coagulation and systemic inflammation. Typical children with HLH are acutely ill with fever, irritability, hepatosplenomegaly, and a purpuric rash from disseminated intravascular coagulation, and this presentation is often mistaken for sepsis with multiorgan dysfunction occurring in severe cases. HLH can be either primary and caused by genetic defects in molecules important for cytotoxic granule release in natural killer (NK) cells and cytotoxic T cells, or it can be secondary to infection or to an underlying inflammatory disease such as systemic onset juvenile idiopathic arthritis (SOJIA) or systemic lupus erythematosus (SLE). Secondary HLH associated with an underlying inflammatory disease is referred to as macrophage activation syndrome (MAS) and typically presents less severely and at a later age than primary HLH. Most patients with primary HLH become symptomatic in the first few years of life, although some present at school age or later.

Approximately 50% of affected patients develop neurologic involvement, either as a primary manifestation or later in the course of the disease, with symptoms including irritability, alteration of consciousness, psychomotor retardation, ataxia, spasticity, hypotonia, hemiparesis, seizures, or meningismus.[25,26] Rarely, HLH presents with isolated neurologic involvement preceding systemic illness by years.[27–38] HLH has been reported to present with isolated ataxia and cerebellar involvement,[29,38–40] encephalopathy,[41,42] focal neurologic deficits,[30,32,33,40] seizures,[34] mass lesions,[33] and demyelinating lesions.[30,35] In many cases, patients were treated with steroids for suspected acute disseminated encephalomyelitis, but later relapsed on withdrawal of steroid therapy. HLH must be considered in young patients with neurologic disease without a clear explanation, especially if they show other diagnostic criteria for HLH (**Box 1**).

Diagnosis of HLH is based on the HLH 2004 guidelines, which require either demonstration of a known genetic cause of HLH or fulfilment of 5 of 8 diagnostic criteria (see **Box 1**).[43] Macrophage activation syndrome can be diagnosed using similar criteria qualitatively, although, in practice, because MAS tends to be less severe, patients with MAS might not meet the strict numeric criteria for HLH. For example, a patient with MAS may be cytopenic relative to their level of inflammation and show a progressive trend downward, but not meet the numeric cutoffs for cytopenia in the HLH 2004 guidelines. This possibility is reflected in the recently published guidelines for

---

Box 1
Hemophagocytic lymphohistiocytosis 2004 criteria

A molecular diagnosis consistent with HLH

OR

Five out of the eight HLH diagnostic criteria in the absence of malignancy:
  Initial diagnostic criteria (to be evaluated in all patients with HLH)
  1. Fever
  2. Splenomegaly
  3. Cytopenias (affecting 2 of 3 lineages in the peripheral blood): hemoglobin less than 90 g/L (in infants <4 weeks, hemoglobin <100 g/L), platelets less than 100×10^9/L, neutrophils less than 1.0×10^9/L
  4. Hypertriglyceridemia and/or hypofibrinogenemia: fasting triglycerides greater than 3.0 mmol/L (ie, >265 mg/dL) and/or fibrinogen <1.5 g/L
  5. Hemophagocytosis in bone marrow or spleen or lymph nodes
  New diagnostic criteria
  1. Low or absent NK-cell activity (according to local laboratory reference)
  2. Ferritin level greater than 500 mg/L
  3. Soluble CD25 (ie, soluble interleukin-2 receptor) level greater than 2400 U/mL

Adapted from Henter J-I, Horne A, Aricó M, et al. HLH-2004: diagnostic and therapeutic guidelines for hemophagocytic lymphohistiocytosis. Pediat Blood Cancer 2007;48:124–31; with permission.

---

diagnosing MAS in patients with known SOJIA, the most common rheumatic cause of MAS. The criteria used in these guidelines are similar to the HLH 2004 criteria, but with less stringent cutoffs for the laboratory criteria.[44]

Imaging findings of HLH are nonspecific and change throughout the course of the disease. CT of the head may show hypoattenuating parenchymal lesions or calcifications, both of which are most commonly located at the gray-white junction.[45] MRI of the brain has a higher sensitivity for parenchymal lesions, which may be supratentorial and/or infratentorial, and may involve the gray and/or white matter with a predominance at the gray-white matter junction. The parenchymal lesions are typically laminated, nodular areas of increased signal intensity on T2-weighted and FLAIR sequences. The laminated signal refers to central increased signal surrounded by a rim of low signal intensity.[45] These lesions may become confluent as the disease progresses (**Fig. 1**). Postcontrast T1-weighted images may show nodular, linear, or rim enhancement of the parenchymal lesions. Leptomeningeal enhancement may also be seen on postcontrast images but is not present in all cases. Follow-up images may show cerebral atrophy (see **Fig. 1**D) and hemorrhage within parenchymal lesions.[45] Imaging findings outside of the CNS can also be seen in children with HLH. Abdominal ultrasonography may show hepatosplenomegaly, gallbladder wall thickening, and ascites.

PRESENTATIONS WITH ACUTE-ONSET FOCAL NEUROLOGIC DEFICITS

The acute onset of focal neurologic deficits should cause concern for acute ischemic or hemorrhagic stroke. In this setting, neuroimaging is the highest yield diagnostic modality and can identify restricted diffusion and ischemic damage that should prompt consideration for an underlying risk factor for acute stroke or cerebrovascular disease in children or adolescents. Patients lacking identifiable risk factors for stroke should be investigated for possible immune-mediated disorders that can lead to focal neurologic

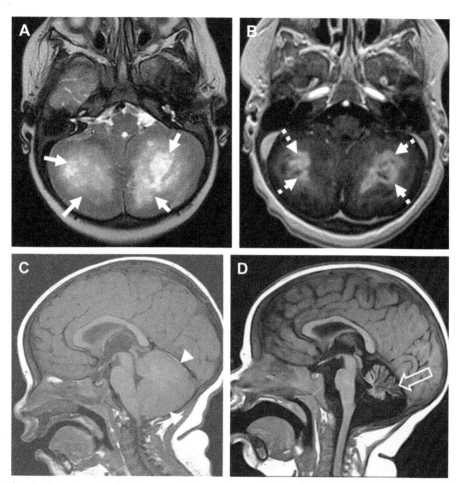

Fig. 1. A 16-month-old boy with hemophagocytic lymphohistiocytosis. (*A*) Axial T2-weighted MR image shows diffuse increased signal intensity throughout the cerebellar white matter (*arrows*). (*B*) Axial postcontrast T1-weighted MR image shows patchy areas of enhancement throughout the cerebellar white matter lesions (*dashed arrows*). (*C, D*) Sagittal T1-weighted MR images obtained at 16 months (*C*) and 22 months (*D*) of age. On the initial MRI (*C*) there was cerebellar swelling (*arrowheads*); on the follow-up MRI (*D*) there is marked cerebellar atrophy (*open arrow*).

deficits, which include primary angiitis of the CNS and the antiphospholipid antibody syndrome (APLS).

Angiography-Positive Primary Angiitis of the Central Nervous System

Primary angiitis of the CNS (PACNS) is an idiopathic granulomatous vasculitis of CNS vessels that presents with focal neurologic deficits, but can also present with seizures, cognitive dysfunction, and behavioral changes.[46–48] Focal neurologic signs in PACNS stem from ischemia secondary to vessel narrowing or to thromboembolic events from damaged and therefore thrombogenic vascular endothelium. A more diffuse presentation is more likely to occur with angiography-negative PACNS and may be caused by smaller ischemic foci or by vasculitic disruption of the blood-brain barrier with resultant local disruption of neuronal function. Angiography-negative PACNS is discussed in more detail in the context of conditions presenting with encephalopathy.

In children, PACNS is broadly divided into angiography-positive and angiography-negative disease based on findings on conventional angiography, which is the gold standard imaging test. An acute stroke presentation with focal neurologic findings is more likely to occur with angiography-positive disease. In addition, patients presenting with a symptom cluster consisting of paresis, speech difficulties, and imaging findings consistent with ischemia are more likely to have angiography-positive PACNS.[49] Therefore, the initial evaluation of focal neurologic signs should include vascular imaging, usually magnetic resonance (MR) angiography of the brain, along with conventional brain MRI.

More than half of adult patients with PACNS show multifocal infarcts.[50] The findings in children are similar, although multifocal infarcts are more likely to occur unilaterally and affect territories supplied by the anterior circulation, especially the lateral lenticulostriate territory and the basal ganglia.[51] MRI findings in PACNS include areas of high diffusion-weighted imaging signal with associated low absolute diffusion coefficient signal indicating acute to subacute infarction (**Figs. 2** and **3**). In addition, white matter T2/FLAIR lesions, mass lesions, meningeal enhancement, and hemorrhages can be seen but are less specific for PACNS.[50,52] If MRI and MR angiography are not diagnostic, diagnosis may require conventional angiography, which has a higher resolution and therefore higher sensitivity for small vessel lesions, but entails higher risk to the patient. Conventional angiography may show segmental irregularity, or narrowing or occlusion of small and medium-sized parenchymal and leptomeningeal arteries. The classic sign on any type of angiography is multiple adjacent areas of focal narrowing giving the appearance of "beads on a string".

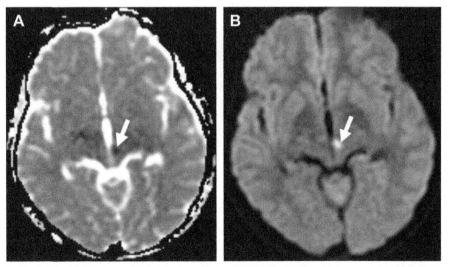

Fig. 2. A 15-year-old boy with primary angiitis of the CNS. Axial diffusion-weighted imaging (DWI) (*A*), and apparent diffusion coefficient (ADC) (*B*) sequences from brain MRI at the time of initial presentation. There is a focal area of abnormal signal intensity in the medial, inferior aspect of the left basal ganglia (*solid arrows*) that is increased signal intensity on the DWI and low signal intensity on the ADC sequences, consistent with restrictive diffusion caused by an acute infarct.

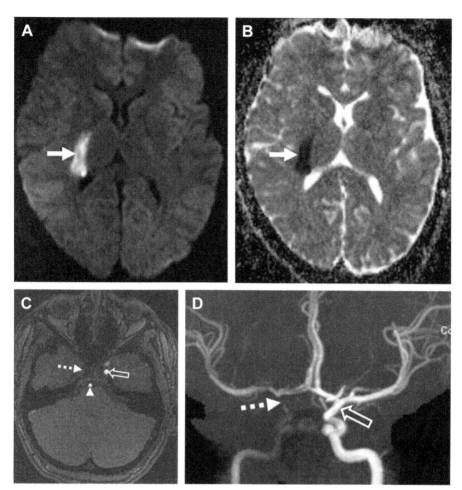

Fig. 3. A 12-year-old boy with primary angiitis of the CNS. Axial DWI (*A*) and ADC (*B*) sequences at the time of initial presentation show an area within the region of the right external capsule (*arrows*) that is increased signal intensity on the DWI and low signal intensity on the ADC sequences. This finding is consistent with an acute stroke. Axial (*C*) and three-dimensional (3D) reformatted (*D*) images from time-of-flight (TOF) MR angiography (MRA) shows absence of flow within the distal right internal carotid artery (*dashed arrows*). The left internal carotid (*open arrows*) and basilar (*arrowhead*) arteries show normal flow.

Antiphospholipid Antibody Syndrome and Neuropsychiatric Systemic Lupus Erythematosus

APLS is characterized by a propensity for venous or arterial thrombosis or for recurrent miscarriages in the setting of positive serum antiphospholipid antibodies. The syndrome can occur as a primary phenomenon or as secondary to systemic autoimmune disease, usually SLE. Because up to 30% of patients initially diagnosed with APLS go on to develop criteria for SLE, some investigators have suggested that APLS may be a precursor to SLE.[53,54] SLE is itself a risk factor for clotting and therefore, antiphospholipid antibodies in the setting of SLE can be particularly problematic. Diagnosis of APLS is based on the Sydney criteria (**Box 2**),[55] which require demonstration of either

> **Box 2**
> **Revised classification criteria for antiphospholipid antibody syndrome**
>
> Requires at least 1 clinical criterion and 1 laboratory criterion
>
> Clinical criteria
> 1. Vascular thrombosis
> 2. Pregnancy morbidity (1 of the following)
>   a. One or more unexplained deaths of a morphologically normal fetus at or beyond the 10th week of gestation
>   b. One or more premature births of a morphologically normal neonate before the 34th week of gestation because of (1 of the following)
>   i. Eclampsia or severe preeclampsia
>   ii. Recognized features of placental insufficiency
>   c. Three or more unexplained consecutive spontaneous abortions before the 10th week of gestation, with maternal anatomic or hormonal abnormalities and paternal and maternal chromosomal causes excluded.
>
> Laboratory criteria
> 1. Lupus anticoagulant present in plasma, on 2 or more occasions at least 12 weeks apart
> 2. Anticardiolipin antibody of immunoglobulin (Ig) G and/or IgM isotype in serum or plasma, present in medium or high titer (ie, >40 GPL or MPL [IgG or IgM phospholipid units, respectively], or >99th percentile), on 2 or more occasions, at least 12 weeks apart, measured by a standardized enzyme-linked immunosorbent assay (ELISA)
> 3. Anti–β2-glycoprotein-I antibody of IgG and/or IgM isotype in serum or plasma (in titer >99th percentile), present on 2 or more occasions, at least 12 weeks apart, measured by a standardized ELISA
>
> *Adapted from* Miyakis S, Lockshin MD, Atsumi T, et al. International consensus statement on an update of the classification criteria for definite antiphospholipid syndrome (APS). J Thromb Haemost 2006;4:295–306.

thrombosis or pregnancy-related morbidity (eg, recurrent miscarriages) and at least 1 laboratory criterion showing antiphospholipid antibodies (eg, lupus anticoagulant, anticardiolipin antibody or anti–β2-glycoprotein antibody).

Neurologic symptoms in APLS arise through several different mechanisms. Arterial thrombosis can lead to transient ischemic attacks and stroke, cerebral venous sinus thrombosis can cause both focal and diffuse neurologic symptoms, and nonthrombotic sequelae have been proposed to be caused by APLS as well. Up to 26% of patients with primary or secondary APLS present with acute arterial ischemic stroke.[54] Acute stroke in APLS presents in a manner similar to strokes of other causes, with focal neurologic symptoms localizable to the thrombosed vascular territory, most often in the anterior circulation, and MRI findings that indicate cerebral ischemia. In the context of SLE, embolic stroke may also occur because of SLE-associated cardiac valvulitis, either alone or in combination with APLS.[56]

Cerebral venous sinus thrombosis is the initial manifestation of APLS in 7% of patients and can present with focal neurologic findings caused by parenchymal lesions, most commonly monoparesis or hemiparesis. Venous sinus thrombosis can also present with more diffuse neurologic findings related to decreased cerebrospinal fluid resorption and increased intracranial pressure, such as headache, vomiting, papilledema, and the Cushing triad. Alternatively, decreased cerebral perfusion pressure can cause diffuse cerebral dysfunction and symptoms of encephalopathy with mental status change, stupor, or coma. MRI of the brain with venography shows reduced flow within the affected sinus (**Fig. 4**). Ultrasonography can be used in the detection of peripheral venous and arterial thrombosis (see **Fig. 4**D). Conventional venography and

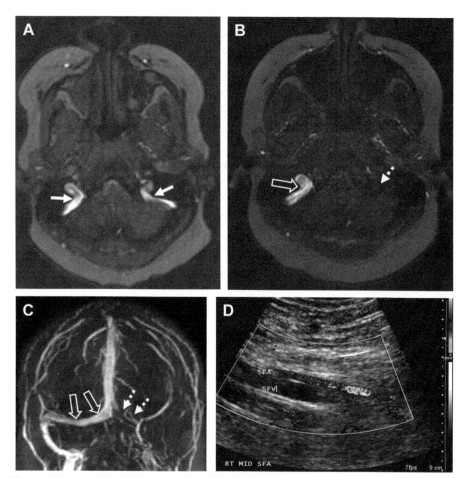

Fig. 4. A 16-year-old with lupus and antiphospholipid antibody syndrome. (*A*) Axial TOF MR venography (MRV) of the head shows normal flow in the sagittal sinuses (*solid arrows*). Axial (*B*) and 3D reformatted (*C*) images from TOF MRV performed the following year show lack of flow within the right sagittal sinus (*dashed arrows*) with preserved flow in the right sagittal sinus (*open arrows*). (*D*) Color Doppler ultrasonography image of the left superficial femoral vein (SFV) in the same patient performed shortly after the MRV in *B* shows lack of color Doppler signal in the SFV consistent with occlusive thrombus. Flow is present in the adjacent superficial femoral artery (SFA).

angiography are still considered the gold standard for the detection and characterization of thrombus and are typically used in cases in which catheter-directed thrombolysis is indicated.

The other most common findings on MRI in lupus involving the CNS are small focal subcortical and periventricular white matter lesions with increased signal intensity in T2-weighted and FLAIR sequences (**Fig. 5**).[57] Areas of acute and subacute infarction show increased signal intensity on diffusion-weighted imaging and low signal intensity on apparent diffusion coefficient (ADC) sequences (see **Fig. 5**). Intracranial hemorrhage may manifest as parenchymal hemorrhage, subarachnoid hemorrhage, or subdural hematoma. The appearance of hemorrhage on CT and MRI depends on the

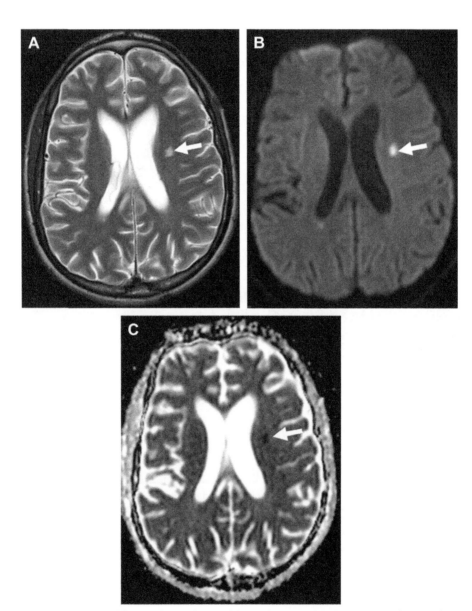

Fig. 5. A 15-year-old boy with CNS lupus. (*A*) Axial T2-weighted MR image shows a focal area of increased signal intensity within the right periventricular white matter (*arrow*). Axial DWI (*B*) and ADC (*C*) sequences show that this lesion (*arrows*) has increased signal intensity on the DWI and low signal on the ADC sequences, consistent with restrictive diffusion seen with an acute infarct.

chronicity of the bleed. Cerebral atrophy is seen in slightly less than half the patients affected.[57] CT, MR, and conventional angiography may show narrowing or occlusion of the carotid arteries.[57] Coexisting myelopathy is rare in children with CNS involvement of lupus but, if present, shows increased signal intensity within the central spinal cord on T2-weighted MR sequences.[57,58]

APLS is associated with a variety of nonthrombotic neurologic complications, such as seizures, chorea, transverse myelitis, dementia, migraine, cognitive dysfunction, and psychiatric symptoms, although some of these associations are controversial.[59,60] Chorea, other movement disorders, and transverse myelitis are particularly associated with antiphospholipid antibodies in the setting of SLE.[61] Some of these manifestations may be related to infarcts that are too small to be seen on neuroimaging, such as multi-infarct dementia or seizures secondary to small infarct-related epileptic foci, although some studies have suggested that antiphospholipid antibodies may target specific neuronal antigens or may simply indicate a propensity for developing CNS autoimmunity.[62–65] Antiphospholipid antibodies are known to have more subtle effects on endothelial function and it is interesting to speculate that they might be altering the function of the blood-brain barrier.

When nonthrombotic complications of APLS predominate, the disorder may not enter the differential diagnosis; however, subtle systemic findings may reorient the clinician to the possibility of antiphospholipid antibody-mediated disease. Systemic findings suggestive of APLS include livedo racemosa, a lacy or netlike rash similar to cutis marmorata that can occur in approximately one-fourth of patients with APLS.[54] In contrast with the more physiologic cutis marmorata, livedo racemosa associated with APLS has more broken circles, does not resolve as well with rewarming, and does not respond to changes in position. Patients with APLS can also develop vasculopathic lesions and ulcers. In addition, patients with APLS commonly develop thrombocytopenia and autoimmune hemolytic anemia. In patients with thrombotic and nonthrombotic neurologic sequelae of APLS, these findings alert clinicians to the possibility of antiphospholipid antibodies underlying the patient's symptoms. However, no specific therapy, such as anticoagulation or immune therapy, has been clearly shown to be beneficial for the nonthrombotic manifestations of APLS, and treatment is limited to symptomatic management.

PRESENTATIONS CHARACTERIZED BY ENCEPHALOPATHY OR BEHAVIORAL DISTURBANCES

The primary differential diagnostic considerations in patients presenting with encephalopathy or behavioral disturbances include infection, toxic ingestion, and psychiatric disturbances. Frank encephalitis appropriately directs much of the initial diagnostic momentum toward infectious causes, particularly when patients present with fever, neurologic changes, and cerebrospinal fluid pleocytosis. Initial diagnostic assays focus on establishing or excluding the presence of pathogenic organisms (**Box 3**),[66,67] and patients are often treated with empiric antiinfective medications while these assays are pending. Patients with behavioral changes may be evaluated for psychiatric disorders or toxic or metabolic encephalopathies. For subtle behavior or cognitive changes that might present in the outpatient setting, clinicians must rely on history obtained from family members, caregivers, and teachers who know the patient well to determine whether new symptoms represent a significant deviation from the prior baseline behaviors and development, and the input of neurologists, psychiatrists, psychologists, and neuropsychologists may assist further in this assessment. The lack of a response to antiinfective or psychiatric therapies can be an additional indication that the symptoms have another underlying cause. Recognizing which symptom constellations suggest immune-mediated disease allows clinicians to obtain appropriate diagnostic assays for these disorders while simultaneously focusing initial diagnostic and therapeutic effort on infectious, toxic, or metabolic causes.[2,4,9,68,69]

Box 3
Diagnostic evaluation of patients with possible autoimmune encephalopathy

Neuroimaging
- MRI of the brain
- MR angiography/MR venography if clinical presentation or MRI suggests stroke

Cerebrospinal fluid studies
- Opening pressure
- Cell count
- Glucose
- Protein
- Infectious studies
  - Bacterial culture and Gram stain
  - Polymerase chain reaction (PCR) assays for varicella-zoster virus, herpes simplex virus
  - In May through October, add West Nile virus IgM, arbovirus antibody
- Immune studies
  - Oligoclonal bands
  - Neuromyelitis optica antibody
  - Autoimmune encephalopathy panel (includes antibodies to GAD65, VGKC, ANNA-1, ANNA-2, ANNA-3, PCA-1, PCA-2, PCA-Tr, amphiphysin, CRM-5 Ig, AGNA-1, N-methyl-D-aspartate [NMDA] receptor, alpha-amino-3-hydroxy-5-methyl-4-isoxazolepropionic acid receptor, gamma-aminobutyric acid-B receptor)
- Set aside extra cerebrospinal fluid for future studies

Blood
- Erythrocyte sedimentation rate, C-reactive protein
- Infectious studies
  - Blood culture
  - Enterovirus and Parechovirus PCR
  - Varicella-zoster antibody panel
  - Epstein-Barr virus (EBV) antibody panel. If positive, send EBV PCR on cerebrospinal fluid
  - HIV-1 RNA
  - Lyme ELISA with reflex Western blot; if positive, send Lyme ELISA on cerebrospinal fluid
  - Bartonella and West Nile virus antibody titers (blood/cerebrospinal fluid)
  - Brucella antibody; if positive, send *Brucella* antibodies on cerebrospinal fluid
  - In May through October, add tick-borne PCR panel and Powassan virus antibody
- Autoimmune serologies
  - Antinuclear antibody (ANA) with reflex extractable nuclear antigen (ENA) antibody panel (anti-SS-A, anti-SS-B, anti-ribonucleoprotein [RNP], and anti-Smith antibodies) and anti–double-stranded DNA (dsDNA)
  - Complement C3, C4
  - Antithyroid antibodies
- Set aside extra serum for future studies

Nasopharyngeal swabs
- Adenovirus PCR
- *C pneumoniae* PCR
- *Mycoplasma* PCR; if positive send *Mycoplasma* PCR on cerebrospinal fluid
- In November through April, send influenza A and B PCR

Adapted from Venkatesan A, Tunkel AR, Bloch KC, et al. Case Definitions, Diagnostic Algorithms, and Priorities in Encephalitis: Consensus Statement of the International Encephalitis Consortium Clin Infect Dis 2013;57:1114–28 and Kneen R, Michael BD, Menson E, et al. Management of suspected viral encephalitis in children - Association of British Neurologists and British Paediatric Allergy, Immunology and Infection Group National Guidelines. J Infect 2012;64:449–77.

Autoimmune Encephalitis

Encephalitis in general is a rapidly progressive, potentially serious disorder conventionally characterized by altered mental status, fever, cerebrospinal fluid pleocytosis (in most), and diffuse cerebral dysfunction on electroencephalography. Because many commonly recognized causes are infectious, initial diagnostic effort is often placed on identifying specific pathogens for which targeted antiinfective medications can be prescribed; however, there has been increasing recognition of noninfectious, often immune-mediated, causes of encephalitis.[6] These immune-mediated conditions, associated with antibodies directed against neuronal cell surface or synaptic protein antigens, can evolve similarly to infectious encephalitis, with reduced levels of consciousness, fever, cerebrospinal fluid pleocytosis, characteristic imaging findings, and encephalopathic tracings on electroencephalography. However, these inflammatory symptoms need not always be present or overt, and manifestations may be subtle or atypical, favoring alterations in behavior, memory, or sleep.[4,8,68]

Given this phenotypic heterogeneity, it may be challenging for clinicians to recognize the varied and sometimes subtle signs of neurologic dysfunction as being secondary to autoimmune encephalitis, although clinically useful criteria for the early diagnosis of possible autoimmune encephalitis have recently been proposed.[70] The diagnosis is considered as possible based on the subacute onset and rapid progression of short-term memory loss, decreased or altered levels of consciousness, personality change, and lethargy.[68] In addition, new focal findings on neurologic examination, new-onset idiopathic epilepsy, cerebrospinal fluid pleocytosis, and suggestive MRI findings are supportive, although not all of these supportive criteria need be present. Neuroimaging findings in autoimmune encephalitis vary depending on the cause. Most imaging findings are nonspecific, although they may narrow the differential diagnosis when combined with clinical information. CT scans in many of these conditions are normal, with the exception of nonspecific hypoattenuating white matter lesions in steroid-responsive encephalopathy associated with autoimmune thyroiditis. Initial brain MRI in these conditions may be normal.[70,71] Many of these entities show increased signal intensity on T2-weighted and FLAIR sequences in various areas, including the mesial temporal lobes, hippocampus, amygdala, cingulate gyrus, pyriform cortex, subfrontal cortex, and insula.[72] These findings may be unilateral or bilateral and can mimic the appearance of herpes encephalitis on imaging. Gradient echo and other MRI sequences that are sensitive for detecting hemorrhage are useful, because finding areas of hemorrhage favors a diagnosis of herpes rather than an autoimmune cause of encephalitis.

When considering the diagnosis of autoimmune encephalitis, reasonable exclusion of other infectious, toxic, and metabolic causes should be established. Prompt recognition of autoimmune encephalitis allows earlier initiation of immunomodulatory therapy and a greater potential for minimizing morbidity and mortality. Distinguishing among various causes of autoimmune encephalitis on clinical grounds is challenging, although several syndromes have well-described phenotypes.[2,70]

Anti–N-methyl-D-aspartate receptor encephalitis

Perhaps the best characterized of these disorders is secondary to antibodies directed against the N-methyl-D-aspartate (NMDA) receptor. Anti–NMDA receptor encephalitis (NMDARe) was first described in 2005 in a group of 4 young women presenting with acute psychiatric symptoms, seizures, memory loss, and encephalopathy associated with an ovarian teratoma,[69,73] although the syndrome has since been recognized to occur often in children without malignancy.[3] NMDARe affects young individuals, with 37% of identified patients being less than 18 years of age. A female predominance exists, especially in patients between the ages of 12 and 45 years. An identified tumor occurs in less than 5% of children younger than 12 years, although in more than half of woman more than 18 years of age.[6,8,9,74]

The disorder frequently presents with a recognizable constellation of cognitive and behavioral symptoms, as well as with speech dysfunction, movement disorders, decreased or variable levels of consciousness, central hypoventilation, dysautonomia, and seizures. There are age-related differences in presenting symptoms. Children typically present with movement disorders and seizures. Teenagers and adults present with a stereotypical progression of psychosis (consisting of hallucinations, paranoia, and delusions), mood volatility, aggression, and sleep disturbances (eg, insomnia, lethargy). These symptoms are then followed by speech difficulties, involuntary movements, amnesia, and autonomic instability. Despite these age-related differences in symptom progression, after 4 weeks children and adults tend to show the same behavioral and cognitive disturbances, memory deficits, speech abnormalities, seizures, abnormal movements, autonomic dysfunction, and focal motor or cerebellar deficits.[3,4,8,68]

Electroencephalographic abnormalities are variable and include interictal epileptiform discharges, disorganization, focal or generalized slowing, and the pathognomonic extreme delta brush. Cerebrospinal fluid analysis may reveal a lymphocyte-predominant pleocytosis in approximately 90% of patients that is typically mild (<200 cells/mm^3),[68,73,75] and oligoclonal bands may be present in up to half of patients as well.[68,76] These patients express antineuronal cell surface antibodies targeting NR1 and NR2 NMDA glutamate receptors in the cerebrospinal fluid, which are diagnostic of the condition.[77] Presence of these antibodies in the serum is suggestive, although is less specific.[4]

In addition to patients presenting with the typical symptom constellation and progression, patients presenting with relapsing herpes simplex encephalitis should undergo investigation for cerebrospinal fluid anti-NMDA receptor (NMDAR) antibodies. Rarely, patients with NMDARe simultaneously or subsequently develop demyelinating disorders, and as such, the presence of demyelinating changes on neuroimaging should not preclude consideration of NMDARe.[78]

Limbic encephalitis

Limbic encephalitis is a clinical syndrome comprising seizures, episodic memory loss, and suggestive but nonspecific changes on MRI. The disorder can be classified by pathogenesis as being associated either with onconeuronal antibodies or with antibodies directed against neuronal cell surface antigens. Paraneoplastic limbic encephalitis is most often associated with neoplasms of adult onset, is generally less responsive to immunotherapy, and is beyond the scope of this article. Neuronal cell surface antigens in nonparaneoplastic limbic encephalitis include components of the voltage-gated potassium channel complex (VGKC) (anti–VGKC complex antibodies), including leucine-rich glioma inactivated 1 (LGI1) and contactin-associated protein 2 (CASPR2). Antibodies to alpha-amino-3-hydroxy-5-methyl-4-isoxazolepropionic acid receptor, gamma-aminobutyric acid receptor (GABAR), and the metabotropic glutamate receptor have also been associated with the clinical syndrome of limbic encephalitis.[79] Similar to NMDARe, the cerebrospinal fluid in patients with limbic encephalitis may show a moderate lymphocytic pleocytosis, although it does so less frequently than in NMDARe.[76] Symptoms can be restricted to the limbic system, although many patients also present with limbic, diencephalic, and brainstem symptoms and signs. Accordingly, in addition to the typical symptoms of confusion, affective dysregulation, short-term memory impairment, and seizures, patients with this expanded presentation of limbic encephalitis may have sleep dysfunction, oculomotor disturbances (eg, supranuclear gaze palsy), autonomic dysfunction, movement disorders, and the syndrome of inappropriate antidiuretic hormone secretion.[2,69,80]

Rasmussen encephalitis

Rasmussen encephalitis is a chronic progressive inflammatory encephalopathy characterized by impaired cortical function caused by immune-mediated regional, lobar, or hemispheric atrophy. The disease typically begins with characteristic seizure patterns, the most common of which include medically refractory focal sensorimotor seizures, focal dyscognitive seizures, and epilepsia partialis continua, which consists of continuous facial or distal extremity myoclonic seizures of at least an hour in duration, with no pauses in seizure activity lasting longer than 10 seconds. Some patients present with a prodromal phase during which seizures are rare and lateralized, and in which focal neurologic deficits are subtle or minimal. Following the appearance of seizures, the disease progresses across the involved hemisphere, leading to contralateral hemiparesis, hemianopia, cognitive impairment, and dysphasia. If the involved hemisphere is dominant for language, then speech is compromised.[81–83]

Diagnosis is based on clinical and radiologic findings. Rasmussen encephalitis typically shows unilateral areas of increased signal on T2-weighted and FLAIR sequences in the cortex and adjacent white matter.[83] Initially, there may be cortical swelling but atrophy is characteristic of later stages, usually with associated atrophy of the head of the ipsilateral caudate nucleus (**Fig. 6**).[83] There may also be atrophy of the ipsilateral hippocampus and contralateral cerebellar hemisphere.[83] MR spectroscopy can show a decreased *N*-acetyl aspartate/choline ratio and an increased lactate level, suggestive of neuronal loss or dysfunction.[72] ^{18}F-fluorodeoxyglucose (FDG-PET) can show hypometabolism of involved areas when there is only minimal MRI atrophy.

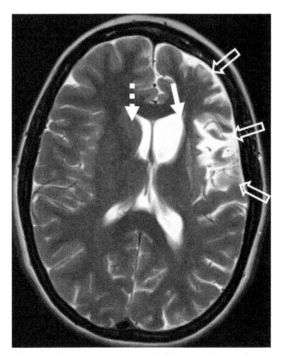

Fig. 6. A 15-year-old girl with Rasmussen encephalitis. Axial T2-weighted MR image shows left frontal, temporal atrophy (*open arrows*). There is associated atrophy of the head of the left caudate nucleus (*solid arrow*), compared with the normal head of the right caudate nucleus (*dashed arrow*).

Steroid-responsive encephalopathy associated with autoimmune thyroiditis

Steroid-responsive encephalopathy associated with autoimmune thyroiditis (SREAT), also referred to as Hashimoto encephalitis, is characterized by broad, nonspecific clinical manifestations. This phenotypic heterogeneity has led to difficulty establishing a description of a typical clinical presentation, systematically investigating pathogenesis, and providing evidence-based diagnostic and therapeutic recommendations.[84] As such, SREAT is often a diagnosis of exclusion, which requires ruling out infectious and other autoimmune causes of encephalitis. Alterations in mentation or levels of consciousness are an essential characteristic, with seizures, psychosis, and myoclonus being the next most common manifestations.[84,85] In addition to hypoattenuating periventricular and subcortical white matter lesions seen on head CT scans in some patients with SREAT, the MRI findings in SREAT are variable and also nonspecific, ranging from unilateral or bilateral patchy to confluent periventricular and subcortical white matter lesions.[72] These lesions typically do not enhance on postcontrast imaging. Additional evidence supporting a diagnosis of SREAT includes abnormal thyroid studies and the presence of antithyroid antibodies, as well as a clinical response to corticosteroid therapy. Less common manifestations include sleep disturbances, tremors, dysphasia, and ataxia.[84]

Because antithyroid antibody titers are frequently and nonspecifically increased in a variety of autoimmune diseases, and because a causal link between the presence of these antibodies and encephalopathy has not been definitively established, the designation of SREAT as a distinct entity is controversial.[84] Because the clinical features are shared with other autoimmune encephalitides, it is possible that many proposed cases of SREAT may have been caused by these other autoimmune disorders. As such, the responsiveness of noninfectious encephalopathy to treatment with corticosteroids or immunomodulation in patients with abnormal thyroid studies and antithyroid antibodies may be insufficient evidence to support a diagnosis of SREAT.[86,87]

Acute Disseminated Encephalomyelitis

The primary hallmark of acute disseminated encephalomyelitis (ADEM) is the sudden and first-time onset of multifocal immune-mediated inflammatory CNS demyelination in the setting of an encephalopathy that cannot be explained by fever. The disorder affects primarily school-aged children with a slight female predominance and is usually preceded by a systemic viral infection in the weeks before symptom onset, although some patients have presented following vaccination or without an identifiable antecedent event.[88,89] In addition to encephalopathy, clinical features include fever, gait disturbance, and speech impairment, whereas laboratory features include cerebrospinal fluid pleocytosis and increased protein levels, and electroencephalogram typically reveals diffuse slowing.[89] Clinical and radiographic features are variable, including the degree of encephalopathy, which can make differentiation from other demyelinating processes, such as multiple sclerosis and neuromyelitis optica, challenging. One characteristic distinguishing ADEM from both multiple sclerosis and neuromyelitis optica is its monophasic course: although ADEM by definition shows no new clinical or radiographic features 3 months after symptom onset, both multiple sclerosis and neuromyelitis optica are characterized by their episodic, relapsing courses.[90] Although this diagnostic feature requires long-term prospective follow-up after an initial episode of inflammatory demyelination, certain biomarkers can refine the diagnostic impression during the initial episode. The presence of intrathecal oligoclonal bands that are distinct from bands present in the patient's serum is more strongly associated with multiple sclerosis (present in up to 95% of patients with multiple sclerosis but only 30% of patients with ADEM), intrathecal antibodies to the water channel aquaporin 4 are seen in neuromyelitis optica and intrathecal antibodies to myelin oligodendrocyte glycoprotein are seen in both multiple sclerosis and neuromyelitis optica, although neither is present in ADEM.[91] The presence of demyelinating changes on neuroimaging and the lack of antibodies and other biomarkers (eg, antithyroid antibodies in SREAT) specifically associated with the autoimmune encephalitides differentiates ADEM from these conditions.[88]

The diagnosis of ADEM requires all of the following: (1) a first polyfocal, clinical CNS event with presumed inflammatory demyelinating cause; (2) encephalopathy that cannot be explained by fever; (3) no new clinical and MRI findings 3 months or more after the onset; and (4) abnormal brain MRI during the acute (3-month) phase.[90] Typical MRI findings include diffuse, poorly demarcated, large (>1–2 cm) lesions involving predominantly the cerebral white matter, although hypointense white matter lesions on T1-weighted imaging and deep gray matter lesions in areas such as the basal ganglia or thalamus may rarely be seen.[90] Up to 2% of patients with ADEM have a second monophasic episode that meets these criteria and subsequently have no further episodes, a phenomenon termed multiphasic ADEM. In contrast, up to 10% of patients whose initial episode of demyelination is most consistent with ADEM have subsequent episodes that ultimately meet diagnostic criteria for multiple sclerosis, with the primary determinants of this diagnostic distinction most often being that subsequent episodes lack encephalopathy or show new findings on neuroimaging consistent with dissemination in time and space.[90]

Treatment modalities are designed to curb aberrant immunologic activity and consist of corticosteroids, intravenous immunoglobulin, and even plasmapheresis.[88] Most patients recover without identifiable sequelae, although up to 20% of patients have subtle neurocognitive or neuropsychiatric deficits despite receiving appropriate therapy.[92]

Neuropsychiatric Manifestations of Childhood Systemic Lupus Erythematosus

SLE is a chronic multisystem immune-mediated disease that commonly affects the central and peripheral nervous systems. The pathophysiology of SLE involves the development of autoantibodies that activate complement and form soluble immune complexes that deposit in target tissues, causing organ dysfunction. Children and adults have similar organ system involvement, although children show greater frequency and severity of systemic disease than do adults. The American College of Rheumatology defines 12 distinct central syndromes that can be associated with SLE, as well as 7 syndromes involving the peripheral nervous system (**Box 4**).[93] Depending on which neuropsychiatric manifestations are studied, the estimate of the incidence of neuropsychiatric disease in SLE can vary widely. This variation is further complicated by the nonspecific symptoms such as headache, fatigue, mild cognitive deficits, anxiety, and depression that are common in SLE, but are also common in the general population, making it difficult to ascertain whether these are directly related to the underlying disease. In addition, many manifestations may be secondary to disease-related end organ dysfunction or caused by treatment of the disease. For example, cortical blindness can result from hypertension-related posterior reversible encephalopathy syndrome, and the hypertension can be secondary to SLE-related renal disease or to corticosteroid therapy used to treat SLE. Psychosis may be a direct manifestation of neuropsychiatric SLE or may be steroid induced. Here, the spectrum of behavioral manifestations of SLE is discussed. Stroke, seizures, and movement disorders associated with SLE are discussed elsewhere in the article.

Box 4
Neuropsychiatric syndromes observed in systemic lupus erythematosus

CNS
  Aseptic meningitis
  Cerebrovascular disease
  Demyelinating syndrome
  Headache (including migraine and benign intracranial hypertension)
  Movement disorder (chorea)
  Myelopathy
  Seizure disorders
  Acute confusional state
  Anxiety disorder
  Cognitive dysfunction
  Mood disorder
  Psychosis

Peripheral nervous system
  Acute inflammatory demyelinating polyradiculoneuropathy (Guillain-Barré syndrome)
  Autonomic disorder
  Mononeuropathy, single/multiplex
  Myasthenia gravis
  Neuropathy, cranial
  Plexopathy
  Polyneuropathy

Adapted from ACR Ad Hoc Committee on Neuropsychiatric Lupus Nomenclature. The American College of Rheumatology nomenclature and case definitions for neuropsychiatric lupus syndromes. Arthritis Rheum 1999;42:599–608.

Behavioral disturbances in SLE can range from delirium and psychosis to mild cognitive defects, and can include mood and anxiety disorders. Key to establishing whether these symptoms are caused by underlying SLE is establishing a diagnosis of SLE through the recently revised Systemic Lupus International Collaborating Clinics (SLICC) criteria (**Box 5**),[94] which are divided into 11 clinical criteria and 6 immunologic criteria. Diagnosis of SLE requires the presence of a total of 4 criteria, with at least 1 clinical criterion and 1 immunologic criterion. Alternatively, by itself, a renal biopsy consistent with SLE nephritis can suffice to classify a patient as having SLE. In addition to active features of SLE, general biomarkers of SLE such as complements C3 and C4 and anti–double-stranded DNA antibody are consistent with active disease.

In addition to these clinical and immunologic criteria, other diagnostic assays may provide more specificity for the identification of SLE-related CNS disease. Cerebrospinal fluid studies may show pleocytosis, increased protein levels, oligoclonal bands, and an increased immunoglobulin synthesis index, but any of these individually or in combination does not have sufficient sensitivity or specificity to accurately diagnose CNS SLE distinct from other CNS inflammatory diseases.[95–99] Both serum and cerebrospinal fluid antibodies to ribosomal phosphoproteins (anti–ribosomal P antibody) have been suggested to be risk factors for CNS disease in SLE but also have varying sensitivity and specificity.[100,101] Antiphospholipid antibodies have clearly been implicated in SLE-associated stroke in both adults and children,[102] but have only been associated with more diffuse disease in adults.[103–106] Cerebrospinal fluid antibodies to neuroblastoma cell lines have been associated with CNS SLE, but have shown mixed success in accurately detecting neuropsychiatric SLE.[107] Thus far, these autoantibodies have only been shown to be risk factors for CNS disease in SLE, and titers

---

Box 5
Systemic Lupus International Collaborating Clinics classification criteria for systemic lupus erythematosus

Classification of SLE requires either a renal biopsy consistent with SLE nephritis or 4 of the following clinical and immunologic criteria, with at least 1 from each.

Clinical criteria
1. Acute cutaneous lupus or subacute cutaneous lupus
   a. Acute cutaneous lupus
   b. Subacute cutaneous lupus (nonindurated psoriasiform and/or annular polycyclic lesions that resolve without scarring, although occasionally with postinflammatory dyspigmentation or telangiectasias)
2. Chronic cutaneous lupus
3. Oral/nasal ulcer (in the absence of other causes, such as vasculitis, Behçet disease, infection [herpesvirus], inflammatory bowel disease, reactive arthritis, and acidic foods)
4. Nonscarring alopecia (diffuse thinning or hair fragility with visible broken hairs) in the absence of other causes, such as alopecia areata, drugs, iron deficiency, and androgenic alopecia
5. Synovitis involving 2 or more joints, characterized by swelling or effusion, or tenderness in 2 or more joints and at least 30 minutes of morning stiffness
6. Serositis (in the absence of other causes, such as infection, uremia, and Dressler pericarditis)
7. Renal disease on urinalysis (proteinuria or hematuria)
8. Neurologic involvement (seizures, psychosis, acute confusional state, mononeuritis multiplex, myelitis, peripheral or cranial neuropathy)
9. Hemolytic anemia
10. Leukopenia (<4000/mm^3 at least once) or lymphopenia (<1000/mm^3 at least once)
11. Thrombocytopenia (<100,000/mm^3) at least once

Immunologic criteria
1. ANA level greater than laboratory reference range
2. Anti-dsDNA antibody level greater than laboratory reference range (or >2-fold the reference range if tested by ELISA)
3. Anti-Smith: presence of antibody to Smith nuclear antigen
4. Antiphospholipid antibody positivity as determined by any of the following:
   a. Positive test result for lupus anticoagulant
   b. False-positive test result for rapid plasma reagin (RPR)
   c. Medium-titer or high-titer anticardiolipin antibody level (IgA, IgG, or IgM)
   d. Positive test result for anti–ß2-glycoprotein-I (IgA, IgG, or IgM)
5. Low C3, C4, or CH50
6. Direct Coombs test in the absence of hemolytic anemia

Adapted from Petri M, Orbai AM, Alarcón GS, et al. Derivation and validation of the Systemic Lupus International Collaborating Clinics classification criteria for systemic lupus erythematosus. Arthritis Rheum 2012;64:2677–86.

---

have not been shown to correlate with disease activity. In general, none of these tests alone is sufficient to distinguish neuropsychiatric SLE from other inflammatory causes of CNS dysfunction and they must be interpreted in the broader clinical context of history, examination, and other diagnostic studies.

Other markers have been under investigation for their ability to predict CNS disease in SLE.[107] Certain anti–double-stranded DNA antibodies have been shown to cross react with NMDAR. In some studies, anti-NMDAR antibodies in the cerebrospinal fluid were strongly associated with neuropsychiatric SLE. Autoantibodies to other neuronal components, antiendothelial antibodies, chemokines, and markers of blood-brain barrier integrity are also being investigated for their ability to detect neuropsychiatric SLE.

Angiography-Negative Primary Angiitis of the Central Nervous System

Although, at the microscopic level, angiography-positive and angiography-negative PACNS both involve granulomatous vasculitis of cerebral vessels, angiography-positive PACNS presents with focal neurologic deficits, whereas angiography-negative PACNS affects small vessels and presents with cognitive, behavioral, or psychiatric symptoms. Although these symptoms are often dramatic by the time the patient seeks medical attention, in retrospect, patients and their families often note subtle changes in behavior in the preceding weeks or months. Similar to patients with angiography-positive PACNS, patients with angiography-negative PACNS have no other symptoms or physical findings apart from their neurologic signs and symptoms, and their diagnostic evaluation is otherwise negative, except for perhaps some increase in the levels of inflammatory markers. The cerebrospinal fluid may show a moderate lymphocytic pleocytosis, moderate increases in protein levels, or both, although it is more likely to be abnormal in angiography-negative disease than in angiography-positive disease.[47,52,108,109] However, this cerebrospinal fluid profile can also be seen in other immune-mediated disorders of the CNS and should not be considered specific. In addition, by definition, vascular imaging performed as part of the initial work-up for PACNS is also negative.

Angiography-negative PACNS requires brain biopsy to confirm the diagnosis. Ideally, biopsy should be targeted to lesions shown on MRI, but if there are no MRI lesions or the lesions are in areas too risky to biopsy, then the nondominant temporal lobe and the overlying meninges should be biopsied.[52] Histology shows transmural infiltrate dominated by lymphocytes, plasma cells, and histiocytes, with some organized into ill-defined granulomas containing giant cells, causing necrosis of the vessel wall. Less invasive but sufficiently sensitive and specific tests are lacking for angiography-negative PACNS. One promising finding is that von Willebrand factor antigen (vWF Ag) was increased in 65% of patients with either angiography-confirmed or biopsy-confirmed CNS vasculitis, and, when combined with increased erythrocyte sedimentation rate and C-reactive protein, increased sensitivity to 81%.[110] In addition, vWF Ag correlated with relapse of disease. vWF is synthesized by endothelial cells and is released into the serum by endothelial damage, such as that seen in vasculitis.

PRESENTATIONS CHARACTERIZED BY SEIZURES AS THE PRIMARY MANIFESTATION

The hallmark of immune-mediated epilepsy is its refractory nature, particularly in the absence of overt structural or metabolic derangements. Patients with SLE may also manifest with seizures, without other apparent signs of multisystemic involvement.

Immune-Mediated Epilepsies

Antibody-mediated epilepsy is most typically diagnosed in the setting of autoimmune encephalitis, although it is increasingly recognized in individuals with medically refractory cryptogenic epilepsy that is independent of encephalopathy.[111] Immune-mediated mechanisms are also identified in children with common encephalopathic epilepsies such as Lennox-Gastaut syndrome, as well as refractory and super-refractory status epilepticus.[112] In addition, immune-mediated pathogenesis is speculated to underlie certain presentations of postictal psychosis, as well as mesial temporal sclerosis with concomitant refractory focal seizures.[113] Given this wide spectrum of clinical presentations, the identification of pathogenic autoantibodies directed against neuronal cell surface, synaptic protein, or intracellular antigens is of both therapeutic and prognostic importance in patients presenting with unusual or difficult-to-control seizures.[114] The most commonly identified immune-mediated epilepsies are associated with antibodies targeting the VGKC complex proteins, including LGI1 and CASPR2, as well as the NMDAR, GABAR, and the intracellular enzyme glutamic acid decarboxylase (GAD).[3,111,112,115,116]

Immune-mediated mechanisms should be considered in children presenting with cryptogenic, treatment-resistant status epilepticus, encephalopathic epilepsy syndromes, fulminant inexplicable refractory focal epilepsy, or atypical interictal or postictal psychosis, particularly in the absence of indicators of an infectious process. In those children whose seizures evolve in a less overt fashion, symptom progression may provide some clues to the presence of an immune-mediated mechanism, with psychiatric symptoms, amnestic syndromes, frontal lobe dysexecutive behaviors, and temporal lobe seizures generally developing before the development of movement disorders, dysautonomia, and sleep disorders.[2,4,9,69]

There is considerable overlap and minimal specificity in the neuropsychiatric symptoms and other presenting manifestations of immune-mediated epilepsies. Despite this lack of specificity, certain presentations may suggest specific disorders. Characteristic focal faciobrachial dystonic paroxysms with subsequent amnesia, disorientation, and progressive encephalopathy distinguish VGKC-complex disease secondary to antibodies against LGI1. Hyponatremia is common. Distinctive features of NMDAR-mediated disease include dyskinesias, choreoathetoid and ticlike movements, mutism, and catatonia. GAD antibody–mediated disease has no consistent specific features but may associate with ataxia or stiff-person syndrome. Nonspecific affective and amnestic symptoms, as well as complex partial seizures, may be seen.

Seizure as a Manifestation of Neuropsychiatric Systemic Lupus Erythematosus

Seizures occur in 2% to 10% of patients with SLE and are one of the diagnostic criteria for SLE. Other causes of seizures, such as posterior reversible encephalopathy syndrome, must be ruled out. Recurrence is observed in 12% to 22%. Seizures can be generalized tonic-clonic, focal, or partial onset with secondary generalization. Less than half of patients have interictal epileptiform discharges predictive of recurrences. Risk factors for recurrence include brain MRI structural abnormalities, focal neurologic deficits, antiphospholipid antibodies, and epileptiform discharges on electroencephalography. Seizure prophylaxis should take into consideration risk factors and may be deferred in the absence of structural abnormalities on MRI or interictal epileptiform discharges.

PRESENTATIONS CHARACTERIZED BY MOVEMENT DISORDERS

Patients with neuropsychiatric SLE may have chorea and other movement disorders, although rarely as the sole manifestation, and the presence of other signs and symptoms often suggests the appropriate diagnosis. Similarly, the presenting features of opsoclonus-myoclonus-ataxia syndrome (OMAS) are typically sufficiently characteristic that a focused diagnostic and therapeutic strategy does not prove elusive.[117,118]

Chorea in Neuropsychiatric Systemic Lupus Erythematosus

Movement disorders are rare in neuropsychiatric SLE, occurring in less than 5% of patients, with chorea being the most common movement disorder.[117,118] Athetosis, hemiballismus, and cerebellar ataxia are less frequent. Chorea is characterized by involuntary purposeless movements that are rapid, jerky, and forceful. Usually discrete, if numerous, they can consistently flow and resemble athetosis. When chorea is suppressed, strength is normal, limbs are hypotonic, reflexes are pendular, and voluntary movements are quick and unsustained. Pathologic findings at autopsy include arteriolar microinfarcts and various other vascular lesions.[119] Nonvascular immune-mediated mechanisms are suggested by the lack of consistent lesions involving the basal ganglia.

Opsoclonus-Myoclonus-Ataxia Syndrome (OMAS)

OMAS is a rare, presumably immune-mediated disorder with a predilection for toddlers and a slight female predominance. The condition is characterized by abnormal eye movements, myoclonic jerks, ataxia, dysarthria, and behavioral manifestations. The syndrome occurs fulminantly or subacutely. The neurologic features may occur simultaneously or sequentially.[11]

Opsoclonus is characterized by random, multidirectional conjugate subtle or dramatic pendular saccades (saccadomania). These abnormal eye movements persist but are diminished by sleep and visual fixation. Myoclonus consists of generalized jerks, affecting proximal more than distal muscle groups, as well as axial and abdominal muscles. The myoclonic jerks are not stimulus sensitive and are not abolished by sleep. Head titubation, dysarthria, dysmetria, and tremor are frequently observed and localize to cerebellar structures and pathways. Although weakness is not clearly present, corticospinal (pyramidal) tract manifestations include brisk reflexes, sustained clonus, and extensor plantar responses.[12] Cognitive, behavioral, and sleep problems occur more often than not, often necessitating curriculum adjustment, behavioral therapies, family counseling, and psychopharmacologic treatment.

OMAS may be challenging to diagnose when the complete clinical triad and cerebellar findings are initially absent. Because opsoclonus can be subtle or not present at onset, posterior fossa tumors, acute cerebellar ataxia, and postinfectious cerebellar ataxia are understandably initially considered. Delayed oculomotor control in otherwise normally developing infants can mistakenly be attributed to OMAS. Epileptic myoclonus may be diagnosed, but is distinguished by time-locked scalp electroencephalogram ictal correlates with distal synergistic muscle emphasis. In OMAS, coactivation of proximal agonists and antagonists and axial muscular involvement and normal ictal electroencephalogram are contrasting aspects.[11,12]

Diagnostic evaluation includes screening for extracranial neuroblastoma, 24-hour urine collection for catecholamine metabolites, and cerebrospinal fluid analysis to exclude meningitis and to sample for oligoclonal bands present in a third of children with OMAS. In most cases of OMAS, CT and MRI of the brain are normal.[120] When OMAS is suspected a search for an occult neuroblastoma should be initiated. Initial radiologic screening for neuroblastoma can be done with chest radiographs and abdominal ultrasonography.[120] If these are negative, a metaiodobenzylguanidine (MIBG) nuclear medicine scan can be performed.[120,121] Abnormalities detected on these tests can focus subsequent cross-sectional imaging, but, if negative, cross-sectional imaging with MRI or CT of the neck, chest, abdomen, and pelvis will still be needed for a more sensitive evaluation.[121] If the initial search for neuroblastoma is negative, the evaluation should be repeated after several months (**Fig. 7**).[120] Neuroblastoma associated with OMAS has an appreciable rate of spontaneous remission without treatment. In patients who show no evidence of neuroblastoma in long-term follow-up, it is hypothesized that the primary tumor regressed before diagnosis, leaving behind the autoimmunity that drives the neurologic syndrome.

The prognosis for this condition may be related to several factors, including onset age, disease severity at onset, duration between symptom onset and treatment, whether full remission is achieved or not, and relapse rate and duration. The presence of an identified tumor does not seem to predict favorable or poor outcomes.[12,122]

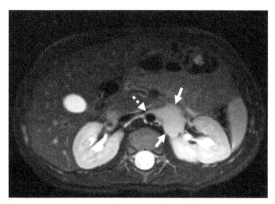

Fig. 7. A 2-year-old boy with OMAS. Axial T2-weighted fat-saturated MRI of the abdomen shows a right retroperitoneal mass (*solid arrows*) that partially encases the aorta (*dashed arrow*). MRI and MIBG studies performed 6 months earlier (not shown) were normal, emphasizing the importance of reimaging if the initial search for occult neuroblastoma is negative.

DEVELOPING A DIAGNOSTIC STRATEGY

The wide scope of manifestations related to immune-mediated CNS dysfunction can make the task of developing a targeted diagnostic evaluation strategy seem daunting. However, when evaluating patients with neurologic complaints, the process is aided by first defining the patient's neuroanatomic and functional phenotype in as specific a manner as possible and then maintaining a broad differential diagnosis that includes immune-mediated CNS disease. Recognizing particular presentations or symptom clusters as potentially indicating immune-mediated disease allows clinicians to perform diagnostic and therapeutic interventions designed to stabilize the patient and exclude broad categories of pathophysiology while simultaneously obtaining diagnostic assays that allow the identification of an immunologic mechanism underlying the patient's symptoms. Neuroimaging may help refine the differential diagnosis when specific findings are present (**Table 1**). For example, in the evaluation of neonates presenting with neurologic findings and multiorgan dysfunction, initial interventions appropriately include investigations for congenital and acquired infections and empiric antiinfective therapy. Neuroimaging may provide clues to a diagnosis of AGS, and if infectious assays return negative, the persistence of cerebrospinal fluid pleocytosis and the evolution of cutaneous and systemic findings reorient the diagnostic evaluation toward this disorder. Similarly, patients presenting with encephalitis typically undergo a broad infectious evaluation and are often started on empiric antiinfective medications while this evaluation is pending. The presence of characteristic neuropsychiatric symptoms may provide indications of an autoimmune mechanism, or characteristic imaging findings, such as unilateral atrophic changes, may suggest specific diagnoses, such as Rasmussen encephalitis. Many patients at our institution presenting with encephalitis and lacking a clear infectious cause undergo simultaneous evaluations for infection and autoimmune causes. However, presentations are often more subtle or insidious, and immune-mediated disease may only be considered following exhaustive investigations for alternative causes. To minimize such unfocused diagnostic evaluations, clinicians should recognize the circumstances under which a patient's neurologic symptoms may be secondary to immune-mediated disease and evaluate accordingly.

Table 1
Imaging findings of autoimmune central nervous system diseases

Diagnosis	Head CT Findings	Brain MRI Findings	Other Imaging

Autoimmune encephalitis	• Early: often normal
	 • Late: nonspecific hypoattenuation, atrophy
	 • Hypoattenuating subcortical, periventricular white matter lesions may be present in SREAT
		• Initial MRI may be normal
		 • Unilateral or bilateral mesotemporal lobe, cingulate gyrus, pyriform cortex, subfrontal and insular cortex SI T2W/FLAIR, ± contrast enhancement
		 • Can mimic HSV encephalitis (hemorrhage favors HSV)
		 • Rasmussen
		   ○ Unilateral SI T2W/FLAIR in frontal/insula
		   ○ Initial cortical swelling/atrophy
		   ○ ±Ipsilateral caudate, hippocampal atrophy
			• NMDAR encephalitis: pelvic ultrasonography or MRI to evaluate for associated ovarian tumor
			 • Rasmussen: FDG-PET, hypometabolism of involved area even when minimal MRI findings

Opsoclonus-myoclonus ataxia	Typically normal	Typically normal	• Search for occult neuroblastoma • MRI or CT of neck to pelvis and MIBG scan • Repeat if initial search is normal

Primary angiitis of the CNS	May show hypoattenuating infarcts	• Infarcts typically unilateral, multifocal, and supratentorial
		 • Usually lateral lenticulostriate territory, basal ganglia
		 • DWI most sensitive evaluation for acute infarcts:
		   ○ SI DWI/SI ADC
		 • SI on FLAIR after 6–12 h
			• Brain CTA/MRA:
			   ○ Narrowing, irregularity, or occlusion of small to medium arteries
			   ○ Terminal carotid, proximal ACA/MCA
			 • Conventional angiography gold standard
			 • Body CTA/MRA to rule out systemic vasculitis

CNS lupus and antiphospholipid syndrome	• Small focal subcortical/ periventricular hypodensities
	 • Hemorrhage
	   ○ Parenchymal
	   ○ Subarachnoid
	   ○ Subdural
		• Small focal subcortical/periventricular SI T2W/FLAIR
		 • Hemorrhage
		   ○ Parenchymal
		   ○ Subarachnoid
		   ○ Subdural
			• Brain CTA/CTV, MRA/MRV: narrowing or occlusion of carotid arteries and sinus thrombosis
			 • Spinal MRI: coexisting myelopathy (rare in children), central cord SI T2W/FLAIR
			 • If antiphospholipid antibodies present: US, CTA/ CTV, MRA/MRV to evaluate peripheral arterial and venous thrombosis

Aicardi-Goutieres Syndrome (AGS)	• Calcifications in basal ganglia, white matter, dentate nuclei ○ May not be on initial scan • Hypoattenuating white matter lesions • Cerebral atrophy	• Calcifications (less apparent than on CT) • SI T2W/FLAIR, lobar white matter lesions ○ Diffuse or anteroposterior gradient (greater frontal lobe involvement) ○ May progress to cystic lesions and cerebral atrophy	
Cerebral folate deficiency	• Atrophy	• SI T2W/FLAIR in basal ganglia, brainstem, cerebral/cerebellar white matter, corpus callosum • Atrophy	
Hemophagocytic lymphohistiocytosis (HLH) and macrophage activation syndrome (MAS)	• Hypoattenuating parenchymal lesions or calcifications • Typically at gray-white junction • Diffuse cerebral edema	• Parenchymal lesions typically at gray-white junction • Supratentorial and/or infratentorial SI T2W/FLAIR lesions ○ Nodular or laminated (SI rim) • Postcontrast T1W ○ Nodular or rim enhancement of lesions ○ ± Leptomeningeal enhancement • Hemorrhage may be seen in parenchymal lesions at follow-up and cerebral atrophy	Abdominal US: • Hepatosplenomegaly • Gallbladder wall thickening • Ascites

Abbreviations: ACA, anterior cerebral artery; ADC, apparent diffusion coefficient MRI sequence; CTA, CT angiography; CTV, CT venography; DWI, diffusion-weighted imaging MRI sequence; HSV, herpes simplex virus; MCA, middle cerebral artery; MRA, MR angiography; MRV, MR venography; SI, signal intensity; T1W, T1-weighted MRI sequence; T2W, T2-weighted MRI sequence; US, ultrasonography.

REFERENCES

1. Bigi S, Hladio M, Twilt M, et al. The growing spectrum of antibody-associated inflammatory brain diseases in children. Neurol Neuroimmunol Neuroinflamm 2015;2:e92.
2. Rubio-Agusti I, Salavert M, Bataller L. Limbic encephalitis and related cortical syndromes. Curr Treat Options Neurol 2013;15:169–84.
3. Peery HE, Day GS, Doja A, et al. Anti-NMDA receptor encephalitis in children: the disorder, its diagnosis, and treatment. Handb Clin Neurol 2013;112: 1229–33.
4. Hacohen Y, Wright S, Waters P, et al. Paediatric autoimmune encephalopathies: clinical features, laboratory investigations and outcomes in patients with or without antibodies to known central nervous system autoantigens. J Neurol Neurosurg Psychiatry 2013;84:748–55.
5. Titulaer MJ, McCracken L, Gabilondo I, et al. Treatment and prognostic factors for long-term outcome in patients with anti-N-methyl-D-aspartate (NMDA) receptor encephalitis: a cohort study. Lancet Neurol 2013;12:157–65.
6. Van Mater H. Pediatric inflammatory brain diseases: a diagnostic approach. Curr Opin Rheumatol 2014;26:553–61.
7. Goodman A. News from the AAN annual meeting: aggressive treatment, team approach and patience needed for anti-NMDA receptor encephalitis. Neurol Today 2012;12:4–5.
8. Florance-Ryan N, Dalmau J. Update on anti-N-methyl-D-aspartate receptor encephalitis in children and adolescents. Curr Opin Pediatr 2010;22:739–44.
9. Chapman MR, Vause HE. Anti-NMDA receptor encephalitis: diagnosis, psychiatric presentation, and treatment. Am J Psychiatry 2011;168:245–51.
10. Lebon S, Mayor-Dubois C, Popea I, et al. Anti-N-methyl-D-aspartate (NMDA) receptor encephalitis mimicking a primary psychiatric disorder in an adolescent. J Child Neurol 2012;27:1607–10.
11. Wells EM, Dalmau J. Paraneoplastic neurologic disorders in children. Curr Neurol Neurosci Rep 2011;11:187–94.
12. Tate ED, Allison TJ, Pranzatelli MR, et al. Neuroepidemiologic Trends in 105 US cases of pediatric opsoclonus-myoclonus syndrome. J Pediatr Oncol Nurs 2005;22:8–19.
13. Crow YJ. Aicardi-Goutières syndrome. Handb Clin Neurol 2013;113:1629–35.
14. Rice GI, Kasher PR, Forte GM, et al. Mutations in ADAR1 cause Aicardi-Goutières syndrome associated with a type I interferon signature. Nat Genet 2012;44:1243–8.
15. Rice GI, del Toro Duany Y, Jenkinson EM, et al. Gain-of-function mutations in IFIH1 cause a spectrum of human disease phenotypes associated with upregulated type I interferon signaling. Nat Genet 2014;46:503–9.
16. Crow YJ, Rehwinkel J. Aicardi-Goutieres syndrome and related phenotypes: linking nucleic acid metabolism with autoimmunity. Hum Mol Genet 2009;18: R130–6.
17. Stephenson JB. Aicardi-Goutières syndrome (AGS). Eur J Paediatr Neurol 2008; 12:355–8.
18. D'Arrigo S, Riva D, Bulgheroni S, et al. Aicardi-Goutières syndrome: description of a late onset case. Dev Med Child Neurol 2008;50:631–4.
19. Rice G, Patrick T, Parmar R, et al. Clinical and molecular phenotype of Aicardi-Goutieres syndrome. Am J Hum Genet 2007;81:713–25.
20. Uggetti C, La Piana R, Orcesi S, et al. Aicardi-Goutieres syndrome: neuroradiologic findings and follow-up. AJNR Am J Neuroradiol 2009;30:1971–6.

21. Ramaekers VT, Blau N. Cerebral folate deficiency. Dev Med Child Neurol 2004; 46:843–51.
22. Ramaekers VT, Rothenberg SP, Sequeira JM, et al. Autoantibodies to folate receptors in the cerebral folate deficiency syndrome. N Engl J Med 2005;352: 1985–91.
23. Djukic A. Folate-responsive neurologic diseases. Pediatr Neurol 2007;37: 387–97.
24. Hyland K, Shoffner J, Heales SJ. Cerebral folate deficiency. J Inherit Metab Dis 2010;33:563–70.
25. Meeths M, Horne A, Sabel M, et al. Incidence and clinical presentation of primary hemophagocytic lymphohistiocytosis in Sweden. Pediatr Blood Cancer 2014. http://dx.doi.org/10.1002/pbc.25308.
26. Horne A, Trottestam H, Aricò M, et al. Frequency and spectrum of central nervous system involvement in 193 children with haemophagocytic lymphohistiocytosis. Br J Haematol 2008;140:327–35.
27. Deiva K, Mahlaoui N, Beaudonnet F, et al. CNS involvement at the onset of primary hemophagocytic lymphohistiocytosis. Neurology 2012;78:1150–6.
28. Anderson TL, Carr CM, Kaufmann TJ. Central nervous system imaging findings of hemophagocytic syndrome. Clin Imaging 2015;39:1090–4.
29. Aksu Uzunhan T, Çalışkan M, Karaman S, et al. A rare cause of acute cerebellar ataxia: familial hemophagocytic lymphohistiocytosis. Pediatr Neurol 2014;51: 465–6.
30. Weisfeld-Adams JD, Frank Y, Havalad V, et al. Diagnostic challenges in a child with familial hemophagocytic lymphohistiocytosis type 3 (FHLH3) presenting with fulminant neurological disease. Childs Nerv Syst 2009;25:153–9.
31. van Egmond ME, Vermeulen RJ, Peeters-Scholte CM, et al. Familial hemophagocytic lymphohistiocytosis in a pediatric patient diagnosed by brain magnetic resonance imaging. Neuropediatrics 2011;42:191–3.
32. Turtzo LC, Lin DD, Hartung H, et al. A neurologic presentation of familial hemophagocytic lymphohistiocytosis which mimicked septic emboli to the brain. J Child Neurol 2007;22:863–8.
33. Shinoda J, Murase S, Takenaka K, et al. Isolated central nervous system hemophagocytic lymphohistiocytosis: case report. Neurosurgery 2005;56:187.
34. Chong KW, Lee JH, Choong CT, et al. Hemophagocytic lymphohistiocytosis with isolated central nervous system reactivation and optic nerve involvement. J Child Neurol 2012;27:1336–9.
35. Beaty AD, Weller C, Levy B, et al. A teenage boy with late onset hemophagocytic lymphohistiocytosis with predominant neurologic disease and perforin deficiency. Pediatr Blood Cancer 2008;50:1070–2.
36. Astigarraga I, Prats JM, Navajas A, et al. Near fatal cerebellar swelling in familial hemophagocytic lymphohistiocytosis. Pediatr Neurol 2004;30:361–4.
37. Akbayram S, Akgun C, Dogan M, et al. Central nervous system involvement in a case of familial hemophagocytic lymphohistiocytosis with perforin mutation. Genet Couns 2011;22:281–5.
38. Chiapparini L, Uziel G, Vallinoto C, et al. Hemophagocytic lymphohistiocytosis with neurological presentation: MRI findings and a nearly miss diagnosis. Neurol Sci 2011;32:473–7.
39. Khan SG, Binmahfoodh M, Alali M, et al. Cerebellar swelling due to familial hemophagocytic lymphohistiocytosis: an unusual presentation. Eur J Paediatr Neurol 2015;19:603–6.

40. Rostasy K, Kolb R, Pohl D, et al. CNS disease as the main manifestation of hemophagocytic lymphohistiocytosis in two children. Neuropediatrics 2004;35:45–9.
41. Kieslich M, Vecchi M, Driever PH, et al. Acute encephalopathy as a primary manifestation of haemophagocytic lymphohistiocytosis. Dev Med Child Neurol 2001;43:555–8.
42. Feldmann J, Ménasché G, Callebaut I, et al. Severe and progressive encephalitis as a presenting manifestation of a novel missense perforin mutation and impaired cytolytic activity. Blood 2005;105:2658–63.
43. Henter JI, Horne A, Aricó M, et al. HLH-2004: diagnostic and therapeutic guidelines for hemophagocytic lymphohistiocytosis. Pediatr Blood Cancer 2007;48:124–31.
44. Ravelli A, Minoia F, Davì S, et al. 2016 classification criteria for macrophage activation syndrome complicating systemic juvenile idiopathic arthritis: a European League against Rheumatism/American College of Rheumatology/Paediatric Rheumatology International Trials Organisation collaborative initiative. Arthritis Rheumatol 2016;68:566–76.
45. Goo HW, Weon YC. A spectrum of neuroradiological findings in children with haemophagocytic lymphohistiocytosis. Pediatr Radiol 2007;37:1110–7.
46. Tiège XD, Van Bogaert P, Aeby A, et al. Primary angiitis of the central nervous system: neurologic deterioration despite treatment. Pediatrics 2011;127:e1086–90.
47. Cellucci T, Tyrrell PN, Sheikh S, et al. Childhood primary angiitis of the central nervous system: identifying disease trajectories and early risk factors for persistently higher disease activity. Arthritis Rheum 2012;64:1665–72.
48. Rodriguez-Pla A, Monach PA. Primary angiitis of the central nervous system in adults and children. Rheum Dis Clin North Am 2015;41:47–62.
49. Cellucci T, Tyrrell PN, Twilt M, et al. Distinct phenotype clusters in childhood inflammatory brain diseases: implications for diagnostic evaluation. Arthritis Rheumatol 2014;66:750–6.
50. Salvarani C, Brown RD Jr, Calamia KT, et al. Primary central nervous system vasculitis: analysis of 101 patients. Ann Neurol 2007;62:442–51.
51. Aviv RI, Benseler SM, DeVeber G, et al. Angiography of primary central nervous system angiitis of childhood: conventional angiography versus magnetic resonance angiography at presentation. AJNR Am J Neuroradiol 2007;28:9–15.
52. Hajj-Ali RA, Calabrese LH. Diagnosis and classification of central nervous system vasculitis. J Autoimmun 2014;48–49:149–52.
53. Gattorno M, Falcini F, Ravelli A, et al. Outcome of primary antiphospholipid syndrome in childhood. Lupus 2003;12:449–53.
54. Avčin T, Cimaz R, Silverman ED, et al. Pediatric antiphospholipid syndrome: clinical and immunologic features of 121 patients in an international registry. Pediatrics 2008;122:e1100–7.
55. Miyakis S, Lockshin MD, Atsumi T, et al. International consensus statement on an update of the classification criteria for definite antiphospholipid syndrome (APS). J Thromb Haemost 2006;4:295–306.
56. Roldan CA, Gelgand EA, Qualls CR, et al. Valvular heart disease as a cause of cerebrovascular disease in patients with systemic lupus erythematosus. Am J Cardiol 2005;95:1441–7.
57. Abdel Razek AA, Alvarez H, Bagg S, et al. Imaging spectrum of CNS vasculitis. Radiographics 2014;34:873–94.
58. Vieira JP, Ortet O, Barata D, et al. Lupus myelopathy in a child. Pediatr Neurol 2002;27:303–6.

59. Muscal E, Brey RL. Antiphospholipid syndrome and the brain in pediatric and adult patients. Lupus 2010;19:406–11.
60. Yelnik CM, Kozora E, Appenzeller S. Non-stroke central neurologic manifestations in antiphospholipid syndrome. Curr Rheumatol Rep 2016;18:11.
61. Carecchio M, Cantello R, Comi C. Revisiting the molecular mechanism of neurological manifestations in antiphospholipid syndrome: beyond vascular damage. J Immunol Res 2014;2014:239398.
62. Mackworth-Young CG. Antiphospholipid syndrome: multiple mechanisms. Clin Exp Immunol 2004;136:393–401.
63. Chapman J, Cohen-Armon M, Shoenfeld Y, et al. Antiphospholipid antibodies permeabilize and depolarize brain synaptoneurosomes. Lupus 1999;8:127–33.
64. Chapman J, Soloveichick L, Shavit S, et al. Antiphospholipid antibodies bind ATP: a putative mechanism for the pathogenesis of neuronal dysfunction. Clin Dev Immunol 2005;12:175–80.
65. Hanly JG, Fisk JD, Sherwood G, et al. Cognitive impairment in patients with systemic lupus erythematosus. J Rheumatol 1992;19:562–7.
66. Kneen R, Michael BD, Menson E, et al. Management of suspected viral encephalitis in children – Association of British Neurologists and British Paediatric Allergy, Immunology and Infection Group national guidelines. J Infect 2012;64: 449–77.
67. Venkatesan A, Tunkel AR, Bloch KC, et al. Case definitions, diagnostic algorithms, and priorities in encephalitis: consensus statement of the international encephalitis consortium. Clin Infect Dis 2013;57:1114–28.
68. Dalmau J, Gleichman AJ, Hughes EG, et al. Anti-NMDA-receptor encephalitis: case series and analysis of the effects of antibodies. Lancet Neurol 2008;7:1091–8.
69. Vitaliani R, Mason W, Ances B, et al. Paraneoplastic encephalitis, psychiatric symptoms, and hypoventilation in ovarian teratoma. Ann Neurol 2005;58: 594–604.
70. Graus F, Titulaer MJ, Balu R, et al. A clinical approach to diagnosis of autoimmune encephalitis. Lancet Neurol 2016;15:391–404.
71. Wingfield T, McHugh C, Vas A, et al. Autoimmune encephalitis: a case series and comprehensive review of the literature. QJM 2011;104:921–31.
72. Vargas MI, Gariani J, Lovblad KO. Imaging of autoimmune epilepsies. Epileptologie 2014;31:39–43.
73. Florance NR, Davis RL, Lam C, et al. Anti–N-methyl-D-aspartate receptor (NMDAR) encephalitis in children and adolescents. Ann Neurol 2009;66:11–8.
74. Millichap JG, Millichap JJ. Clinical features of NMDAR Ab-mediated encephalitis. Pediatr Neurol Briefs 2015;29:48.
75. Jones KC, Benseler SM, Moharir M. Anti-NMDA receptor encephalitis. Neuroimaging Clin N Am 2013;23:309–20.
76. Malter MP, Elger CE, Surges R. Diagnostic value of CSF findings in antibody-associated limbic and anti-NMDAR-encephalitis. Seizure 2013;22:136–40.
77. Dalmau J, Tüzün E, Wu HY, et al. Paraneoplastic anti–N-methyl-D-aspartate receptor encephalitis associated with ovarian teratoma. Ann Neurol 2007;61:25–36.
78. Hacohen Y, Absoud M, Hemingway C, et al. NMDA receptor antibodies associated with distinct white matter syndromes. Neurol Neuroimmunol Neuroinflammation 2014;1:e2.
79. Lim M, Hacohen Y, Vincent A. Autoimmune encephalopathies. Pediatr Clin North Am 2015;62:667–85.

80. Gultekin SH, Rosenfeld MR, Voltz R, et al. Paraneoplastic limbic encephalitis: neurological symptoms, immunological findings and tumour association in 50 patients. Brain 2000;123:1481–94.

81. Wiendl H, Bien CG, Bernasconi P, et al. GluR3 antibodies: prevalence in focal epilepsy but no specificity for Rasmussen's encephalitis. Neurology 2001;57:1511–4.

82. Watson R, Jiang Y, Bermudez I, et al. Absence of antibodies to glutamate receptor type 3 (GluR3) in Rasmussen encephalitis. Neurology 2004;63:43–50.

83. Varadkar S, Bien CG, Kruse CA, et al. Rasmussen's encephalitis: clinical features, pathobiology, and treatment advances. Lancet Neurol 2014;13:195–205.

84. Ferracci F, Moretto G, Candeago RM, et al. Antithyroid antibodies in the CSF their role in the pathogenesis of Hashimoto's encephalopathy. Neurology 2003;60:712–4.

85. Ferracci F, Bertiato G, Moretto G. Hashimoto's encephalopathy: epidemiologic data and pathogenetic considerations. J Neurol Sci 2004;217:165–8.

86. Chong JY, Rowland LP, Utiger RD. Hashimoto encephalopathy: syndrome or myth? Arch Neurol 2003;60:164–71.

87. Castillo P, Woodruff B, Caselli R, et al. Steroid-responsive encephalopathy associated with autoimmune thyroiditis. Arch Neurol 2006;63:197–202.

88. Esposito S, Di Pietro GM, Madini B, et al. A spectrum of inflammation and demyelination in acute disseminated encephalomyelitis (ADEM) of children. Autoimmun Rev 2015;14:923–9.

89. Sanz-Monllor A, Alcaraz-Saura M, Martínez-Fernández C, et al. Acute disseminated encephalomyelitis. A fourteen years review. Neurology 2016;86(16 Suppl):P5.139.

90. Krupp LB, Tardieu M, Amato MP, et al. International Pediatric Multiple Sclerosis Study Group criteria for pediatric multiple sclerosis and immune-mediated central nervous system demyelinating disorders: revisions to the 2007 definitions. Mult Scler 2013;19:1261–7.

91. Kezuka T, Usui Y, Yamakawa N, et al. Relationship between NMO-antibody and anti-MOG antibody in optic neuritis. J Neuroophthalmol 2012;32:107–10.

92. Beatty C, Bowler RA, Farooq O, et al. Long-term neurocognitive, psychosocial, and magnetic resonance imaging outcomes in pediatric-onset acute disseminated encephalomyelitis. Pediatr Neurol 2016;57:64–73.

93. The American College of Rheumatology nomenclature and case definitions for neuropsychiatric lupus syndromes. Arthritis Rheum 1999;42:599–608.

94. Petri M, Orbai AM, Alarcón GS, et al. Derivation and validation of the Systemic Lupus International Collaborating Clinics classification criteria for systemic lupus erythematosus. Arthritis Rheum 2012;64:2677–86.

95. Yu HH, Lee JH, Wang LC, et al. Neuropsychiatric manifestations in pediatric systemic lupus erythematosus: a 20-year study. Lupus 2006;15:651–7.

96. West SG, Emlen W, Wener MH, et al. Neuropsychiatric lupus erythematosus: a 10-year prospective study on the value of diagnostic tests. Am J Med 1995;99:153–63.

97. Olfat MO, Al-Mayouf SM, Muzaffer MA. Pattern of neuropsychiatric manifestations and outcome in juvenile systemic lupus erythematosus. Clin Rheumatol 2004;23:395–9.

98. Lim LS, Lefebvre A, Benseler S, et al. Psychiatric illness of systemic lupus erythematosus in childhood: spectrum of clinically important manifestations. J Rheumatol 2013;40:506–12.

99. Joseph FG, Lammie GA, Scolding NJ. CNS lupus: a study of 41 patients. Neurology 2007;69:644–54.
100. Arnett FC, Reveille JD, Moutsopoulos HM, et al. Ribosomal P autoantibodies in systemic lupus erythematosus. Frequencies in different ethnic groups and clinical and immunogenetic associations. Arthritis Rheum 1996;39:1833–9.
101. Haddouk S, Marzouk S, Jallouli M, et al. Clinical and diagnostic value of ribosomal P autoantibodies in systemic lupus erythematosus. Rheumatology (Oxford) 2009;48:953–7.
102. Harel L, Sandborg C, Lee T, et al. Neuropsychiatric manifestations in pediatric systemic lupus erythematosus and association with antiphospholipid antibodies. J Rheumatol 2006;33:1873–7.
103. Whitelaw DA, Spangenberg JJ, Rickman R, et al. The association between the antiphospholipid antibody syndrome and neuropsychological impairment in SLE. Lupus 1999;8:444–8.
104. Menon S, Jameson-Shortall E, Newman SP, et al. A longitudinal study of anticardiolipin antibody levels and cognitive functioning in systemic lupus erythematosus. Arthritis Rheum 1999;42:735–41.
105. Hanly JG, Hong C, Smith S, et al. A prospective analysis of cognitive function and anticardiolipin antibodies in systemic lupus erythematosus. Arthritis Rheum 1999;42:728–34.
106. Denburg SD, Denburg JA. Cognitive dysfunction and antiphospholipid antibodies in systemic lupus erythematosus. Lupus 2003;12:883–90.
107. Rubinstein TB, Putterman C, Goilav B. Biomarkers for CNS involvement in pediatric lupus. Biomark Med 2015;9:545–58.
108. de Boysson H, Zuber M, Naggara O, et al. Primary angiitis of the central nervous system: description of the first fifty-two adults enrolled in the French cohort of patients with primary vasculitis of the central nervous system. Arthritis Rheumatol 2014;66:1315–26.
109. Hajj-Ali RA, Singhal AB, Benseler S, et al. Primary angiitis of the CNS. Lancet Neurol 2011;10:561–72.
110. Cellucci T, Tyrrell PN, Pullenayegum E, et al. von Willebrand factor antigen—a possible biomarker of disease activity in childhood central nervous system vasculitis? Rheumatology 2012;51:1838–45.
111. Irani SR, Bien CG, Lang B. Autoimmune epilepsies. Curr Opin Neurol 2011;24:146–53.
112. Wright S, Geerts AT, Jol-van der Zijde CM, et al. Neuronal antibodies in pediatric epilepsy: clinical features and long-term outcomes of a historical cohort not treated with immunotherapy. Epilepsia 2016;57:823–31.
113. Pollak TA, Nicholson TR, Mellers JD, et al. Epilepsy-related psychosis: a role for autoimmunity? Epilepsy Behav 2014;36:33–8.
114. Vincent A, Irani SR, Lang B. The growing recognition of immunotherapy-responsive seizure disorders with autoantibodies to specific neuronal proteins. Curr Opin Neurol 2010;23:144–50.
115. Irani SR, Michell AW, Lang B, et al. Faciobrachial dystonic seizures precede Lgi1 antibody limbic encephalitis. Ann Neurol 2011;69:892–900.
116. Lai M, Huijbers MG, Lancaster E, et al. Investigation of LGI1 as the antigen in limbic encephalitis previously attributed to potassium channels: a case series. Lancet Neurol 2010;9:776–85.
117. Besbas N, Damarguc I, Ozen S, et al. Association of antiphospholipid antibodies with systemic lupus erythematosus in a child presenting with chorea: a case report. Eur J Pediatr 1994;153:891–3.

118. Herd JK, Medhi M, Uzendoski DM, et al. Chorea associated with systemic lupus erythematosus: report of two cases and review of the literature. Pediatrics 1978; 61:308–15.
119. Hanly JG, Walsh NM, Sangalang V. Brain pathology in systemic lupus erythematosus. J Rheumatol 1992;19:732–41.
120. Wong A. An update on opsoclonus. Curr Opin Neurol 2007;20:25–31.
121. Gorman MP. Update on diagnosis, treatment, and prognosis in opsoclonus-myoclonus-ataxia syndrome. Curr Opin Pediatr 2010;22:745–50.
122. Pranzatelli MR, Tate ED, Travelstead AL, et al. Rituximab (anti-CD20) adjunctive therapy for opsoclonus-myoclonus syndrome. J Pediatr Hematol Oncol 2006;28: 585–93.

Usual and Unusual Manifestations of Familial Hemophagocytic Lymphohistiocytosis and Langerhans Cell Histiocytosis

Craig Erker, MD, Paul Harker-Murray, MD, PhD, Julie-An Talano, MD*

KEYWORDS

- Hemophagocytic lymphohistiocytosis (HLH)
- Familial hemophagocytic lymphohistiocytosis (FHL)
- Langerhans cell histiocytosis (LCH) • Histiocytic disorders

KEY POINTS

- Familial hemophagocytic lymphohistiocytosis (FHL) is a life-threatening autosomal recessive condition of young children caused by many different gene mutations that affect cytotoxic lymphocytes and lead to a variety of clinical presentations.
- FHL is treated with hematopoietic stem cell transplant and cure rates continue to improve, with overall survival rates ranging from 54% to 91%.
- Langerhans cell histiocytosis (LCH) is recognized as a myeloid-derived dendritic cell neoplasm with an inflammatory component and can affect almost any system of the body, with bone and skin being most common.

Continued

Disclosure: This work was supported by the Midwest Athletes Against Cancer (MACC) Fund and the Medical College of Wisconsin High-Risk Hematologic Malignancy Program.
This publication was supported by the National Center for Advancing Translational Sciences, National Institutes of Health, through grant number UL1TR001436. Its contents are solely the responsibility of the authors and do not necessarily represent the official views of the National Institutes of Health.
The authors have no other relevant affiliations or financial involvement with any organization or entity with a financial interest in or financial conflict with the subject matter or materials discussed in this article apart from those disclosed. No writing assistance was received in the production of this article.
Division of Pediatric Hematology/Oncology/Blood and Marrow Transplant, Medical College of Wisconsin, 8701 Watertown Plank Road, MFRC 3018, Milwaukee, WI 53226, USA
* Corresponding author.
E-mail address: jtalano@mcw.edu

Pediatr Clin N Am 64 (2017) 91–109
http://dx.doi.org/10.1016/j.pcl.2016.08.006
0031-3955/17/© 2016 Elsevier Inc. All rights reserved.

pediatric.theclinics.com

Continued

- Treatments and outcomes for LCH are as varied as its clinical presentations and new findings in LCH bring hope for the possibility of active targeted therapies.
- Both FHL and LCH may mimic several diseases, leading to delays in diagnosis and treatment. LCH and FHL should be considered as differential diagnoses for many unusual case presentations.

FAMILIAL HEMOPHAGOCYTIC LYMPHOHISTIOCYTOSIS
Introduction

Hemophagocytic lymphohistiocytosis (HLH) is a life-threatening syndrome of uncontrolled inflammation and abnormal immune regulation.[1] A spectrum of clinical presentations may occur depending on triggers and genetics. HLH can be broadly divided into primary HLH or familial HLH (FHLH) and secondary forms. This article focuses on FHLH that is caused by lymphocyte defects inherited in an autosomal recessive manner. FHLH is most common in the first year of life, with an incidence in infants less than 1 year old of 1.1 per 100,000 (median age of onset, 5.1 months).[2] Most children are asymptomatic at birth, although a small subset may be symptomatic within the first weeks of life.[3]

Case 1

A 2-month-old boy presented with 3 days of fever up to 39.2°C (102.6°F), sleepiness, and poor feeding. Past medical history was significant for a sibling stillborn at 37 weeks with fetal hydrops and neonatal hemochromatosis. The mother was treated with intravenous immunoglobulin (IVIG) during pregnancy to abrogate neonatal hemochromatosis. The infant was born at 36 weeks without signs of liver disease and was clinically well until admission. On admission, the patient had pancytopenia, hepatitis, hypoalbuminemia, coagulopathy, hyperferritinemia, hepatosplenomegaly, and respiratory failure requiring mechanical ventilation. Septic work-up and infectious studies were negative. MRI of the abdomen revealed low signal intensity in liver consistent with suspected primary hemochromatosis. Two attempts for biopsy of salivary gland tissue to evaluate for iron deposition were inadequate. However, because of this atypical presentation and continued clinical deterioration, further laboratory studies were obtained.

Further work-up revealed hemophagocytosis in his bone marrow, increased soluble interleukin-2 receptor (sIL-2R) level (38,872 U/mL) and CD8 lacking perforin. Genetic testing revealed a compound heterozygote MUNC13-4 gene mutation diagnostic for FHLH. He was started on dexamethasone, cyclosporine, and etoposide per the HLH-2004 protocol. He responded well to induction therapy and ultimately underwent myeloablative hematopoietic stem cell transplant (HSCT). He is currently well 4 years after transplant.

Further studies were performed on the stillborn infant's genetic tissue, confirming a MUNC13-4 gene mutation and ruling out the previous diagnosis of neonatal hemochromatosis. This misdiagnosis led to delay in treatment of the current patient and shows that neonatal hemochromatosis may mimic FHLH.

Case 2

A 16-month-old boy presented with mild hepatomegaly and 3 months of generalized tremors, truncal ataxia, and generalized motor regression with loss of the ability to ambulate. Initial differential diagnosis included hereditary ataxias, inborn errors of metabolism (including lysosomal storage disorders and mitochondrial disorders), spinal muscular atrophy, as well as autoimmune and inflammatory conditions.

He was initially treated with high-dose steroids for presumed central nervous system (CNS) inflammatory disease and had improvement. However, when steroids were discontinued, his tremors, ataxia, and motor regression recurred. He ultimately had 3 prolonged hospitalizations involving multiple subspecialists over a 5-month period (summarized here).

	Admission 1	Admission 2	Admission 3
Signs and Symptoms on Admission	Truncal ataxia, regression of motor skills, papilledema, and mild hepatosplenomegaly	Increasing ataxia and generalized tremors, no hepatosplenomegaly	High fevers, vomiting, worsening ataxia, and motor regression
CBC	WBC 8.8 × 10³/μL Hb 10.1 g/dL Plt 259 × 10³/μL ANC 1056/μL	WBC 11.5 × 10³/μL Hb 11.9 g/dL Plt 475 × 10³/μL ANC 4900/μL	WBC 12.3 × 10³/μL Hb 11 g/dL Plt 221 × 10³/μL ANC 3000/μL
Coagulation Panel	PT 13.5 s PTT 27.4 s	PT 13.6 s PTT 28 s	PT 13.4s, PTT 34.8s, D-dimer 1.12 μg/mL, fibrinogen 291 mg/dL
CSF	No increase in cellularity, protein, and no hemophagocytosis	Moderate cellularity with inflammatory lymphocytes and macrophages, no hemophagocytosis	NA
Bone Marrow	Occasional hemophagocytosis	NA	NA
Ferritin	180 ng/mL	NA	83 ng/mL
Liver Enzymes	AST 348 iU/L, ALT 457 iU/L	AST 35 iU/L, ALT 63 iU/L	AST 73 iU/L, ALT 70 iU/L
MRI Brain	Cerebellitis and mild hydrocephalus	Worsening cerebellitis on left with new-onset frontal lobe and parieto-occipital lesions	Hyperintense periventricular white matter and increased enhancement of cerebellar lesions
Treatment in Hospital	Steroids and temporary external ventricular drain	Steroids and IVIG	Steroids, IVIG, and plasma exchange
Discharge	Diagnosis of CNS inflammatory disease, likely infectious. Home on steroid taper	Concern for inflammatory demyelinating disease. Home on steroid taper	Home on hydrocortisone wean because of adrenal suppression

Abbreviations: ALT, alanine aminotransferase; ANC, absolute neutrophil count; AST, aspartate aminotransferase; CBC, complete blood count; CSF, cerebrospinal fluid; Hb, hemoglobin; NA, not available; Plt, platelet count; PT, prothrombin time; PTT, partial thromboplastin time; WBC, white blood cell.

Because of the uncertainty of his diagnosis, he ultimately underwent whole-exome sequencing. Sequencing was positive for 2 heterozygous autosomal recessive mutations in the perforin gene (c.755A > G and c.1066C > T), diagnostic for FHLH. He began treatment with dexamethasone, cyclosporine, and etoposide and work-up for HSCT was initiated. He developed new language regression and had progression of disease noted on cranial MRI. At time of transplant he had no hemophagocytosis in his bone marrow but had occasional CNS hemophagocytosis in his CSF with stabilized motor symptoms. He received a matched unrelated donor with a reduced-intensity conditioning regimen. His post-HSCT course was complicated with 2 CNS reactivations noted by hemophagocytosis in the CSF and worsening tremors. Both of these CNS reactivations were treated successfully with oral dexamethasone. He is currently off steroids and clinically well 2 years after HSCT.

Pathogenesis of Familial Hemophagocytic Lymphohistiocytosis

Cytotoxic lymphocytes such as natural killer (NK) cells and cytotoxic T lymphocytes (CTLs) are important components of a working immune system. Normally, infected or abnormal cells are targeted and destroyed by NK cells and CTLs. In HLH, the infected or abnormal cells are overactive and are unable to undergo apoptosis. An impaired granule exocytosis cytotoxicity pathway incites a positive feedback loop in which antigen-presenting cells (APCs) overproduce proinflammatory cytokines, including tumor necrosis factor (TNF) alpha, interferon (IFN) gamma, interleukin (IL) 1b, IL-6, IL-8, IL-12, and IL-18, which then further activate APCs (**Fig. 1**).[4,5] This process then leads to tissue necrosis, hemophagocytosis (mediated by CD163 heme-scavenging receptor), and ultimately multiorgan failure.

Genotype and Phenotype Correlations in Familial Hemophagocytic Lymphohistiocytosis

There are at least 12 genetic mutations currently associated with FHLH (**Table 1**).[28] The most common mutations are in the fHLH-2 and fHLH-3 genes. Mutations that

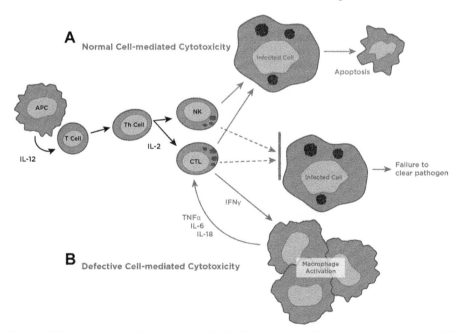

Fig. 1. (A) Normal cell-mediated cytotoxicity leading to appropriate target cell apoptosis. (B) Defective cell-mediated cytotoxicity in HLH triggered by an inciting event (eg virus, malignancy, or rheumatologic disease) leading to a positive cytokine feedback loop further stimulating APC activation. Th, T helper.

Table 1
Hemophagocytic lymphohistiocytosis

Disease	Gene	Protein	Percentage of FHLH	Immune Impairment	Unique Clinical Characteristics
fHLH-1[6]	Unknown 9q21.3–22		Rare		
fHLH-2	PRF1	Perforin	~20–37,[7–9] 50delT mainly in African American/African descent[10]	Cytotoxicity; forms pores in APCs[11]	
fHLH-3	UNC13D	Munc13–4	20–33[9]	Cytotoxicity; vesicle priming[12]	Increased incidence of CNS HLH[9]
fHLH-4	STX11	Syntaxin 11	<5[9]	Cytotoxicity; vesicle fusion[13]	Mild, recurrent HLH, and colitis
fHLH-5	STXBP2	Syntaxin binding protein 2	5–20[9]	Cytotoxicity; vesicle fusion[14]	Colitis and hypogammaglobulinemia
Syndromes with Partial Oculocutaneous Albinism					
Griscelli syndrome	RAB27A	Rab27A	~5[9]	Cytotoxicity; vesicle docking[15]	Partial albinism and silver-gray hair
Chédiak-Higashi syndrome	LYST	Lyst	~2[9]	Cytotoxicity; heterogeneous defects in NK cells[16]	Partial albinism, bleeding tendency, and recurrent infections
Hermansky-Pudlak syndrome type II	AP3B1	AP-3 complex subunit beta-1	Rare	Cytotoxicity; vesicle trafficking	Partial albinism and bleeding tendency
EBV-driven and Rare Causes					
XLP1	SH2D1A	SAP	~7[9]	Signaling in cytotoxic NK and T cells[17,18]	Hypogammaglobulinemia and lymphoma[19]
XLP2	BIRC4	XIAP	~2[9]	NK T-cell survival and NF-κB signaling[20,21]	Mild, recurrent HLH and colitis
ITK deficiency	ITK	ITK	Rare	IL-2 signaling in T cells	Hypogammaglobulinemia, autoimmunity and Hodgkin lymphoma[22]
CD27 deficiency	CD27	CD27	Rare	Signal transduction in lymphocytes	Combined immunodeficiency and lymphoma[23]
XMEN syndrome	MAGT1	MAGT1	Rare	Magnesium transporter, induced by TCR stimulation	Lymphoma, recurrent infections, and CD4 T-cell lymphopenia[24]

Abbreviations: EBV, Epstein-Barr virus; ITK, IL-2-inducible T-cell kinase; NF-κB, nuclear factor kappa-B; TCR, to cell receptor.
Data from Refs.[25–27]

render these proteins nonfunctional result in early disease onset, whereas missense mutations and splice-site sequence variants can have adult onset.[29,30] Also, FHLH phenotypes in childhood can occur with bigenic heterozygous mutations in which 2 separate FHLH genes have mutations.[31] Although patients with a single heterozygous mutation in genes of the granule exocytosis pathway can develop HLH, it is often considered secondary HLH, because patients often respond to immunosuppression alone.[32]

The first genetic defect discovered in association with HLH was a perforin deficiency. Perforin is a cytolytic mediator produced by cytotoxic lymphocytes and released from cytoplasmic granules when the effector cells are activated. Perforin produces holes in the target cell membranes on activation. The effector molecule, granzyme B, a serine protease also found in cytolytic cells, is delivered into target cells (predominantly cancerous or pathogen-infected cells) via the porelike structures, which are generated on activation of NK cells and cytotoxic T cells. Granzyme B then induces programmed cell death in target cells. Decreased levels or absence of perforin or granzyme results in HLH.

Other HLH-related syndromes are associated with vesicle priming, fusion, docking, or trafficking (see **Table 1**). Three diseases that can lead to HLH-like reactions are X linked (see **Table 1**) and have a propensity to develop HLH-like symptoms after exposure to Epstein-Barr virus (EBV). Other symptoms frequently seen include immunodeficiency (most often hypogammaglobulinemia or dysgammaglobulinemia), colitis, and lymphoproliferative disorders. Recently described and rare disorders related to persistent or recurrent EBV infection include IL-2–inducible T-cell kinase (ITK) deficiency and CD27 deficiency.

Common Findings and Diagnosis of Familial Hemophagocytic Lymphohistiocytosis

Almost all patients with FHLH have findings of fever, bicytopenia/pancytopenia,[33] and increased soluble CD25 levels. Other common findings include splenomegaly (95%), hepatomegaly (94%), hyperferritinemia (90%), hypertriglyceridemia (85%), hemophagocytosis (85%), (**Fig. 2**) hypofibrinogenemia (79%), and CNS disease in 30% to 76% with CSF pleocytosis and/or neurologic symptoms such as seizures or coma.[2,34] Not all signs and symptoms are present when a patient first encounters medical care, but with time FHLH progresses if untreated.[35]

Diagnostic criteria for HLH have been created by consensus and last revised in 2004 by the Histiocyte Society (**Table 2**). At presentation, FHLH is often diagnosed clinically but genetic testing alone is also sufficient and often used in siblings and diagnostic confirmation. Often young children are misdiagnosed with sepsis. If FHLH is unrecognized or untreated dismal outcomes occur, with an estimated survival of less than 10%.[25]

Central Nervous System Hemophagocytic Lymphohistiocytosis

CNS disease is noted clinically or by examination of the CSF or neuroradiologic imaging. It can occur at initial presentation or may develop later in the disease course and is associated with increased mortality.[29,31,39] Suspicion of CNS disease should prompt MRI and diagnostic lumbar puncture. In a patient cohort from the HLH-94 trial of 193 patients, 70 patients had documented neurologic symptoms; irritability was found in 24 patients (34%); seizures (focal or generalized) in 23 patients (33%); meningeal findings, including neck stiffness, opisthotonus, bulging fontanel, and papilledema, were seen in 17 patients (24%); and altered levels of consciousness in 8 patients (11%).[40] Furthermore, findings on brain MRI parallel the severity of neurologic impairment. About half of patients with CNS pleocytosis have abnormal MRI with white matter

Table 2
Hemophagocytic lymphohistiocytosis diagnostic criteria

HLH can be Established if Either A or B is Fulfilled	
A A molecular diagnosis is consistent with HLH (see **Table 1**)	
B Diagnostic criteria (5 out of the 8 criteria below)	Cause
1 Fever	Increased IL-1 and IL-6 levels
2 Splenomegaly	Organ infiltration by lymphocytes and histiocytes

3   Cytopenias (affecting 2 of 3 lineages on peripheral blood)
     Hemoglobin <9 g/dL (or infants <4 wk old, use <10 g/dL)
     Platelets <100 × 10⁹/L
     Neutrophils <1 × 10⁹/L
	Increased TNF-α and IFN-γ

4   Hypertriglyceridemia and/or hypofibrinogenemia
     Fasting triglycerides $\geq$265 mg/dL
     Fibrinogen $\leq$1.5 g/L
	Increased TNF-α inhibits lipoprotein lipase
	Activated macrophages secrete plasminogen activator, which results in high plasmin levels and hyperfibrinolysis

5 Hemophagocytosis in bone marrow or spleen or lymph nodes	Activated macrophages
6 Low or absent NK-cell activity (using local laboratory reference)	
7 Ferritin $\geq$500 mg/L[a]	Activated macrophages secrete ferritin
8 Soluble CD25 (ie, soluble IL-2 receptor) $\geq$ 2400 U/mL	From activated lymphocytes (sIL-2R)

[a] A ferritin level of greater than 500 ng/mL is nonspecific and can be seen in a variety of diseases, including shock, chronic transfusions, immunodeficiency, liver disease, cystic fibrosis, malignancy, after transplant, and autoimmune diseases. Experts often use ferritin level of greater than 2000 ng/mL[25] as concerning and greater than 10,000 ng/mL as highly suspicious for HLH. The sensitivity and specificity for HLH with a ferritin level greater than 10,000 ng/mL are ~90% and greater than 95% respectively.[38]

Data from Refs.[25,36,37]

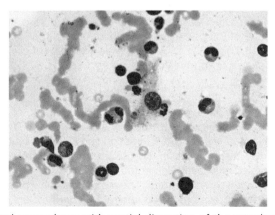

Fig. 2. An activated macrophage with partial disruption of the cytoplasm, with phagocytosed neutrophils and abundant iron/hemosiderin granules (wright giesma, original magnification ×100). (*Courtesy of* Sara Szabo, MD, PhD, Children's Hospital of Wisconsin, Milwaukee, WI.)

changes, whereas patients with neurologic symptoms often have necrotic lesions and cerebral atrophy.[34]

Treatment

All patients with primary or secondary HLH are treated with 8 weeks of cytotoxic induction therapy (dexamethasone, etoposide with or without cyclosporine). Patients with FHLH require an HSCT for cure and correction of their genetic abnormality. Patients with presumed secondary HLH often do not require further therapy after induction unless they develop recurrence, for which HSCT is often needed.

In the HLH-2004 protocol, cyclosporine was moved to up-front treatment compared with the HLH-1994 protocol in which cyclosporine started in week 9 of continuation therapy. There is some concern that cyclosporine may increase neurotoxicity, including risk of posterior reversible encephalopathy syndrome.[41,42] Other complications, including early morality before transplant, HSCT-related mortality, and neurologic late effects, are areas of difficulty and ongoing research.[39] The HLH-94 trial reported a 5-year overall survival of 54% ± 6% for all patients, whereas those who underwent HSCT had a 5-year overall survival of 66% ± 8%.[39] This trial also showed that patients with active HLH at the time of transplant have worse outcomes. Results for the HLH-2004 trial with early initiation of cyclosporine are not yet available.

Recently, reduced-intensity conditioning regimens with alemtuzumab, fludarabine, and melphalan have shown improvements in overall survival. One report in patients with XLP-1 showed an estimated 71% long-term survival, whereas other types of FHLH have shown 92% 3-year overall survival.[19,43] Furthermore, promising results from a retrospective study using antithymocyte globulin during induction have led to a hybrid immunotherapy-HLH phase II clinical trial (NCT01104025).[44] Ongoing HLH research and collaboration is needed for ongoing improvements in FHLH care and outcomes.

LANGERHANS CELL HISTIOCYTOSIS
Introduction

Langerhans cell histiocytosis (LCH), once thought of as a reactive clonal proliferation, has recently become recognized as a myeloid-derived dendritic cell neoplasm with a strong inflammatory component.[45] It is a clonal disease of CD1a+/CD207+ myeloid dendritic cells that can affect all age groups.[46] In children less than 15 years old, LCH has an incidence of 8.9 per 1 million children, with a median age of 3.8 years (range, 2 months to 13.7 years).[47] LCH has a wide spectrum of clinical presentations and outcomes despite its uniform histologic nature.

Case 1

An 18-month-old boy presented with a pink papular rash on his scrotum and edematous circumferential painful papules on the corona of his penis.[48] Topical clotrimazole was initiated for presumed tinea corporis infection and antibiotic ointment for possible impetigo. He was also diagnosed with molluscum contagiosum lesions on his face. Further history revealed that hypopigmented lesions on his trunk and extremities had existed since about 6 months of age. The remainder of his physical examination was normal. Failure to improve prompted referral to a dermatologist who prescribed topical steroids for presumed allergic dermatitis. His lesions worsened and a skin biopsy confirmed LCH. Skeletal survey was normal, he had no hepatosplenomegaly, and had a normal complete blood count (CBC) and liver function tests. He was diagnosed with LCH isolated to the skin; however, his treatment course was complicated by multiple recurrences and required various treatment regimens that included weekly vinblastine with steroid bursts, cytarabine, methotrexate, and phototherapy. At present his disease is under control with weekly oral dosing of methotrexate.

Case 2

A 2-year-old boy presented with a limp and CBC showed a normal WBC count and differential, hemoglobin level of 7.1 g/dL, and platelet count of 534,000/μL. His mean corpuscular volume was low at 60.5 fL, ferritin level was 84 ng/mL, and erythrocyte sedimentation rate was 8 times the upper limit of normal. He began ferrous sulfate for iron deficiency anemia; however, his limp progressively worsened over the next couple of months. During this time, medical care was sought on multiple occasions. Eventually femur and pelvic plain films were completed, noting numerous small lytic lesions. Suspicion was raised for leukemia, prompting oncology referral, where further history elicited intermittent right leg pain, right arm weakness, and gradual decrease in activity. He had no polyuria, polydipsia, chronic ear infections, or skin rashes. His physical examination was remarkable for limited range of motion of his right hip. There was no hepatosplenomegaly or neurologic deficits. His anemia was thought to be caused by iron deficiency, although inflammation and infiltrative processes were possibilities. His oncologic differential included bone disease from neuroblastoma, leukemia, or LCH. A computed tomography (CT) scan of his chest, abdomen, and pelvis was performed, revealing innumerable lytic bone lesions of the skull base, mandible, pelvis, extremities, and vertebral column, along with areas of vertebral collapse. MRI brain was negative for intracranial involvement and initial bone biopsy was nondiagnostic. Diagnoses of Gorham-Stout disease and chronic recurrent multifocal osteomyelitis were entertained because of the extensive and unusual pattern of bony disease including the mandible and calvaria involvement. A second biopsy of the iliac crest was diagnostic for LCH and treatment of multifocal bone LCH with weekly vinblastine and twice-daily prednisone began. After completion of initial therapy, disease reactivation occurred 3 months later with new skull lesions and a palpable parietal swelling. Cladribine monotherapy was started and, after 6 months, 2 new parietal skull lesions were found. At this point, single-agent clofarabine was given. After completion of a clofarabine maintenance regimen, skeletal survey revealed normal pelvic and long bones, whereas the skull lesions were improved. He has had no further reactivation of LCH and is now 21 months off therapy (**Fig. 3**).

Clinical Presentations

The spectrum of LCH is vast, ranging from self-limited to fulminant disease. The clinical manifestations largely depend on the number, size, and location of the lesions (**Table 3**).

Previous separation of LCH into distinct diseases of eosinophilic granuloma (single or multiple bone lesions), Hand-Schüller-Christian disease (triad of exophthalmos, skull lesions, and diabetes insipidus), and Abt-Letterer-Siwe disease (systemic disease, often with fevers, lymphadenopathy, hepatosplenomegaly, bone marrow involvement, and bone lesions) is outdated. The current classification of LCH is divided into 2 broad categories for treatment purposes: single-system (SS) and multisystem (MS) disease. SS disease involves only 1 organ system, such as single or multiple bones, skin, lymph node, or lung. SS disease accounts for up to 69% of LCH at diagnosis, and 25% later develop into MS disease.[47] MS disease involves 2 or more organs or systems with or without risk organ involvement (**Table 4**).

Bone lesions are the hallmark of LCH, occurring in up to 75% of LCH cases.[50] Skeletal involvement occurs most commonly in the cranium (73%), followed by femur

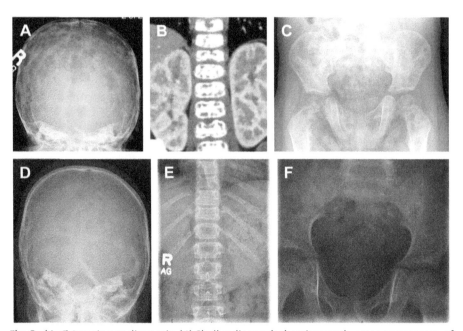

Fig. 3. (*A–C*) Imaging at diagnosis. (*A*) Skull radiograph showing moth-eaten appearance of skull. (*B*) CT chest, abdomen, and pelvis with close-up of the thoracic spine lytic lesions. (*C*) Plain film of the pelvis with multiple lytic lesions. Imaging at completion of clofarabine therapy shows skeletal survey improvement in skull (*D*), vertebral (*E*), and pelvic lesions (*F*).

(23%), facial bones (13%), vertebra (7%), and pelvis (7%).[51] Unifocal bone lesions are generally more common than multifocal bone lesions, for which one study found 57% of 79 skeletally involved patients to have unifocal lesions.[52] However, children less than 24 months of age are more likely to have multiple bone lesions at diagnosis.[53,54]

Table 3	
Symptoms of Langerhans cell histiocytosis	
Location of LCH	**Associated Symptoms**
Skin	Rash (may mimic several disease processes)[49]
Ears	Chronic drainage
Bone	Asymptomatic, pain, limp, pathologic fractures, swelling, or soft tissue mass
Pituitary stalk	Polyuria, polydipsia, growth hormone deficiency
CNS	Cerebellar ataxia, proptosis, neurodegeneration
Disseminated	Fevers, ill appearance
Dental	Floating or loose teeth
Hematologic	Pallor, bleeding, bruising, infections
Pulmonary	Respiratory distress
Hepatic	Icterus, coagulation abnormalities, hepatomegaly

Data from Totadri S, Bansal D, Trehan A, et al. The 5-year EFS of multisystem LCH with risk-organ involvement is suboptimal: a single-center experience from India. J Pediatr Hematol Oncol 2016;38(1):e1–5; and Arkader A, Glotzbecker M, Hosalkar HS, et al. Primary musculoskeletal Langerhans cell histiocytosis in children: an analysis for a 3-decade period. J Pediatr Orthop 2009;29(2):201–7.

Table 4
Clinical classification of Langerhans cell histiocytosis according to the Histiocyte Society LCH-III Trial

Involved System	Involved Organs
Multisystem high risk	Any risk[a] organ involvement
Multisystem low risk	≥2 Organs without risk[a] organ involvement
SS • Multifocal bone or • Special site[b]	≥2 Lesions in 1 organ or in special site[b]
SS unifocal/localized	1 Lesion in 1 organ

[a] Risk organs consist of liver, spleen, bone marrow, or hematologic dysfunction.
[b] Special sites are intracranial soft tissue extension or vertebral lesions with intraspinal soft tissue extension.
Data from Monsereenusorn C, Rodriguez-Galindo C. Clinical characteristics and treatment of Langerhans cell histiocytosis. Hematol Oncol Clin North Am 2015;29(5):853–73.

Epiphyseal lesions with LCH are uncommon and should be differentiated from other lesions, especially chondroblastoma.[52] About 73% of patients with MS LCH have bone involvement.[55] Bone is the most common location of reactivation, occurring in up to 18% of patients with initial SS bone disease (range, 3 weeks to 25 months after initial disease resolution).[53,54] Orthopedic abnormalities, including vertebral collapse, facial asymmetry, jaw problems, scoliosis, and limb asymmetry, are common long-term consequences of LCH and occur in up to 24% of patients.[56] Craniofacial bone involvement may be termed CNS-risk lesions when the skull base is involved, including the orbital, zygomatic, sphenoidal, temporal, mastoid, petrous, palatal, maxillary, or mandibular bones. Independent of disease extent, these bones have been found to increase the risk of developing diabetes insipidus, with a relative hazard rate of 1.7.[57] Skeletal survey is the current standard for detecting bone lesions.[53]

Skin is the second most common system and is affected in up to 34% of cases, including about 11% and 53% of those with SS and MS disease respectively.[50,53,58–60] Neonates with skin-limited LCH soon after birth may have so-called self-healing reticulohistiocytosis and spontaneous regression of solitary or multiple skin lesions often occurs in weeks to months.[61] Resolution of skin-only disease without therapy for patients not in infancy may also occur but is less common.[62] Importantly, any patient with LCH skin involvement requires a thorough initial evaluation and long-term follow-up because prediction of disease extent and further progression to MS disease is not possible based on physical examination, histology, or molecular testing.[59,63–65] Skin LCH is widely variable in appearance and may include necrotic or non-necrotic papules, nodules, macules, crusts, vesicles, or petechiae, and may or may not have mucosal involvement.[59]

The involvement of certain organs with LCH is associated with poor prognosis, and these are termed risk organs. These organs include liver, spleen, and the hematopoietic system.[66,67] Lung was previously considered a risk organ but has since been removed from this category.[55,68] Liver/spleen and hematologic dysfunction have been noted to occur in 4% and 5% of patients with LCH, respectively.

Isolated CNS LCH is uncommon and occurs in only 3% of cases; however, 19% of MS LCH has CNS involvement. LCH cell infiltration of the hypothalamic-pituitary region may result in diabetes insipidus (DI) or anterior pituitary hormone deficiency and is the classic feature of LCH CNS involvement. The risk of DI in SS LCH is 7% at 10 years and 7% to 17% in MS LCH, whereas another 8% to 12% of patients develop DI during therapy.[57,66] The risk of DI secondary to LCH increases with the duration of disease activity and disease reactivation.[57] Aside from hypothalamic-pituitary involvement, other CNS involvement can occur and is grouped into neurodegenerative LCH (ND-LCH) and tumor like LCH (TN-LCH).[69] ND-LCH is a serious and irreversible condition and occurs in up to 3.4% of patients.[70] The exact pathophysiology of ND-LCH is unknown but it may be caused by direct LCH cell infiltration or may resemble a paraneoplastic process with neuron and axonal damage.[71] Patients with DI have increased risk for ND-LCH.[72] ND-LCH has characteristic MRI and clinical findings, in which image changes can be detected earlier with bilateral symmetric lesions in the dentate nuclei of the cerebellum and/or basal ganglia.[73] Patients with radiographic findings of ND-LCH may not develop clinical ND-LCH but should be followed closely.[73] Clinically, ND-LCH shows progressive cerebellar ataxia and may be associated with severe disability, such as cognitive decline and spastic tetrapareses.[69,70] TN-LCH is caused by LCH cell infiltration, is not limited to any specific location, and carries a better prognosis than ND-LCH.[70,71]

Diagnosis

LCH is diagnosed based on characteristic clinical features and confirmed by histology and immunohistochemistry. Histologic tissue analysis shows LCH cells with abundant eosinophilic cytoplasm in a background of inflammatory cells. Immunophenotypic expression of CD1a and/or Langerin (CD207) in LCH cells is required for definitive diagnosis. Positive staining with S100 is also characteristic.[74] Electron microscopy shows classic Birbeck granules, which are elongated zipper-shaped cytoplasmic structures. Demonstration of Birbeck granules is no longer necessary for diagnosis because Langerin confirms their presence.[75,76]

Histologic diagnosis is essential before treating and only rare circumstances occur in which risk of biopsy outweighs benefits. Cases that are high risk to biopsy and warrant careful thought include those with isolated vertebra plana disease without a soft tissue component and those with isolated odontoid peg involvement.[77,78]

Mutational Analysis

Advancements in the understanding of LCH were made in 1994, when 2 landmark studies confirmed LCH to be a clonal disease using X-inactivation polymerase chain reaction–based assays.[79,80] Later, recurrent BRAFV600E mutations were shown in 35 of 61 (57%) patient samples.[81] The BRAFV600E mutation does not correlate with disease site or stage, but the mutation is more common in young individuals, with a median age of 9 years versus 31 years in those who did not have the mutation. Subsequently, mutually exclusive *MAP2K1* mutations were found in 7 of 21 (33%) LCH samples.[82] Both of these mutations activate the mitogen-activated protein kinase (MAPK) pathway resulting extracellular signal-regulated kinases (ERK) phosphorylation.[81,82] Note that the *BRAF-V600E* point mutation has been shown in hematopoietic stem cells in patients with risk organ involvement, whereas the mutation is restricted to tissue-specific dendritic cell precursors in those with non–risk organ disease.[83] Targeting these mutations is a current area of interest, and small adult studies are promising. However, prospective clinical trials are needed to assess their efficacy and safety.[84,85] These mutations may also be used to assess response to therapy.[86]

CURRENT TREATMENTS AND OUTCOMES
Single-system Skeletal

Unifocal bone disease varies by treating provider and anatomic location of the lesion. Often surgical curettage with or without intralesional steroids are used versus observation. Optimal treatment of single-bone lesions in CNS-risk locations using systemic chemotherapy (vincristine and steroids) versus local therapy (biopsy, curettage with or without intralesional steroids) is debated.[87] One retrospective study comparing the two approaches showed no difference in 5-year event-free survival or overall survival.[87]

SS multifocal bone involvement also has a survival rate approaching 100%, although has high probability of reactivation and progression.[88,89] Treatment of SS multifocal bone disease uses 6 weeks of intensive therapy followed by 12 months of vinblastine and prednisone continuation therapy.[66]

Single-system Cutaneous

Similarly to unifocal bone disease, patients with skin-only disease, may not need systemic therapy and can regress spontaneously. Some cases of nonresolving or complicated skin-only LCH may benefit from topical corticosteroids or topical nitrogen mustard, and rarely systemic therapy may need to be considered with steroids with or without vinblastine or low-dose methotrexate.[90,91]

Multisystem Involvement

Multisystem disease is currently treated with 6 to 12 weeks of intensive therapy with vinblastine and prednisone followed by 12 months of continuation therapy.[66] Current 5-year overall survival for patients with MS high-risk disease is 87%, whereas for those with MS low-risk disease it approaches 100%.[66] The 5-year reactivation for patients with MS high risk and low risk is ~25% and ~37% respectively.

Central Nervous System Langerhans Cell Histiocytosis

The use of systemic chemotherapy in LCH with an attempt to prevent DI has not been shown to be superior to the wait-and-see approach or local control.[72,87] However, disease duration and reactivation increase the development of DI. ND-LCH has a poor prognosis, although case reports and case series have shown possible benefit with cytarabine and vincristine with or without dexamethasone.[70,92,93] IVIG has beneficial effects on inflammatory diseases of the CNS and has been recommended by the Japan LCH Study Group to help treat and prevent progression of ND-LCH.[94] Patients with TN-LCH should be approached by resection when possible but may respond to systemic chemotherapy.[70,95]

Salvage Therapy

Although overall survival for LCH is generally high, long-term consequences and survival of MS high-risk patients is suboptimal.[56,66] LCH reactivations often occur in the first 2 years[96] after diagnosis and predispose patients to significant morbidities like pituitary dysfunction, growth retardation, hearing loss, sclerosing cholangitis, and progressive neurodegenerative disease.[56] Patients with disease progression, reactivation, or no response during initial therapy may be treated with salvage therapy. Cytarabine and cladribine use in refractory MS high-risk patients has been found to have an overall response rate of 92% with an 85% 5-year overall survival rate.[97] Also, clofarabine has shown to be an effective salvage therapy in 11 previously heavily pretreated patients with LCH, achieving a 64% complete response rate and 76% progression-free survival.[98] In rare cases, HSCT has been used with success after failure of other salvage therapies, although transplant-related morbidity is high.[99,100]

An ongoing international trial, LCH-IV, is assessing treatment and treatment response. Also, targeted therapies inhibiting MAPK activation are attractive therapies, and a targeted trial in pediatrics is currently underway (NCT01677741).

SUMMARY

LCH and FHLH are histiocytic disorders with widely diverse clinical presentations and disease-causing mutations have been identified for most cases. LCH and FHLH can have serious outcomes and long-term sequelae.

FHLH is caused by several mutations that disrupt genes necessary for the granule exocytosis pathways of cytolytic lymphocytes. In order to diagnose FHLH, patients must meet at least 5 of 8 clinical and laboratory criteria or have genetic diagnosis. FHLH can simulate many diagnoses, including neonatal hemochromatosis, Kawasaki disease, sepsis, CNS inflammatory diseases, and autoimmune diseases. It is important to have HLH in the differential for children with fever, cytopenias, hepatospleno-megaly, and coagulopathy. Patients with FHLH continue to progress over time, often rapidly, and ultimately require aggressive treatment and HSCT.

LCH is a myeloid neoplasm and can mimic several diseases, making it difficult to diagnose. Skin disease may be confused with infectious causes, contact dermatitis, eczema, and/or seborrheic dermatitis. Bone disease may be focal or diffuse, leading to pathologic fractures and long-term deformities. Differentials for bone disease include infections, metastatic deposits from cancer, bone cysts, or in extreme cases Gorham-Stout disease. CNS disease can also mimic a variety of diseases, including malignancies or CNS autoimmune diseases. Diagnosis is confirmed by biopsy of affected tissue. Current treatments vary depending on site and extent of disease, and, despite the high survival rates of patients with LCH, morbidity and disease reactivation continue to be problematic. Advances in the molecular understanding of LCH (*BRAFV600E* and *MAP2K1* mutations) have prompted hope for improvements through targeted therapies. Despite the many differences of these two histiocytic disorders, morbidity and mortality continue to be alarming and ongoing collaborative initiatives are needed.

REFERENCES

1. Filipovich AH, Chandrakasan S. Pathogenesis of hemophagocytic lymphohistio-cytosis. Hematol Oncol Clin North Am 2015;29(5):895–902.
2. Meeths M, Horne A, Sabel M, et al. Incidence and clinical presentation of pri-mary hemophagocytic lymphohistiocytosis in Sweden. Pediatr Blood Cancer 2015;62(2):346–52.
3. Janka GE. Familial and acquired hemophagocytic lymphohistiocytosis. Eur J Pediatr 2007;166(2):95–109.
4. Zhang L, Zhou J, Sokol L. Hereditary and acquired hemophagocytic lymphohis-tiocytosis. Cancer Control 2014;21(4):301–12.
5. Henter J, Ehrnst A, Andersson J, et al. Familial hemophagocytic lymphohistiocy-tosis and viral infections. Acta Paediatr 1993;82(4):369–72.
6. Ohadi M, Lalloz MR, Sham P, et al. Localization of a gene for familial hemopha-gocytic lymphohistiocytosis at chromosome 9q21.3-22 by homozygosity map-ping. Am J Hum Genet 1999;64(1):165–71.
7. Ericson KG, Fadeel B, Nilsson-Ardnor S, et al. Spectrum of perforin gene muta-tions in familial hemophagocytic lymphohistiocytosis. Am J Hum Genet 2001; 68(3):590–7.
8. Suga N, Takada H, Nomura A, et al. Perforin defects of primary haemophago-cytic lymphohistiocytosis in japan. Br J Haematol 2002;116(2):346–9.
9. Cetica V, Sieni E, Pende D, et al. Genetic predisposition to hemophagocytic lym-phohistiocytosis: report on 500 patients from the Italian registry. J Allergy Clin Immunol 2016;137(1):188–96.e4.

10. Lee SM, Sumegi J, Villanueva J, et al. Patients of African ancestry with hemophagocytic lymphohistiocytosis share a common haplotype of PRF1 with a 50delT mutation. J Pediatr 2006;149(1):134–7.
11. Podack ER, Lowrey DM, Lichtenheld M, et al. Structure, function and expression of murine and human perforin 1 (P1). Immunol Rev 1988;103(1):203–11.
12. Feldmann J, Callebaut I, Raposo G, et al. Munc13-4 is essential for cytolytic granules fusion and is mutated in a form of familial hemophagocytic lymphohistiocytosis (FHL3). Cell 2003;115(4):461–73.
13. zur Stadt U, Schmidt S, Kasper B, et al. Linkage of familial hemophagocytic lymphohistiocytosis (FHL) type-4 to chromosome 6q24 and identification of mutations in syntaxin 11. Hum Mol Genet 2005;14(6):827–34.
14. zur Stadt U, Rohr J, Seifert W, et al. Familial hemophagocytic lymphohistiocytosis type 5 (FHL-5) is caused by mutations in Munc18-2 and impaired binding to syntaxin 11. Am J Hum Genet 2009;85(4):482–92.
15. Menasche G, Menager MM, Lefebvre JM, et al. A newly identified isoform of Slp2a associates with Rab27a in cytotoxic T cells and participates to cytotoxic granule secretion. Blood 2008;112(13):5052–62.
16. Gil-Krzewska A, Wood SM, Murakami Y, et al. Chediak-Higashi syndrome: Lysosomal trafficking regulator domains regulate exocytosis of lytic granules but not cytokine secretion by natural killer cells. J Allergy Clin Immunol 2015;137(4):1165–77.
17. Sayos J, Wu C, Morra M, et al. The X-linked lymphoproliferative-disease gene product SAP regulates signals induced through the co-receptor SLAM. Nature 1998;395(6701):462–9.
18. Parolini S, Bottino C, Falco M, et al. X-linked lymphoproliferative disease. 2B4 molecules displaying inhibitory rather than activating function are responsible for the inability of natural killer cells to kill Epstein-Barr virus-infected cells. J Exp Med 2000;192(3):337–46.
19. Marsh RA, Bleesing JJ, Chandrakasan S, et al. Reduced-intensity conditioning hematopoietic cell transplantation is an effective treatment for patients with SLAM-associated protein deficiency/X-linked lymphoproliferative disease type 1. Biol Blood Marrow Transplant 2014;20(10):1641–5.
20. Tang G, Minemoto Y, Dibling B, et al. Inhibition of JNK activation through NF-κB target genes. Nature 2001;414(6861):313–7.
21. Rigaud S, Fondanèche M, Lambert N, et al. XIAP deficiency in humans causes an X-linked lymphoproliferative syndrome. Nature 2006;444(7115):110–4.
22. Ghosh S, Bienemann K, Boztug K, et al. Interleukin-2-inducible T-cell kinase (ITK) deficiency-clinical and molecular aspects. J Clin Immunol 2014;34(8):892–9.
23. Alkhairy OK, Perez-Becker R, Driessen GJ, et al. Novel mutations in TNFRSF7/CD27: clinical, immunologic, and genetic characterization of human CD27 deficiency. J Allergy Clin Immunol 2015;136(3):703–12.e10.
24. Li FY, Chaigne-Delalande B, Su H, et al. XMEN disease: a new primary immunodeficiency affecting Mg2+ regulation of immunity against Epstein-Barr virus. Blood 2014;123(14):2148–52.
25. Allen CE, McClain KL. Pathophysiology and epidemiology of hemophagocytic lymphohistiocytosis. Hematology Am Soc Hematol Educ Program 2015;2015(1):177–82.
26. Zhang K, Filipovich AH, Johnson J, et al. Hemophagocytic lymphohistiocytosis, familial. In: Pagon RA, Adam MP, Ardinger HH, et al, editors. GeneReviews® [Internet]. Seattle (WA): University of Washington; 2013. p. 1993–2016.

27. Chandrakasan S, Filipovich AH. Hemophagocytic lymphohistiocytosis: advances in pathophysiology, diagnosis, and treatment. J Pediatr 2013;163(5): 1253–9.
28. Tesi B, Lagerstedt-Robinson K, Chiang SC, et al. Targeted high-throughput sequencing for genetic diagnostics of hemophagocytic lymphohistiocytosis. Genome Med 2015;7(1):1–13.
29. Zhang K, Jordan MB, Marsh RA, et al. Hypomorphic mutations in PRF1, MUNC13-4, and STXBP2 are associated with adult-onset familial HLH. Blood 2011;118(22):5794–8.
30. Sieni E, Cetica V, Santoro A, et al. Genotype-phenotype study of familial haemophagocytic lymphohistiocytosis type 3. J Med Genet 2011;48(5):343–52.
31. Zhang K, Chandrakasan S, Chapman H, et al. Synergistic defects of different molecules in the cytotoxic pathway lead to clinical familial hemophagocytic lymphohistiocytosis. Blood 2014;124(8):1331–4.
32. Zhang M, Bracaglia C, Prencipe G, et al. A heterozygous RAB27A mutation associated with delayed cytolytic granule polarization and hemophagocytic lymphohistiocytosis. J Immunol 2016;196(6):2492–503.
33. Feldmann J, Le Deist F, Ouachée-Chardin M, et al. Functional consequences of perforin gene mutations in 22 patients with familial haemophagocytic lymphohistiocytosis. Br J Haematol 2002;117(4):965–72.
34. Haddad E, Sulis ML, Jabado N, et al. Frequency and severity of central nervous system lesions in hemophagocytic lymphohistiocytosis. Blood 1997;89(3): 794–800.
35. Janka G. Familial and acquired hemophagocytic lymphohistiocytosis. Annu Rev Med 2012;63:233–46.
36. Janka GE. Hemophagocytic syndromes. Blood Rev 2007;21(5):245–53.
37. Henter J, Horne A, Aricó M, et al. HLH-2004: diagnostic and therapeutic guidelines for hemophagocytic lymphohistiocytosis. Pediatr Blood Cancer 2007; 48(2):124–31.
38. Allen CE, Yu X, Kozinetz CA, et al. Highly elevated ferritin levels and the diagnosis of hemophagocytic lymphohistiocytosis. Pediatr Blood Cancer 2008; 50(6):1227–35.
39. Trottestam H, Horne A, Arico M, et al. Chemoimmunotherapy for hemophagocytic lymphohistiocytosis: Long-term results of the HLH-94 treatment protocol. Blood 2011;118(17):4577–84.
40. Horne A, Trottestam H, Aricò M, et al. Frequency and spectrum of central nervous system involvement in 193 children with haemophagocytic lymphohistiocytosis. Br J Haematol 2008;140(3):327–35.
41. Lee G, Lee SE, Ryu K, et al. Posterior reversible encephalopathy syndrome in pediatric patients undergoing treatment for hemophagocytic lymphohistiocytosis: clinical outcomes and putative risk factors. Blood Res 2013;48(4):258–65.
42. Thompson PA, Allen CE, Horton T, et al. Severe neurologic side effects in patients being treated for hemophagocytic lymphohistiocytosis. Pediatr Blood Cancer 2009;52(5):621–5.
43. Marsh RA, Vaughn G, Kim MO, et al. Reduced-intensity conditioning significantly improves survival of patients with hemophagocytic lymphohistiocytosis undergoing allogeneic hematopoietic cell transplantation. Blood 2010;116(26): 5824–31.
44. Mahlaoui N, Ouachee-Chardin M, de Saint Basile G, et al. Immunotherapy of familial hemophagocytic lymphohistiocytosis with antithymocyte globulins: a single-center retrospective report of 38 patients. Pediatrics 2007;120(3):e622–8.

45. Abla O, Weitzman S. Treatment of Langerhans cell histiocytosis: role of BRAF/ MAPK inhibition. Hematology Am Soc Hematol Educ Program 2015;2015(1): 565–70.

46. Monsereenusorn C, Rodriguez-Galindo C. Clinical characteristics and treatment of Langerhans cell histiocytosis. Hematol Oncol Clin North Am 2015;29(5): 853–73.

47. Stålemark H, Laurencikas E, Karis J, et al. Incidence of Langerhans cell histiocytosis in children: a population-based study. Pediatr Blood Cancer 2008;51(1): 76–81.

48. Ehrhardt MJ, Humphrey SR, Kelly ME, et al. The natural history of skin-limited Langerhans cell histiocytosis: a single-institution experience. J Pediatr Hematol Oncol 2014;36(8):613–6.

49. Simko SJ, Garmezy B, Abhyankar H, et al. Differentiating skin-limited and multisystem Langerhans cell histiocytosis. J Pediatr 2014;165(5):990–6.

50. Guyot-Goubin A, Donadieu J, Barkaoui M, et al. Descriptive epidemiology of childhood Langerhans cell histiocytosis in France, 2000–2004. Pediatr Blood Cancer 2008;51(1):71–5.

51. Totadri S, Bansal D, Trehan A, et al. The 5-year EFS of multisystem LCH with risk-organ involvement is suboptimal: a single-center experience from India. J Pediatr Hematol Oncol 2016;38(1):e1–5.

52. Arkader A, Glotzbecker M, Hosalkar HS, et al. Primary musculoskeletal Langerhans cell histiocytosis in children: an analysis for a 3-decade period. J Pediatr Orthop 2009;29(2):201–7.

53. Titgemeyer C, Grois N, Minkov M, et al. Pattern and course of single-system disease in Langerhans cell histiocytosis data from the DAL-HX 83-and 90-study. Med Pediatr Oncol 2001;37(2):108–14.

54. Kamath S, Arkader A, Jubran RF. Outcomes of children younger than 24 months with Langerhans cell histiocytosis and bone involvement: a report from a single institution. J Pediatr Orthop 2014;34(8):825–30.

55. Aricò M, Astigarraga I, Braier J, et al. Lack of bone lesions at diagnosis is associated with inferior outcome in multisystem Langerhans cell histiocytosis of childhood. Br J Haematol 2015;169(2):241–8.

56. Haupt R, Nanduri V, Calevo MG, et al. Permanent consequences in Langerhans cell histiocytosis patients: a pilot study from the Histiocyte Society—Late Effects Study Group. Pediatr Blood Cancer 2004;42(5):438–44.

57. Grois N, Pötschger U, Prosch H, et al. Risk factors for diabetes insipidus in Langerhans cell histiocytosis. Pediatr Blood Cancer 2006;46(2):228–33.

58. Donadieu Jf, Thomas C, Brugieres L, et al. A multicentre retrospective survey of Langerhans' cell histiocytosis: 348 cases observed between 1983 and 1993. Arch Dis Child 1996;75(1):17–24.

59. Morren M, Vanden Broecke K, Vangeebergen L, et al. Diverse cutaneous presentations of Langerhans cell histiocytosis in children: a retrospective cohort study. Pediatr Blood Cancer 2015;63(3):486–92.

60. Gadner H, Heitger A, Grois N, et al. Treatment strategy for disseminated Langerhans cell histiocytosis. Med Pediatr Oncol 1994;23(2):72–80.

61. Kapur P, Erickson C, Rakheja D, et al. Congenital self-healing reticulohistiocytosis (Hashimoto-Pritzker disease): ten-year experience at Dallas Children's Medical Center. J Am Acad Dermatol 2007;56(2):290–4.

62. Nakahigashi K, Ohta M, Sakai R, et al. Late-onset self-healing reticulohistiocytosis: pediatric case of Hashimoto-Pritzker type Langerhans cell histiocytosis. J Dermatol 2007;34(3):205–9.

63. Stein SL, Paller AS, Haut PR, et al. Langerhans cell histiocytosis presenting in the neonatal period: a retrospective case series. Arch Pediatr Adolesc Med 2001;155(7):778–83.

64. Lau L, Krafchik B, Trebo MM, et al. Cutaneous Langerhans cell histiocytosis in children under one year. Pediatr Blood Cancer 2006;46(1):66–71.

65. Battistella M, Fraitag S, Teillac DH, et al. Neonatal and early infantile cutaneous Langerhans cell histiocytosis: comparison of self-regressive and non-self-regressive forms. Arch Dermatol 2010;146(2):149–56.

66. Gadner H, Minkov M, Grois N, et al. Therapy prolongation improves outcome in multisystem Langerhans cell histiocytosis. Blood 2013;121(25):5006–14.

67. Lahey ME. Prognostic factors in histiocytosis X. J Pediatr Hematol /Oncol 1981; 3(1):57–60.

68. Braier J, Latella A, Balancini B, et al. Outcome in children with pulmonary Langerhans cell histiocytosis. Pediatr Blood Cancer 2004;43(7):765–9.

69. Idbaih A, Donadieu J, Barthez M, et al. Retinoic acid therapy in "degenerative-like" neuro-Langerhans cell histiocytosis: a prospective pilot study. Pediatr Blood Cancer 2004;43(1):55–8.

70. Barthez MA, Araujo E, Donadieu J. Langerhans cell histiocytosis and the central nervous system in childhood: evolution and prognostic factors. results of a collaborative study. J Child Neurol 2000;15(3):150–6.

71. Grois N, Prayer D, Prosch H, et al, CNS LCH Co-operative Group. Neuropathology of CNS disease in Langerhans cell histiocytosis. Brain 2005;128(Pt 4): 829–38.

72. Donadieu J, Rolon M, Thomas C, et al. Endocrine involvement in pediatric-onset Langerhans' cell histiocytosis: a population-based study. J Pediatr 2004;144(3): 344–50.

73. Wnorowski M, Prosch H, Prayer D, et al. Pattern and course of neurodegeneration in Langerhans cell histiocytosis. J Pediatr 2008;153(1):127–32.

74. Harmon CM, Brown N. Langerhans cell histiocytosis: a clinicopathologic review and molecular pathogenetic update. Arch Pathol Lab Med 2015;139(10): 1211–4.

75. Mc Dermott R, Ziylan U, Spehner D, et al. Birbeck granules are subdomains of endosomal recycling compartment in human epidermal Langerhans cells, which form where langerin accumulates. Mol Biol Cell 2002;13(1):317–35.

76. Valladeau J, Ravel O, Dezutter-Dambuyant C, et al. Langerin, a novel C-type lectin specific to Langerhans cells, is an endocytic receptor that induces the formation of Birbeck granules. Immunity 2000;12(1):71–81.

77. Yeom J, Lee C, Shin HY, et al. Langerhans' cell histiocytosis of the spine: analysis of twenty-three cases. Spine 1999;24(16):1740.

78. Huang WD, Yang XH, Wu ZP, et al. Langerhans cell histiocytosis of spine: a comparative study of clinical, imaging features, and diagnosis in children, adolescents, and adults. Spine J 2013;13(9):1108–17.

79. Willman CL, Busque L, Griffith BB, et al. Langerhans'-cell histiocytosis (histiocytosis X)–a clonal proliferative disease. N Engl J Med 1994;331(3):154–60.

80. Yu R, Chu A, Chu C, et al. Clonal proliferation of Langerhans cells in Langerhans cell histiocytosis. Lancet 1994;343(8900):767–8.

81. Badalian-Very G, Vergilio JA, Degar BA, et al. Recurrent BRAF mutations in Langerhans cell histiocytosis. Blood 2010;116(11):1919–23.

82. Chakraborty R, Hampton OA, Shen X, et al. Mutually exclusive recurrent somatic mutations in MAP2K1 and BRAF support a central role for ERK activation in LCH pathogenesis. Blood 2014;124(19):3007–15.

83. Berres ML, Lim KP, Peters T, et al. BRAF-V600E expression in precursor versus differentiated dendritic cells defines clinically distinct LCH risk groups. J Exp Med 2014;211(4):669–83.
84. Haroche J, Cohen-Aubart F, Emile JF, et al. Dramatic efficacy of vemurafenib in both multisystemic and refractory Erdheim-Chester disease and Langerhans cell histiocytosis harboring the BRAF V600E mutation. Blood 2013;121(9):1495–500.
85. Haroche J, Cohen-Aubart F, Emile JF, et al. Reproducible and sustained efficacy of targeted therapy with vemurafenib in patients with BRAF(V600E)-mutated Erdheim-Chester disease. J Clin Oncol 2015;33(5):411–8.
86. Arceci RJ. Biological and therapeutic implications of the BRAF pathway in histiocytic disorders. Am Soc Clin Oncol Educ Book 2014;e441–5.
87. Chellapandian D, Shaikh F, van den Bos C, et al. Management and outcome of patients with Langerhans cell histiocytosis and single-bone CNS-risk lesions: a multi-institutional retrospective study. Pediatr Blood Cancer 2015;62(12):2162–6.
88. Sessa S, Sommelet D, Lascombes P, et al. Treatment of Langerhans-cell histiocytosis in children. experience at the Children's Hospital of Nancy. J Bone Joint Surg Am 1994;76(10):1513–25.
89. Haupt R, Minkov M, Astigarraga I, et al. Langerhans cell histiocytosis (LCH): guidelines for diagnosis, clinical work-up, and treatment for patients till the age of 18 years. Pediatr Blood Cancer 2013;60(2):175–84.
90. Hadfield PJ, Birchall M, Albert D. Otitis externa in Langerhans' cell histiocytosis—the successful use of topical nitrogen mustard. Int J Pediatr Otorhinolaryngol 1994;30(2):143–9.
91. Steen A, Steen K, Bauer R, et al. Successful treatment of cutaneous Langerhans cell histiocytosis with low-dose methotrexate. Br J Dermatol 2001;145(1):137–40.
92. Allen CE, Flores R, Rauch R, et al. Neurodegenerative central nervous system Langerhans cell histiocytosis and coincident hydrocephalus treated with vincristine/cytosine arabinoside. Pediatr Blood Cancer 2010;54(3):416–23.
93. Ehrhardt MJ, Karst J, Donohoue PA, et al. Recognition and treatment of concurrent active and neurodegenerative Langerhans cell histiocytosis: a case report. J Pediatr Hematol Oncol 2015;37(1):e37–40.
94. Imashuku S, Fujita N, Shioda Y, et al. Follow-up of pediatric patients treated by IVIG for Langerhans cell histiocytosis (LCH)-related neurodegenerative CNS disease. Int J Hematol 2015;101(2):191–7.
95. Allen CE, Ladisch S, McClain KL. How I treat Langerhans cell histiocytosis. Blood 2015;126(1):26–35.
96. Minkov M, Steiner M, Pötschger U, et al. Reactivations in multisystem Langerhans cell histiocytosis: data of the international LCH registry. J Pediatr 2008; 153(5):700–5.e2.
97. Donadieu J, Bernard F, van Noesel M, et al. Cladribine and cytarabine in refractory multisystem Langerhans cell histiocytosis: results of an international phase 2 study. Blood 2015;126(12):1415–23.
98. Simko SJ, Tran HD, Jones J, et al. Clofarabine salvage therapy in refractory multifocal histiocytic disorders, including Langerhans cell histiocytosis, juvenile xanthogranuloma and Rosai-Dorfman disease. Pediatr Blood Cancer 2014;61(3):479–87.
99. Jun Y, Quan QM, Bin W, et al. Haploidentical parental hematopoietic stem cell transplantation in pediatric refractory Langerhans cell histiocytosis. Pediatr Transpl 2014;18(4):E124–9.
100. Veys PA, Nanduri V, Baker KS, et al. Haematopoietic stem cell transplantation for refractory Langerhans cell histiocytosis: outcome by intensity of conditioning. Br J Haematol 2015;169(5):711–8.

When to Suspect Autoinflammatory/ Recurrent Fever Syndromes

James W. Verbsky, MD, PhD

KEYWORDS

- Fever • Autoinflammatory • IL-1beta • TNF-α • Innate immunity

KEY POINTS

- Autoinflammatory disorders result in persistent or recurrent episodes of inflammation due to mutations in innate immune system sensors.
- Autoinflammatory disorders should be considered only after a workup for autoimmune disorders, malignancy, or immune deficiency.
- Once an autoinflammatory disorder is diagnosed, targeted therapies are often available.

BACKGROUND AND PATHOPHYSIOLOGY OF AUTOINFLAMMATORY DISORDERS

Inflammation, the classic quadrad of "rubor (redness), tumor (swelling), calor (heat), and dolor (pain)", is a fundamental concept of immunology and a common observation in clinical medicine. One could add "fever" as a fifth marker of inflammation, although it is not unusual to have inflammation without fever.

Inflammation is central to the function of the innate immune system that has evolved to recognize pathogens of all types, including fungi, bacteria, virus, protozoa, and helminths. This system is highly diverse, with multiple related and unrelated protein family members, likely due to the evolution driven by diverse pathogens. These protein families are often referred to pathogen recognition receptors (PRR) and they have evolved to recognize conserved microbial products, known as pathogen-associated molecular patterns (PAMPs). PAMPs are equally diverse, and include molecules unique to microbes, such as lipopolysaccharide (LPS), lipoteichoic acid (LTA), flagellin, and viral nucleic acids, among others. Because humans do not make these molecules, they are natural targets for recognition by the immune system.

This recognition of pathogens is the first line of defense of the immune system, and recognition by PRRs leads to rapid induction of inflammation. Inflammation by these different pathways is scripted, and thus consistent each time that pathogen is

Pediatric Rheumatology, Medical College of Wisconsin, Children's Corporate Center, Suite C465, 9000 West Wisconsin Avenue, PO Box 1997, Milwaukee, WI 53201-1997, USA
E-mail address: jverbsky@mcw.edu

Pediatr Clin N Am 64 (2017) 111–125
http://dx.doi.org/10.1016/j.pcl.2016.08.008   **pediatric.theclinics.com**
0031-3955/17/© 2016 Elsevier Inc. All rights reserved.

recognized. The response to subsequent challenges is no faster or of greater magnitude than the initial response; that is, the innate immune system does not "learn," but is essential to activate the adaptive immune system (ie, T and B lymphocytes) that does learn, and through the acquisition of memory is much more effective at clearing pathogens than the innate immune system.

Not all inflammation is alike, however, and different PRRs are activated by different PAMPs, resulting in differing responses. For example, antiviral PRRs activate the production of interferons that induce inflammation but also induce changes in stromal cells to help slow viral replication until the adaptive immune system can be activated. PRRs specific for LPS or other bacterial products lead to nuclear factor (NF)-κB activation and the generation of number inflammatory proteins. These pathways promote immune cell recruitment, production of stromal cell factors that aid in slowing microbial infiltration, and activate systemic pathways that help protect the host, such as the acute phase response.

Autoinflammatory syndromes are defined as disorders characterized by persistent or recurrent bouts of inflammation without features of autoimmunity (ie, autoantibodies or autoreactive T cells). These disorders are also referred to as periodic fever syndromes, although this nomenclature is falling out of favor as we learn more about these disorders. Many of these disorders exhibit inflammation without fever, and the inflammation can be persistent rather than episodic. Autoinflammatory disorders typical involve activating mutations in PRRs, or loss of regulatory proteins that regulate signaling of PRRs. Because the innate immune system does not exhibit memory and thus each inflammatory episode is of similar magnitude to past episodes, these bouts of inflammation can persist or recur for years before pathology occurs. In contrast, autoimmune disorders do exhibit memory, and thus autoimmune responses can ramp up quickly leading to serious illness in a relatively short period of time (**Fig. 1**).

When to Consider Autoinflammatory Disorders

When considering the diagnosis of an autoinflammatory syndrome in a child with recurrent fevers or inflammation, it is important to realize that fevers are a part of childhood and are overwhelmingly caused by innocuous infections. Autoinflammatory disorders should not be the first consideration of a child with recurrent fevers, as these are rare disorders. The initial workup of a child with recurrent infections should focus on ruling out more serious conditions, such as autoimmune disease, malignancy, or

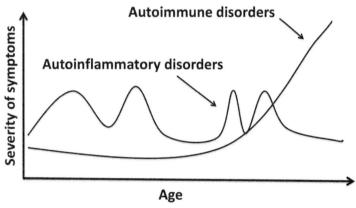

Fig. 1. Graphic representation of symptoms over time of autoinflammatory disorders and autoimmune disorders.

immune deficiency. A conservative workup of a child with recurrent fevers may include the following:

1. Physical examination for signs of autoimmunity or malignancy
2. Infectious workup to determine the organism(s)
3. Imaging or other investigations as indicated (eg, masses on examination, endoscopy to rule out inflammatory bowel disease, bone scan to rule out osteomyelitis)
4. Limited laboratory evaluation
   a. Complete blood count
   b. Immunoglobulin levels
   c. Vaccine titers (diphtheria, tetanus, pneumococcus)
   d. Erythrocyte sedimentation rate (ESR) and C-reactive protein (CRP) (when afebrile)
   e. Uric acid and lactate dehydrogenase (LDH)

Malignancies and autoimmune diseases do not wax and wane, so these would be unlikely with a history of recurrent fevers followed by periods of general well-being. Signs of a characteristic rash, arthritis, or weight loss can be seen juvenile idiopathic arthritis or inflammatory bowel disease. These disorders may have intermittent fevers, but other symptoms typically persist. Inflammatory markers (ie, ESR and CRP) are generally not helpful during febrile episodes, but assessment of these markers between episodes and when fever free may help to rule out autoimmune diseases or malignancy. Persistent inflammation needs to be further evaluated, and this may include endoscopy for inflammatory bowel disease, imaging to rule out vasculitis or masses/malignancies, or a bone scan to look for osteomyelitis. Generally, however, children with recurrent fevers are healthy between these episodes, are growing and developing normally, and have a normal laboratory examination. In these cases, observation is recommended until fevers resolve. If they do not resolve over time, or if symptoms more classically associated with an autoinflammatory disorder appear, genetic testing can be pursued. Because autoinflammatory disorders typically take a long time to cause tissue damage, such as amyloidosis, it is general appropriate to watch and wait to see if the fevers resolve, as long as the patient is generally doing well between episodes.

Autoinflammatory Disorder Overview

Autoinflammatory disorders display stereotypical features that occur during the episodes. These symptoms will occur with each episode. These are varied, and some patients will not present will all of the symptoms of a specific autoinflammatory disorder. Furthermore, young children may present only with fever and it may take some time for other symptoms to occur. Some common symptoms associated with autoinflammatory disorders include the following:

1. Characteristic rash (ie, livedo, erysipelas, granulomas, pustulosis)
2. Serositis (ie, abdominal pain, pericarditis, pleuritis)
3. Arthritis (can be episodic or persistent)
4. Mouth sores/aphthosis
5. Laboratory evidence of inflammation

There are several ways to classify autoinflammatory disorders. They can be organized according to symptoms, although there is considerable overlap of symptoms between these disorders, or by pathophysiology. In this review, we highlight the clinical features of autoinflammatory disorders based on predominant symptoms.

GENETIC DISORDERS WITH PROMINENT ARTHRITIS

Although many of the autoinflammatory disorders have joint symptoms, several present with prominent arthritis.

Familial Mediterranean Fever

Familial Mediterranean fever (FMF) is the most common autoinflammatory syndrome, and is an autosomal recessive disorder due to mutations in the *MEFV* gene that encodes the protein pyrin.[1,2] FMF is characterized by short episodes of fever (ie, 1–3 days), serositis/peritonitis, erysipelas-like rash, and arthritis, although fever can be the only symptom early in life.[3,4] The arthritis is typically monoarticular and predominantly neutrophilic.[5] FMF is treated with daily colchicine, leading to symptomatic relief in 95% of patients with nearly 75% achieving near complete remission, significantly reducing the risk of amyloidosis.[6–11] Amyloidosis prevalence varies considerably among patients, due to ethnicity or more importantly the type of mutation.[7,12] Recently, interleukin (IL)-1 antagonists have been used successfully in patients unresponsive to colchicine.[13–17]

To date, more than 200 variants in the *MEFV* gene have been reported; however, 4 mutations (M680I, M694V, M694I, and V726A) account for most disease-associated alleles in various FMF populations.[18] Pyrin regulates inflammation via interaction with the inflammasome (see later in this article), and thus patients with pyrin mutations exhibit increased processing and secretion of IL-1β and IL-18.[15]

Blau Syndrome

Blau syndrome is an autosomal dominantly inherited disease originally described in 11 family members exhibiting granulomatous inflammation in the skin, joints, and uveal tract.[19–21] Blau syndrome is closely related to sarcoidosis and should be considered in patients with early-onset sarcoidosis, although NOD2 mutations are not found in sarcoidosis, and pulmonary involvement in Blau is unusual. Joint involvement includes boggy synovitis and tenosynovitis, cystic swelling of large joints, campylodactyly, and interphalangeal contractures.[21,22] Skin involvement is described as erythematous maculopapular, lichenoid papules, and biopsy shows noncaseating granulomas.[19,20,23] Less frequent involvement includes granulomatous liver disease, cranial neuropathies, large vessel vasculitis, and interstitial lung disease.[21,23,24]

Gain-of-function mutations in *NOD2/CARD15* cause Blau syndrome and result in spontaneous activation of the NOD2 protein, activation of NF-κB, and production of proinflammatory cytokines.[25] Laboratory studies in Blau syndrome are typically normal, although elevated inflammatory markers (ie, ESR), elevated angiotensin-converting enzyme levels can be seen, and hypergammaglobulinemia can occur.[20,22] Corticosteroids have been used to treat patients with Blau syndrome, although limited reports have shown effectiveness of the tumor necrosis factor (TNF)-α blockers infliximab and etanercept, and IL-1 receptor antagonist (anakinra).[26–30] Ironically, loss-of-function mutations in NOD2 result in Crohn disease, another granulomatous disorder.[31–34] Mutations in NOD2 that cause Crohn disease result in decrease responsiveness to bacterial peptides and decreased NF-κB activation, although how this results in granulomatous disease is not well understood.

Pyogenic Arthritis, Pyoderma Gangrenosum, and Acne

Pyogenic arthritis, pyoderma gangrenosum, and acne (PAPA) syndrome is a rare autosomal dominant disorder presenting in early childhood with recurrent, sterile, monoarticular erosive arthritis.[35–37] By puberty, cystic acne occurs together with ulcerative skin lesions similar to pyoderma gangrenosum. Treatment with intra-articular or systemic steroids have shown benefit in resolving arthritis. Treatment with IL-1 receptor antagonist (anakinra) or TNF-α inhibitors (infliximab and etanercept) has been beneficial.[38–41]

Mutations in *PSTPIP1* were shown to cause PAPA. PSTPIP1 interacts with pyrin, and PSTPIP1 mutations in PAPA cause a gain-of-function effect by increasing the strength of this interaction, resulting in IL-1β activation.[42,43]

GENETIC DISORDERS WITH PROMINENT RASH

Although rash is common in autoinflammatory syndromes, the following present with prominent cutaneous inflammation that if recognized can lead to rapid diagnosis.

Cryopyrin-Associated Periodic Syndrome

Cryopyrin-associated periodic syndrome (CAPS) consists of 3 related disorders due to mutations in *NLRP3/CIAS1*: neonatal-onset multisystem inflammatory disorder (NOMID), Muckle-Wells syndrome (MWS), and familial cold autoinflammatory syndrome (FCAS).[44–46] FCAS is the mildest form of this disorder that only occurs after generalized cold exposure, whereas patients with MWS and NOMID display daily symptoms. The rash is often mistaken for urticaria due to its evanescent nature, but it lacks angioedema, signs of mast cell proliferation or degranulation, and is characterized by neutrophil infiltrates.[20,47,48] Unlike cold urticaria, localized cold challenge (ie, ice cube test) will not precipitate an attack in FCAS, because full-body cold exposure is necessary. NOMID is the most severe variant of CAPS, with patients exhibiting rash at or shortly after birth, aseptic meningitis, cerebral atrophy, uveitis, and hearing loss and mental retardation.[49–51] The chronic arthropathy in NOMID is severe and deforming due to recurrent bouts of inflammation leading to epiphyseal and patellar overgrowth. Approximately 20% of patients with NOMID die before adulthood. MWS presents similar to NOMID but with less severe features. Unlike NOMID and MWS, FCAS does not typically exhibit chronic meningitis and sensorineural hearing loss, arthropathy, or amyloidosis. Laboratory evaluation of MWS and NOMID demonstrate persistent leukocytosis, neutrophilia, anemia, thrombocytosis, and elevated ESR and CRP levels.[46,49,51] Similar abnormalities are seen in patients with FCAS during an attack.

FCAS, NOMID, and MWS are caused by autosomal dominantly inherited mutations in the *CIAS1/NLRP3* gene that encodes for the cryopyrin protein. A lack of a family history is not unusual, because de novo mutations occur, particularly in the most severe cases, and somatic mutations also can occur.[51,52] Mutations in *NLRP3* that cause CAPS occur in an autoinhibitory domain of the cryopyrin protein, leading to spontaneous inflammasome assembly, activation of caspase-1, and cleavage of pro–IL-1β to biologically active IL-1β.

A variety of immunosuppressive treatments have been used in CAPS, including corticosteroids and colchicine, but IL-1 inhibitors are now the treatment of choice.[53] Anakinra (ie, recombinant IL-1 receptor antagonist), rilonacept (ie, IL-1 Trap), and canakinumab (IL-1β monoclonal antibody) have been shown to lead to rapid and sustained improvements in inflammatory markers and symptoms.[54–56] IL-1 inhibitors have been shown to improve long-term morbidity, such as hearing loss, joint deformity, and amyloidosis.[57,58] Patients with FCAS are encouraged to avoid cold exposure.

Deficiency of Interleukin-1 Receptor Antagonist

Because IL-1 receptor antagonist (anakinra) is the effective treatment of several autoinflammatory disorders, it was not surprising that patients with deficiency of

IL-1 receptor antagonist (ie, DIRA) developed an autoinflammatory disorder. DIRA is an autosomal recessive disorder presenting with symptoms shortly after birth with erythroderma, pustular rash, osteopenia with lytic bone lesions, and systemic inflammation.[59,60] Respiratory distress, aphthous ulcers, hepatomegaly, and failure to thrive also occurred, and laboratory abnormalities include elevated ESR and CRP, leukocytosis, anemia, and thrombocytosis. Numerous anti-inflammatory medications have been tried in patients with DIRA with limited efficacy. Corticosteroid showed some benefit, but did not prevent the complications of the disease, and 3 of the original 10 infants died despite treatment.[59] Anakinra treatment results in a rapid and sustained response, with correction of laboratory abnormalities, resolution of rash, and healing of bone lesions.[59,60] IL-1RA binds the IL-1 receptor and competes for binding with IL-1 preventing receptor activation. Monocytes from patients with DIRA stimulated with IL-1β exhibited elevated production of inflammatory cytokines caused by the lack of inhibition of IL-1 receptor antagonist.[59,60]

Guadalupe-Type Fever Syndrome

A group of patients from Guadalupe exhibited symptoms similar to FCAS with fever, rash, arthralgias, and myalgias after generalized cold exposure but without a genetic mutation in CIAS1/NLRP3. Using a candidate gene approach, mutations in the NLRP12 gene were discovered.[61,62] Headache, abdominal pain, lymphadenopathy, and aphthous ulcers also can been seen, whereas sensorineural hearing loss and other central nervous system (CNS) manifestations occurred variably. Laboratory studies reflect an acute phase response with elevated ESR and CRP during the attacks that normalized between attacks. Limiting cold exposure appears effective to prevent attacks, and low-dose steroids, antihistamines, or nonsteroidal anti-inflammatory drugs (NSAIDs) were reported to be somewhat effective. Anakinra was effective in 1 patient, although the response waned over time.[63]

Deficiency of Interleukin-36 Receptor Antagonist

A syndrome of generalized pustular psoriasis was described in 19 individuals from 9 Tunisian families inherited in an autosomal recessive manner due to mutations in the IL-36 receptor antagonist.[64,65] The age of onset varied greatly, but all individuals exhibited episodes characterized by fevers and erythematous skin eruption with pustules. A variety of other symptoms were described, including geographic tongue, nail dystrophy, arthritis, and cholangitis. Episodes were triggered by viral or bacterial infections, menstruation, and pregnancy. White blood cell count, ESR, and CRP are elevated during the attacks. Most patients with this disorder were treated with Acitretin, an oral retinoid, which was beneficial; withdrawal of the medication was associated with recurrence of symptoms. Some patients were also treated with oral and topical steroids, cyclosporine, methotrexate, and TNF antagonists with variable results. IL-36 receptor antagonist is evolutionarily similar to IL-1 receptor antagonist, and the skin manifestations of either disease can appear similar. However, IL-36 receptor antagonist deficiency has no bone or CNS involvement.

Chronic Atypical Neutrophilic Dermatosis with Lipodystrophy and Elevated Temperature

Chronic atypical neutrophilic dermatosis with lipodystrophy and elevated temperature (CANDLE) is an autosomal recessive disease resulting from mutations in the proteasome subunit beta type-8 (PSMB8).[66–69] Patients exhibit early onset of recurrent fevers, purpuric skin plaques with dermal neutrophilic infiltrates, periorbital edema, hepatomegaly, lymphadenopathy, anemia, elevation in acute phase reactants, failure to thrive, and increased level of interferon (IFN)-γ–induced protein (IP-10). Conjunctivitis, myositis, aseptic meningitis, interstitial lung disease, Coombs-positive hemolytic anemia, and hypothyroidism can be seen.[53] PSMB8 is a proteasome subunit involved in protein degradation, and failure to degrade proteins leads to cellular stress, apoptosis, and activation of IFN signaling pathways.[69] Multiple treatment modalities have been attempted, including NSAIDs, colchicine, dapsone, cyclosporine, glucocorticoids, methotrexate, infliximab, etanercept, and anakinra, all of which have minimal success.[53] IL-6 blocking agents normalize inflammatory markers and anemia, but the lipodystrophy appears resistant to therapy.[69] Recent therapeutic developments of specific Janus kinase (JAK) inhibitors (tofacitinib, ruxolitinib, and baricitinib) offer promise in the treatment of this disease and others associated with dysregulated interferon responses (ie, interferonopathies). JAKs are protein tyrosine kinases involved in signaling of many immune cytokines, and JAK1 and JAK2 are important in IFN signaling.

Stimulator of Interferon Genes–Associated Vasculopathy with Onset in Infancy

Patients with stimulator of IFN genes (STING)-associated vasculopathy with onset in infancy (SAVI) present early in life with systemic inflammation, interstitial lung disease, and violaceous scaly skin lesions.[69,70] These lesions worsen over time, can become necrotic, and are caused by leukocytoclastic vasculitis and microthrombotic angiopathy.[70] Affected patients showed that SAVI occurs secondary to a de novo gain-of-function mutation in the *TMEM173* gene that encodes for STING. STING mediates the production of IFN-β, which then signals through the JAK/STAT pathway resulting in production of IFN-responsive genes.[70] Treatment of SAVI is limited, but the development of JAK inhibitors has shown some promise in blocking the transcription of IFN-β and the activation of IFN-response genes.

DISORDERS WITH PROMINENT FEVERS

Fevers can occur in all autoinflammatory syndromes, but the following disorders present with prominent fevers.

Tumor Necrosis Factor Receptor–Associated Periodic Syndrome

Mutations in the extracellular domain of the TNF receptor 1 (TNFR1) results in an autosomal dominant autoinflammatory disease.[71] Patients with TNF receptor–associated periodic syndrome (TRAPS) present with recurrent and often prolonged fevers, abdominal pain, arthralgias, migratory rash with underlying myalgias, and conjunctivitis.[72,73] Febrile flares are generally unprovoked, although stress, exercise, trauma, and hormonal changes are reported triggers.[18] Increased serum levels of CRP, ESR, serum amyloid-A (SAA), and complement often with leukocytosis and thrombocytosis are evident during attacks, and may be detected between attacks.[74] Chronic elevation in SAA can result in systemic amyloidosis and life-threatening organ damage.[75] Sustained SAA above 10 mg/L is associated with the development of amyloidosis.[73,76]

For infrequent attacks, short courses of prednisone at the time of a flare may be effective.[73] For more severe disease, etanercept reduces symptoms of inflammation in a dose-dependent manner, but failure of sustained efficacy and lack of normalization of acute phase reactants has been reported.[77] Infliximab, however, may cause a paradoxic inflammatory response.[78] Beneficial effects of anakinra and the anti–IL-6 receptor antibody tocilizumab have been demonstrated.[79–82]

Mutations that cause TRAPS are primarily located in exons 2 to 4 that encode the first or second cysteine-rich extracellular domains (CRD1 and CRD2). The mutations at cysteine residues are generally associated with a more severe phenotype and a higher incidence of amyloidosis.[73] Initial studies suggested the inflammation associated with TRAPS was due to reduced shedding of the mutant TNFR1, resulting in increased TNF signaling[71] and, understandably, amelioration of disease in a number of cases was provided by anti–TNF-α (etanercept) therapy.[73] Patients with TRAPS may exhibit low serum levels of soluble TNFR1 levels; however, not all patients with TRAPS have low serum TNFR1 levels, and TNF-α inhibition is not completely effective.[83,84] More recent evidence indicates a defect in receptor trafficking and intracellular accumulation of mutant TNF receptors causing increased responsiveness to triggers of innate immunity and the production of proinflammatory cytokines.[85] Although most TRAPS-associated mutations demonstrate full penetrance, 2 variants, P46L and R92Q, have a relatively high allele frequency in the general population (1%–10%). The phenotype of patients with these variants is quite variable and the clinical relevance of these 2 variants is still unclear.[86]

Hyperimmunoglobulin D and Periodic Fever Syndrome

Loss of functions mutations in the gene encoding mevalonate kinase (MVK), an enzyme involved in the biosynthesis of cholesterol and isoprenoids, causes hyperimmunoglobulin D and periodic fever syndrome (HIDS).[87,88] HIDS presents at an early age with recurrent fever, lymphadenopathy, abdominal pain, diarrhea, vomiting, arthralgia or arthritis, a painful macular rash, aphthous ulcers, and splenomegaly.[89] Elevated serum immunoglobulin (Ig)D levels were noted giving the syndrome its name, although a significant percentage of affected individuals exhibit normal IgD levels.[89] Defective MVK enzyme activity results in elevated levels of mevalonic acid in the urine.[87,88] Patients with HIDS have low but detectable mevalonate kinase enzyme activity, whereas patients with mevalonic aciduria, an inborn error of metabolism also due to MVK mutations, have nondetectable enzyme activity and severe symptomatology, including psychomotor retardation, facial dysmorphia, and failure to thrive.[74] Immunizations, infection, trauma, and surgery are noted precipitants of an attack, possibly because MVK loses enzymatic activity at elevated temperature.[90] High-dose corticosteroids started at the beginning of an attack may decrease the severity and duration of symptoms, although reports also have shown beneficial effects with TNF-α and IL-1β inhibitors.[89,91–93] Ex vivo studies indicate a central role of IL-1β in the pathogenesis of disease, although how defects in cholesterol synthesis results in enhanced IL-1β levels is unknown.[94] In addition, simvastatin can be affective in patients with HIDS, and treatment with these agents reduced IL-1 production in vitro.[94,95]

Majeed Syndrome (Chronic Recurrent Multifocal Osteomyelitis, Congenital Dyserythropoietic Anemia, and Dermatosis)

Chronic recurrent multifocal osteomyelitis (CRMO), or sterile osteitis, occurs sporadically or in association with certain autoimmune conditions. CRMO also occurs in an autosomal recessive autoinflammatory disorder named Majeed syndrome.[96] The clinical features of Majeed syndrome consist of early-onset CRMO, fever, lytic/sclerotic bone lesions, dyserythropoietic anemia, and neutrophilic dermatosis.[97,98] Majeed syndrome is caused by recessively inherited mutations in the LPIN2 gene.[99] Corticosteroids and NSAIDs have historically been used with variable results, but a recent report demonstrates effectiveness of IL-1 inhibitors.[100,101]

Deficiency of Adenosine Deaminase 2

Patients with deficiency of adenosine deaminase 2 (DADA2) typically present in childhood with fevers, vasculitis, and CNS stroke.[102] A prominent livedolike rash occurs, with biopsies showing neutrophils, macrophages, and vasculitis in medium-sized vessels. A separate series showed that childhood onset or familial polyarteritis nodosa was caused by mutations in ADA2.[103] Patients with ADA2 deficiency typically exhibit elevated acute phase reactants, neutropenia and lymphopenia, and hypogammaglobulinemia.[102] ADA2 deaminates adenosine and is related to ADA1, a known cause of severe combined immunodeficiency. Patients with DADA2 demonstrate reduced ADA2 activity in the plasma, cell lysates, and macrophage supernatants. ADA2 deficiency compromises endothelial structural integrity while driving monocyte differentiation toward an inflammatory phenotype.[102]

Numerous immunosuppressants have been tried in patients with DADA2, including glucocorticoids and cyclophosphamide. Cytokine inhibitors against TNF-α and IL-1β have been used as well. Macrophages and monocytes are the main sources of ADA2, making stem cell transplantation a possible treatment.[102] One patient successfully underwent a bone marrow transplant for presumed Diamond-Blackfan anemia but was retrospectively diagnosed with ADA2 deficiency.[104]

SUMMARY

Autoinflammatory disorders are rare, typically present in childhood, and exhibit characteristic clinical features. The initial workup of patients with recurrent inflammation should focus on ruling out malignancy, autoimmunity, and immune deficiencies. If this workup is negative and the subject is doing well clinically, observation is warranted. If these symptoms do not resolve, or if symptoms characteristic of autoinflammatory disorders occur, genetic testing should be done. Detection of a genetic defect causing an autoinflammatory disorder can be helpful in guiding specific therapy (**Table 1**).

Table 1		
Mechanisms of disease in autoinflammatory syndromes		
Mechanism/Pathway	**Syndrome**	**Treatment**
IL-1	FMF	Colchicine/IL-1 inhibitors
	CAPS	
	PAPA	
	DIRA	
	NLRP12	
	MVK	
TNF-mediated	TRAPS	TNF-α inhibitors
Interferon-mediated	CANDLE	JAK inhibitors
	SAVI	
Unknown	DADA2 (CECR1)	TNF-α, IL-1 inhibitors

Abbreviations: CANDLE, chronic atypical neutrophilic dermatosis with lipodystrophy and elevated temperature; CAPS, cryopyrin-associated periodic syndrome; DADA2, deficiency of adenosine deaminase 2; DIRA, deficiency of IL-1 receptor antagonist; FMF, familial Mediterranean fever; IL, interleukin; JAK, Janus kinase; MVK, mevalonate kinase; PAPA, pyogenic arthritis, pyoderma gangrenosum, and acne; SAVI, stimulator of interferon genes–associated vasculopathy with onset in infancy; TNF, tumor necrosis factor; TRAPS, TNF receptor–associated periodic syndrome.

REFERENCES

1. Ancient missense mutations in a new member of the roret gene family are likely to cause familial Mediterranean fever. The International FMF Consortium. Cell 1997;90(4):797–807.
2. French FMF Consortium. A candidate gene for familial Mediterranean fever. Nat Genet 1997;17(1):25–31.
3. Brik R, Shinawi M, Kasinetz L, et al. The musculoskeletal manifestations of familial Mediterranean fever in children genetically diagnosed with the disease. Arthritis Rheum 2001;44(6):1416–9.
4. Sohar E, Gafni J, Pras M, et al. Familial Mediterranean fever. A survey of 470 cases and review of the literature. Am J Med 1967;43(2):227–53.
5. Ince E, Cakar N, Tekin M, et al. Arthritis in children with familial Mediterranean fever. Rheumatol Int 2002;21(6):213–7.
6. Ozkaya N, Yalcinkaya F. Colchicine treatment in children with familial Mediterranean fever. Clin Rheumatol 2003;22(4–5):314–7.
7. Ozturk MA, Kanbay M, Kasapoglu B, et al. Therapeutic approach to familial Mediterranean fever: a review update. Clin Exp Rheumatol 2011;29(4 Suppl 67): S77–86.
8. Duzova A, Bakkaloglu A, Besbas N, et al. Role of a-SAA in monitoring subclinical inflammation and in colchicine dosage in familial Mediterranean fever. Clin Exp Rheumatol 2003;21(4):509–14.
9. Majeed HA, Carroll JE, Khuffash FA, et al. Long-term colchicine prophylaxis in children with familial Mediterranean fever (recurrent hereditary polyserositis). J Pediatr 1990;116(6):997–9.
10. Livneh A, Zemer D, Langevitz P, et al. Colchicine treatment of aa amyloidosis of familial Mediterranean fever. An analysis of factors affecting outcome. Arthritis Rheum 1994;37(12):1804–11.
11. Lehman TJ, Peters RS, Hanson V, et al. Long-term colchicine therapy of familial Mediterranean fever. J Pediatr 1978;93(5):876–8.
12. Federici S, Calcagno G, Finetti M, et al. Clinical impact of mefv mutations in children with periodic fever in a prevalent Western European Caucasian population. Ann Rheum Dis 2012;71(12):1961–5.
13. Ozen S, Bilginer Y, Aktay Ayaz N, et al. Anti-interleukin 1 treatment for patients with familial Mediterranean fever resistant to colchicine. J Rheumatol 2011; 38(3):516–8.
14. Meinzer U, Quartier P, Alexandra JF, et al. Interleukin-1 targeting drugs in familial Mediterranean fever: a case series and a review of the literature. Semin Arthritis Rheum 2011;41(2):265–71.
15. Chae JJ, Wood G, Masters SL, et al. The b30.2 domain of pyrin, the familial Mediterranean fever protein, interacts directly with caspase-1 to modulate IL-1beta production. Proc Natl Acad Sci U S A 2006;103(26):9982–7.
16. Belkhir R, Moulonguet-Doleris L, Hachulla E, et al. Treatment of familial Mediterranean fever with anakinra. Ann Intern Med 2007;146(11):825–6.
17. Calligaris L, Marchetti F, Tommasini A, et al. The efficacy of anakinra in an adolescent with colchicine-resistant familial Mediterranean fever. Eur J Pediatr 2008;167(6):695–6.
18. Aksentijevich I, Kastner DL. Genetics of monogenic autoinflammatory diseases: past successes, future challenges. Nat Rev Rheumatol 2011;7(8):469–78.
19. Blau EB. Familial granulomatous arthritis, iritis, and rash. J Pediatr 1985;107(5): 689–93.

20. Pastores GM, Michels VV, Stickler GB, et al. Autosomal dominant granulomatous arthritis, uveitis, skin rash, and synovial cysts. J Pediatr 1990;117(3):403–8.
21. Jabs DA, Houk JL, Bias WB, et al. Familial granulomatous synovitis, uveitis, and cranial neuropathies. Am J Med 1985;78(5):801–4.
22. Raphael SA, Blau EB, Zhang WH, et al. Analysis of a large kindred with Blau syndrome for HLA, autoimmunity, and sarcoidosis. Am J Dis Child 1993; 147(8):842–8.
23. Okafuji I, Nishikomori R, Kanazawa N, et al. Role of the nod2 genotype in the clinical phenotype of Blau syndrome and early-onset sarcoidosis. Arthritis Rheum 2009;60(1):242–50.
24. Saini SK, Rose CD. Liver involvement in familial granulomatous arthritis (Blau syndrome). J Rheumatol 1996;23(2):396–9.
25. Kanazawa N, Okafuji I, Kambe N, et al. Early-onset sarcoidosis and card 15 mutations with constitutive nuclear factor-kappab activation: common genetic etiology with Blau syndrome. Blood 2005;105(3):1195–7.
26. Punzi L, Furlan A, Podswiadek M, et al. Clinical and genetic aspects of Blau syndrome: a 25-year follow-up of one family and a literature review. Autoimmun Rev 2009;8(3):228–32.
27. Milman N, Andersen CB, Hansen A, et al. Favourable effect of TNF-alpha inhibitor (infliximab) on Blau syndrome in monozygotic twins with a de novo card15 mutation. APMIS 2006;114(12):912–9.
28. Arostegui JI, Arnal C, Merino R, et al. Nod2 gene-associated pediatric granulomatous arthritis: clinical diversity, novel and recurrent mutations, and evidence of clinical improvement with interleukin-1 blockade in a Spanish cohort. Arthritis Rheum 2007;56(11):3805–13.
29. Martin TM, Zhang Z, Kurz P, et al. The nod2 defect in Blau syndrome does not result in excess interleukin-1 activity. Arthritis Rheum 2009;60(2):611–8.
30. Yasui K, Yashiro M, Tsuge M, et al. Thalidomide dramatically improves the symptoms of early-onset sarcoidosis/Blau syndrome: its possible action and mechanism. Arthritis Rheum 2010;62(1):250–7.
31. Ogura Y, Bonen DK, Inohara N, et al. A frameshift mutation in nod2 associated with susceptibility to Crohn's disease. Nature 2001;411(6837):603–6.
32. Hugot JP, Chamaillard M, Zouali H, et al. Association of nod2 leucine-rich repeat variants with susceptibility to Crohn's disease. Nature 2001;411(6837):599–603.
33. Chamaillard M, Philpott D, Girardin SE, et al. Gene-environment interaction modulated by allelic heterogeneity in inflammatory diseases. Proc Natl Acad Sci U S A 2003;100(6):3455–60.
34. Kobayashi KS, Chamaillard M, Ogura Y, et al. Nod2-dependent regulation of innate and adaptive immunity in the intestinal tract. Science 2005;307(5710): 731–4.
35. Lindor NM, Arsenault TM, Solomon H, et al. A new autosomal dominant disorder of pyogenic sterile arthritis, pyoderma gangrenosum, and acne: PAPA syndrome. Mayo Clin Proc 1997;72(7):611–5.
36. Wise CA, Bennett LB, Pascual V, et al. Localization of a gene for familial recurrent arthritis. Arthritis Rheum 2000;43(9):2041–5.
37. Demidowich AP, Freeman AF, Kuhns DB, et al. Genotype, phenotype, and clinical course in five patients with pyogenic arthritis, pyoderma gangrenosum, and acne (PAPA) syndrome. Arthritis Rheum 2012;64(6):2022–7.
38. Dierselhuis MP, Frenkel J, Wulffraat NM, et al. Anakinra for flares of pyogenic arthritis in PAPA syndrome. Rheumatology (Oxford) 2005;44(3):406–8.

39. Brenner M, Ruzicka T, Plewig G, et al. Targeted treatment of pyoderma gangrenosum in PAPA (pyogenic arthritis, pyoderma gangrenosum and acne) syndrome with the recombinant human interleukin-1 receptor antagonist anakinra. Br J Dermatol 2009;161(5):1199–201.
40. Tofteland ND, Shaver TS. Clinical efficacy of etanercept for treatment of PAPA syndrome. J Clin Rheumatol 2010;16(5):244–5.
41. Stichweh DS, Punaro M, Pascual V. Dramatic improvement of pyoderma gangrenosum with infliximab in a patient with PAPA syndrome. Pediatr Dermatol 2005;22(3):262–5.
42. Shoham NG, Centola M, Mansfield E, et al. Pyrin binds the pstpip1/cd2bp1 protein, defining familial Mediterranean fever and PAPA syndrome as disorders in the same pathway. Proc Natl Acad Sci U S A 2003;100(23):13501–6.
43. Fernandes-Alnemri T, Yu JW, Datta P, et al. Aim2 activates the inflammasome and cell death in response to cytoplasmic DNA. Nature 2009;458(7237):509–13.
44. Dode C, Le Du N, Cuisset L, et al. New mutations of cias1 that are responsible for Muckle-Wells syndrome and familial cold urticaria: a novel mutation underlies both syndromes. Am J Hum Genet 2002;70(6):1498–506.
45. Hoffman HM, Mueller JL, Broide DH, et al. Mutation of a new gene encoding a putative pyrin-like protein causes familial cold autoinflammatory syndrome and Muckle-Wells syndrome. Nat Genet 2001;29(3):301–5.
46. Arostegui JI, Aldea A, Modesto C, et al. Clinical and genetic heterogeneity among Spanish patients with recurrent autoinflammatory syndromes associated with the cias1/pypaf1/nalp3 gene. Arthritis Rheum 2004;50(12):4045–50.
47. Wanderer AA, Hoffman HM. The spectrum of acquired and familial cold-induced urticaria/urticaria-like syndromes. Immunol Allergy Clin North Am 2004;24(2):259–86, vii.
48. Kolivras A, Theunis A, Ferster A, et al. Cryopyrin-associated periodic syndrome: an autoinflammatory disease manifested as neutrophilic urticarial dermatosis with additional perieccrine involvement. J Cutan Pathol 2011;38(2):202–8.
49. Prieur AM, Griscelli C. Arthropathy with rash, chronic meningitis, eye lesions, and mental retardation. J Pediatr 1981;99(1):79–83.
50. Feldmann J, Prieur AM, Quartier P, et al. Chronic infantile neurological cutaneous and articular syndrome is caused by mutations in cias1, a gene highly expressed in polymorphonuclear cells and chondrocytes. Am J Hum Genet 2002;71(1):198–203.
51. Aksentijevich I, Nowak M, Mallah M, et al. De novo cias1 mutations, cytokine activation, and evidence for genetic heterogeneity in patients with neonatal-onset multisystem inflammatory disease (NOMID): a new member of the expanding family of pyrin-associated autoinflammatory diseases. Arthritis Rheum 2002;46(12):3340–8.
52. Tanaka N, Izawa K, Saito MK, et al. High incidence of nlrp3 somatic mosaicism in patients with chronic infantile neurologic, cutaneous, articular syndrome: results of an international multicenter collaborative study. Arthritis Rheum 2011;63(11):3625–32.
53. Torrelo A, Patel S, Colmenero I, et al. Chronic atypical neutrophilic dermatosis with lipodystrophy and elevated temperature (CANDLE) syndrome. J Am Acad Dermatol 2010;62(3):489–95.
54. Hoffman HM, Rosengren S, Boyle DL, et al. Prevention of cold-associated acute inflammation in familial cold autoinflammatory syndrome by interleukin-1 receptor antagonist. Lancet 2004;364(9447):1779–85.

55. Hawkins PN, Lachmann HJ, McDermott MF. Interleukin-1-receptor antagonist in the Muckle-Wells syndrome. N Engl J Med 2003;348(25):2583–4.

56. Lovell DJ, Bowyer SL, Solinger AM. Interleukin-1 blockade by anakinra improves clinical symptoms in patients with neonatal-onset multisystem inflammatory disease. Arthritis Rheum 2005;52(4):1283–6.

57. Neven B, Marvillet I, Terrada C, et al. Long-term efficacy of the interleukin-1 receptor antagonist anakinra in ten patients with neonatal-onset multisystem inflammatory disease/chronic infantile neurologic, cutaneous, articular syndrome. Arthritis Rheum 2010;62(1):258–67.

58. Sibley CH, Plass N, Snow J, et al. Sustained response and prevention of damage progression in patients with neonatal-onset multisystem inflammatory disease treated with anakinra: a cohort study to determine three- and five-year outcomes. Arthritis Rheum 2012;64(7):2375–86.

59. Aksentijevich I, Masters SL, Ferguson PJ, et al. An autoinflammatory disease with deficiency of the interleukin-1-receptor antagonist. N Engl J Med 2009; 360(23):2426–37.

60. Reddy S, Jia S, Geoffrey R, et al. An autoinflammatory disease due to homozygous deletion of the IL1rn locus. N Engl J Med 2009;360(23):2438–44.

61. Jeru I, Duquesnoy P, Fernandes-Alnemri T, et al. Mutations in nalp12 cause hereditary periodic fever syndromes. Proc Natl Acad Sci U S A 2008;105(5):1614–9.

62. Borghini S, Tassi S, Chiesa S, et al. Clinical presentation and pathogenesis of cold-induced autoinflammatory disease in a family with recurrence of an nlrp12 mutation. Arthritis Rheum 2011;63(3):830–9.

63. Jeru I, Hentgen V, Normand S, et al. Role of interleukin-1beta in nlrp12-associated autoinflammatory disorders and resistance to anti-interleukin-1 therapy. Arthritis Rheum 2011;63(7):2142–8.

64. Marrakchi S, Guigue P, Renshaw BR, et al. Interleukin-36-receptor antagonist deficiency and generalized pustular psoriasis. N Engl J Med 2011;365(7):620–8.

65. Onoufriadis A, Simpson MA, Pink AE, et al. Mutations in IL36RN/IL1F5 are associated with the severe episodic inflammatory skin disease known as generalized pustular psoriasis. Am J Hum Genet 2011;89(3):432–7.

66. Agarwal AK, Xing C, DeMartino GN, et al. Psmb8 encoding the beta5i proteasome subunit is mutated in joint contractures, muscle atrophy, microcytic anemia, and panniculitis-induced lipodystrophy syndrome. Am J Hum Genet 2010;87(6):866–72.

67. Arima K, Kinoshita A, Mishima H, et al. Proteasome assembly defect due to a proteasome subunit beta type 8 (psmb8) mutation causes the autoinflammatory disorder, Nakajo-Nishimura syndrome. Proc Natl Acad Sci U S A 2011;108(36): 14914–9.

68. Kitamura A, Maekawa Y, Uehara H, et al. A mutation in the immunoproteasome subunit psmb8 causes autoinflammation and lipodystrophy in humans. J Clin Invest 2011;121(10):4150–60.

69. Liu Y, Ramot Y, Torrelo A, et al. Mutations in proteasome subunit beta type 8 cause chronic atypical neutrophilic dermatosis with lipodystrophy and elevated temperature with evidence of genetic and phenotypic heterogeneity. Arthritis Rheum 2012;64(3):895–907.

70. Liu Y, Jesus AA, Marrero B, et al. Activated sting in a vascular and pulmonary syndrome. N Engl J Med 2014;371(6):507–18.

71. McDermott MF, Aksentijevich I, Galon J, et al. Germline mutations in the extracellular domains of the 55 kda TNF receptor, TNFR1, define a family of dominantly inherited autoinflammatory syndromes. Cell 1999;97(1):133–44.

72. Toro JR, Aksentijevich I, Hull K, et al. Tumor necrosis factor receptor-associated periodic syndrome: a novel syndrome with cutaneous manifestations. Arch Dermatol 2000;136(12):1487–94.

73. Hull KM, Drewe E, Aksentijevich I, et al. The TNF receptor-associated periodic syndrome (TRAPS): emerging concepts of an autoinflammatory disorder. Medicine (Baltimore) 2002;81(5):349–68.

74. Stoffels M, Simon A. Hyper-IGd syndrome or mevalonate kinase deficiency. Curr Opin Rheumatol 2011;23(5):419–23.

75. Dode C, Hazenberg BP, Pecheux C, et al. Mutational spectrum in the mefv and tnfrsf1a genes in patients suffering from AA amyloidosis and recurrent inflammatory attacks. Nephrol Dial Transplant 2002;17(7):1212–7.

76. Gillmore JD, Lovat LB, Persey MR, et al. Amyloid load and clinical outcome in AA amyloidosis in relation to circulating concentration of serum amyloid a protein. Lancet 2001;358(9275):24–9.

77. Bulua AC, Mogul DB, Aksentijevich I, et al. Efficacy of etanercept in the tumor necrosis factor receptor-associated periodic syndrome: a prospective, open-label, dose-escalation study. Arthritis Rheum 2012;64(3):908–13.

78. Nedjai B, Quillinan N, Coughlan RJ, et al. Lessons from anti-TNF biologics: infliximab failure in a traps family with the t50m mutation in tnfrsf1a. Adv Exp Med Biol 2011;691:409–19.

79. Gattorno M, Pelagatti MA, Meini A, et al. Persistent efficacy of anakinra in patients with tumor necrosis factor receptor-associated periodic syndrome. Arthritis Rheum 2008;58(5):1516–20.

80. Simon A, Bodar EJ, van der Hilst JC, et al. Beneficial response to interleukin 1 receptor antagonist in traps. Am J Med 2004;117(3):208–10.

81. Sacre K, Brihaye B, Lidove O, et al. Dramatic improvement following interleukin 1beta blockade in tumor necrosis factor receptor-1-associated syndrome (TRAPS) resistant to anti-TNF-alpha therapy. J Rheumatol 2008;35(2):357–8.

82. Vaitla PM, Radford PM, Tighe PJ, et al. Role of interleukin-6 in a patient with tumor necrosis factor receptor-associated periodic syndrome: assessment of outcomes following treatment with the anti-interleukin-6 receptor monoclonal antibody tocilizumab. Arthritis Rheum 2011;63(4):1151–5.

83. Aganna E, Hammond L, Hawkins PN, et al. Heterogeneity among patients with tumor necrosis factor receptor-associated periodic syndrome phenotypes. Arthritis Rheum 2003;48(9):2632–44.

84. Drewe E, McDermott EM, Powell PT, et al. Prospective study of anti-tumour necrosis factor receptor superfamily 1b fusion protein, and case study of anti-tumour necrosis factor receptor superfamily 1a fusion protein, in tumour necrosis factor receptor associated periodic syndrome (TRAPS): clinical and laboratory findings in a series of seven patients. Rheumatology (Oxford) 2003;42(2):235–9.

85. Lobito AA, Kimberley FC, Muppidi JR, et al. Abnormal disulfide-linked oligomerization results in ER retention and altered signaling by TNFR1 mutants in TNFR1-associated periodic fever syndrome (TRAPS). Blood 2006;108(4):1320–7.

86. Ravet N, Rouaghe S, Dode C, et al. Clinical significance of p46l and r92q substitutions in the tumour necrosis factor superfamily 1a gene. Ann Rheum Dis 2006;65(9):1158–62.

87. Drenth JP, Cuisset L, Grateau G, et al. Mutations in the gene encoding mevalonate kinase cause hyper-IGD and periodic fever syndrome. International hyper-IGD study group. Nat Genet 1999;22(2):178–81.

88. Houten SM, Kuis W, Duran M, et al. Mutations in mvk, encoding mevalonate kinase, cause hyperimmunoglobulinaemia d and periodic fever syndrome. Nat Genet 1999;22(2):175–7.
89. van der Hilst JC, Bodar EJ, Barron KS, et al. Long-term follow-up, clinical features, and quality of life in a series of 103 patients with hyperimmunoglobulinemia D syndrome. Medicine 2008;87(6):301–10.
90. Houten SM, Frenkel J, Rijkers GT, et al. Temperature dependence of mutant mevalonate kinase activity as a pathogenic factor in hyper-IGD and periodic fever syndrome. Hum Mol Genet 2002;11(25):3115–24.
91. Bodar EJ, Kuijk LM, Drenth JP, et al. On-demand anakinra treatment is effective in mevalonate kinase deficiency. Ann Rheum Dis 2011;70(12):2155–8.
92. Takada K, Aksentijevich I, Mahadevan V, et al. Favorable preliminary experience with etanercept in two patients with the hyperimmunoglobulinemia D and periodic fever syndrome. Arthritis Rheum 2003;48(9):2645–51.
93. Cailliez M, Garaix F, Rousset-Rouviere C, et al. Anakinra is safe and effective in controlling hyperimmunoglobulinaemia D syndrome-associated febrile crisis. J Inherit Metab Dis 2006;29(6):763.
94. Frenkel J, Rijkers GT, Mandey SH, et al. Lack of isoprenoid products raises ex vivo interleukin-1beta secretion in hyperimmunoglobulinemia D and periodic fever syndrome. Arthritis Rheum 2002;46(10):2794–803.
95. Simon A, Drewe E, van der Meer JW, et al. Simvastatin treatment for inflammatory attacks of the hyperimmunoglobulinemia D and periodic fever syndrome. Clin Pharmacol Ther 2004;75(5):476–83.
96. Majeed HA, Kalaawi M, Mohanty D, et al. Congenital dyserythropoietic anemia and chronic recurrent multifocal osteomyelitis in three related children and the association with sweet syndrome in two siblings. J Pediatr 1989;115(5 Pt 1): 730–4.
97. Ferguson PJ, Sandu M. Current understanding of the pathogenesis and management of chronic recurrent multifocal osteomyelitis. Curr Rheumatol Rep 2012;14(2):130–41.
98. Majeed HA, El-Shanti H, Al-Rimawi H, et al. On mice and men: an autosomal recessive syndrome of chronic recurrent multifocal osteomyelitis and congenital dyserythropoietic anemia. J Pediatr 2000;137(3):441–2.
99. Ferguson PJ, Chen S, Tayeh MK, et al. Homozygous mutations in lpin2 are responsible for the syndrome of chronic recurrent multifocal osteomyelitis and congenital dyserythropoietic anaemia (Majeed syndrome). J Med Genet 2005; 42(7):551–7.
100. Herlin T, Fiirgaard B, Bjerre M, et al. Efficacy of anti-IL-1 treatment in Majeed syndrome. Ann Rheum Dis 2013;72(3):410–3.
101. Herlin T, Bjerre M, Firrgaard B, et al. Novel mutation of the lpin2 gene in Turkish brothers with Majeed syndrome. Response to IL-1 inhibition. Pediatr Rheumatol 2011;9(Suppl 1):300.
102. Zhou Q, Yang D, Ombrello AK, et al. Early-onset stroke and vasculopathy associated with mutations in ada2. N Engl J Med 2014;370(10):911–20.
103. Navon Elkan P, Pierce SB, Segel R, et al. Mutant adenosine deaminase 2 in a polyarteritis nodosa vasculopathy. N Engl J Med 2014;370(10):921–31.
104. Van Montfrans JM, Hartman EA, Braun KP, et al. Phenotypic variability in patients with ada2 deficiency due to identical homozygous r169q mutations. Rheumatology (Oxford) 2016;55(5):902–10.

When Autistic Behavior Suggests a Disease Other than Classic Autism

Mark D. Simms, MD, MPH[a,b,*]

KEYWORDS

- Autism spectrum disorder • Specific language impairment
- Social (pragmatic) communication disorder • Anxiety disorder • Selective mutism

KEY POINTS

- Most neurodevelopmental disorders are defined by their clinical symptoms and many disorders share common features.
- In recent years, there has been an increase in the number of children diagnosed with autism spectrum disorder, although concerns have been raised about the accuracy of the reported prevalence rates.
- This article reviews the essential features of autism spectrum disorder and describes other conditions that may include similar symptoms that may be misdiagnosed as autism spectrum disorder (primary communication disorders, anxiety disorders, attachment disorders, intellectual disability, vision and hearing impairment, and normal variations).
- An approach to differential diagnosis is discussed with particular attention to evaluation of young children.

There has been a significant increase during the past decade in the number of children diagnosed with autism spectrum disorders (ASD). A disorder once thought to be exceedingly rare is now estimated to affect 1 in 45 (2.2%) US children. Public awareness campaigns by advocacy groups, testimonials by celebrities with affected children, and increased funding for treatment programs and research have also contributed to parents' and professionals' better recognition of children with this condition. However, concerns have been raised about the accuracy of the prevalence figures and the dramatic increase in autism diagnoses over time.[1–4]

Most neurodevelopmental and behavior disorders are defined by their clinical symptoms and many disorders share common features. The key to accurate

[a] Section of Developmental Pediatrics, Department of Pediatrics, Medical College of Wisconsin, 8701 Watertown Plank Road, Milwaukee, WI 53226, USA; [b] Child Development Center, Children's Hospital of Wisconsin, PO Box 1997, Mail Station 744, Milwaukee, WI 53226, USA
* Child Development Center, Children's Hospital of Wisconsin, PO Box 1997, Mail Station 744, Milwaukee, WI 53226.
E-mail address: msimms@mcw.edu

Pediatr Clin N Am 64 (2017) 127–138
http://dx.doi.org/10.1016/j.pcl.2016.08.009
0031-3955/17/© 2016 Elsevier Inc. All rights reserved.

pediatric.theclinics.com

differential diagnosis is identifying the core, or essential, symptoms that help distinguish one condition from others that have overlapping symptom manifestations.[5] No single behavior or category of behavior is characteristic (pathognomonic) of ASD. To the contrary, there is evidence that some of the central features of ASD are fractionable (ie, they occur individually at fairly high frequency in the normal population even to the extent seen in individuals with ASD).[6] A further complication arises with the use of the term "spectrum." The American Psychiatric Association Diagnostic and Statistical Manual of Mental Disorders-5 (DSM-5) clearly intended use of this term as a way to account for differences in symptom severity between individuals, and changing manifestations related to developmental level and chronologic age. Thus, it is often the unique clustering of symptoms that defines a specific disorder.

This article provides information about ASD and other disorders that share common symptoms that should be considered as part of the differential diagnosis of a child with a developmental disorder (**Box 1**). It is not sufficient when screening children with early signs of ASD to simply rule in or rule out an ASD diagnosis. The screening must encompass consideration of which diagnoses could best account for the child's symptoms and what interventions or treatments will be most effective.

AUTISM SPECTRUM DISORDER

The most recent revision of the DSM-5 identifies two core domain deficits in ASD. The first involves a persistent impairment in social communication and social interaction across multiple contexts. Individuals with ASD have significant difficulty in three areas of social functioning: (1) social-emotional reciprocity; (2) using nonverbal communicative behaviors for social interaction; and (3) developing, maintaining, and understanding relationships. DSM-5 specifies that deficits must be present in all three areas. The second domain involves restricted, repetitive patterns of behavior, interests, or activities (RRBIs) manifesting in at least two of the following categories of behavior: stereotyped or repetitive motor movements, use of objects, or speech; insistence on sameness, inflexible adherence to routines, or ritualized patterns of verbal or nonverbal behavior; highly restricted, fixated interest that are abnormal in intensity or focus; and hyperactivity or hyporeactivity to sensory input or unusual interest in sensory aspects of the environment. RRBIs must be present in the early

---

Box 1
Conditions commonly misdiagnosed as autism spectrum disorder

Primary communication disorder
- Specific language impairment
- Social (pragmatic) communication disorder

Anxiety disorder
- Selective mutism

Reactive attachment disorder
- Postinstitutional autistic syndrome

Cognitive impairment

Visual impairment

Hearing impairment

Normal behavioral variations

developmental period, but may not become fully manifest until social demands exceed a child's capacity for interaction.

One of the earliest signs of the social deficit characteristic of ASD is impairment in joint attention behaviors that typically appear by 8 to 9 months of age. Joint attention involves sharing experiences, emotions, and intentions with another person through the use of gaze, gestures, and vocalizations. DSM-5 includes this under "deficits in nonverbal communicative behaviors used for social interactions." Other striking characteristics of children with ASD include deficits in imitation and pretend play that are out of proportion to the child's nonverbal cognitive ability.[7,8] Like joint attention, imitation and pretend play are linked to the concept of "theory of mind," which is the capacity to understand what another person is thinking and feeling, and to react and adapt to that person's needs and desires.[9]

Approximately one-third of children diagnosed with ASD have a history of developmental regression occurring between 15 and 30 months of age. The change may be abrupt or slow and insidious, occurring over the course of days or weeks. Loss of previously acquired language skills is accompanied by regression in social skills and the appearance of behaviors that are associated with ASD: decreased eye contact; loss of social smile and interest in others; and the onset of hyperactive, perseverative, and stereotypic behaviors. In some children, slow and incomplete recovery may follow, but long-term outcome is generally poor. No specific cause or explanation for this phenomenon has been identified.[10]

The cause of ASD is multifactorial. Most evidence suggests that it is a structural and functional brain disorder with a strong genetic basis.[11] Nonetheless, proximal causes may include premature birth, known genetic and metabolic disorders (**Box 2**), and as yet unspecified environmental influences on gene expression. A world survey of ASD identified a strong (81%) male predominance.[12]

Several prospective longitudinal studies have documented the persistence of symptoms of ASD over childhood, particularly in the domain of social communication and social interaction.[13,14] In some instances, symptoms of RRBIs may diminish with

---

Box 2
Some genetic and metabolic conditions associated with autism spectrum disorder

Bardet-Biedl syndrome

Congenital rubella

Cornelia de Lange syndrome

Fragile X syndrome

Hypomelanosis of Ito

Möbius syndrome

Neurofibromatosis

Phenylketonuria

Rett syndrome

Smith-Lemli-Opitz syndrome

Smith Magenis syndrome

Trisomy 21 syndrome

Tuberous sclerosis complex

increasing age. Clinical improvement is often associated with increased communication ability. There are also well-documented reports of children who have recovered from ASD.[15,16]

PRIMARY COMMUNICATION DISORDERS

Two types of primary communication disorders are confused with ASD and should be considered in a differential diagnosis: specific language impairment (SLI) and social (pragmatic) communication disorder (SPCD).

SLI often presents as delayed onset of expressive and receptive language abilities. Nonverbal cognitive abilities, social interactions, and play patterns are normal, and delayed verbal development is not caused by oral-motor or speech sound production deficits.[17] Children with SLI are about 2 years delayed in onset of language development but then follow a similar rate of development as their typically developing peers, although they do not seem to catch up over time. Deficits in specific aspects of grammar, semantics, and conversational skills are characteristic of SLI and persist through adulthood. These lingering deficits often lead to academic, social, and adjustment disorders as children progress through school.

SPCD is a form of communication disorder that affects how language is used for social exchanges. This condition was first described in the 1980s as a higher-level language disorder affecting how words and gestures are used to mediate social interactions.[18] Affected individuals have intact structural language abilities but struggle with practical and appropriate aspects of social communication.[19] As described in DSM-5, individuals with SPCD may not know how to initiate conversations or may fail to follow rules of turn taking. They may not adapt their language to match the context or needs of their partner. For example, they may provide too little or too much background information. Additionally, they frequently have difficulty interpreting nonliteral or ambiguous language, such as idioms, humor, metaphors, sarcasm, irony, and so forth.

Communication ability appears as a fractionable component function in several neurodevelopmental disabilities. Thus, children diagnosed with ASD may have normal structural language abilities or present with a profile of deficits that is indistinguishable from SLI.[20] Similarly, pragmatic deficits are seen in children without other features of ASD, and in individuals with attention-deficit/hyperactivity disorder, structural brain anomalies (hydrocephalus), and genetic disorders (Williams syndrome).[21–24]

Distinguishing Specific Language Impairment and Social (Pragmatic) Communication Disorder from Autism Spectrum Disorders

Before development of functional expressive and receptive language skills (<4 years old), children with SLI may resemble those with ASD. For example, they may fail to engage with strangers and demonstrate poor eye contact, rely strongly on structured routines (RRBIs), and manifest sensory difficulties in response to change and new environments. As language abilities improve, most of these symptoms improve, although peer interactions may continue be affected by persisting communication deficits.[25]

Differential diagnosis depends on identifying a broader profile of functioning. In contrast to individuals with ASD, those with SLI and SPCD demonstrate a typical social drive to communicate and interact with others but lack the necessary skill set to be successful.[26] In addition, there is a lifetime absence of RRBIs in individuals who have SPCD.

ANXIETY DISORDERS

Anxiety disorders are common in typically developing children and those with ASD. These disorders are characterized by persistent symptoms that are excessive or out-of-proportion to the situation. Several types of disorders are recognized including generalized anxiety disorder, social anxiety disorder, and panic disorder, and a variety of specific phobias. Lifetime prevalence of any type of anxiety disorder in children or adolescents is estimated to be 15% to 20%.[27] Symptoms may be present early in life and manifest as disturbances of sensory regulation (excessive irritability, colic or feeding difficulty, overstimulation), or behavioral withdrawal. Behavioral inhibition (the tendency to exhibit quiet withdrawal in response to novel stimuli or strangers) is a temperamental trait seen in toddlers and is often predictive of social anxiety during adolescence.[28–30] Inhibited children may avoid eye contact with others, display social avoidance with peers, and prefer to play alone.

Selective mutism is a unique and uncommon (prevalence 0.18%–1.9%) form of anxiety. Children affected avoid speaking with individuals outside of their immediate family circle.[31] Symptoms appear between 2 and 4 years of age, and selective mutism is more common in boys. Many children are not identified until they enter school for the first time. Two-thirds of children with selective mutism have other symptoms of anxiety, and a strong history of "shyness" and anxiety is usually present in immediate and extended family members. Follow-up studies suggest that the mean duration of symptoms is about 8 years. Selective mutism may dissipate completely, but the persistence of communication problems is associated with elevated rates of school and psychiatric disorders even into adult years.[32]

Anxiety disorders are also a common feature in children with ASD; the prevalence is approximately 42%.[33] Communication difficulties and discomfort in social situations may lead to anxiety, because a child with ASD may be unable to express emotions or negotiate social interactions well. For example, children with ASD are often fearful of intense and unwanted stimulation from medical or dental visits. The sensory stimulation of sound and touch during these visits is most upsetting. Similarly, crowds or unfamiliar settings may trigger extreme reactions in this group of children.[34] Increased stereotyped language (rumination) and stereotyped behaviors (RBBIs) often appear in response to anxiety and may have a soothing and stress relieving effect.

Differential Diagnosis of Anxiety Disorders and Autism Spectrum Disorders

Distinguishing children with anxiety disorders from those in whom anxiety is a facet of ASD can be difficult. A study of children with anxiety and mood disorders who were carefully screened to exclude those with a diagnosis or history of ASD found 62% met ASD symptom cutoff criteria on one of three rating scales (the Social Communication Questionnaire, the Children's Communication Checklist, and the Social Reciprocity Scale). However, only 8% screened positive on all three instruments.[35]

Individuals with ASD have difficulty interpreting verbal (emotional) and nonverbal (facial expression) cues; as a result, they experience generalized discomfort in many social situations. They also have difficulty learning new social skills and developing more functional social behaviors, compared with those who have anxiety disorders.[36] In contrast, individuals with social anxiety are generally accurate in interpretations of verbal and nonverbal cues and can develop age-appropriate friendships. However, they tend to have a strong negative bias and are hypervigilant and engage in active avoidance behaviors when they perceive a situation to be threatening.

REACTIVE ATTACHMENT DISORDER AND POSTINSTITUTIONAL AUTISTIC SYNDROME

Reactive attachment disorder (RAD) in infants and young children results from serious environmental and social neglect in which there has been an inconsistent or emotionally unavailable primary attachment figure. Children with RAD consistently withdraw from adult caregivers and fail to seek or respond to comfort. In addition, they appear unhappy and emotionally fragile, and they derive little pleasure from contact with others. Although some of these behaviors are present in children diagnosed with ASD, those with RAD respond positively when they receive appropriate care.[37]

In the early 1990s, many children who had been living in deplorable orphanage settings in Romania were adopted by European and North American families following the fall of the Ceausescu regime. A quasi-autism syndrome was described in a small proportion of children adopted before the age of 2 years into English homes.[38] When evaluated at age 4, approximately 6% were thought to be autistic because of difficulties in social relationships and in communication skills. Their scores on the Autism Diagnostic Interview-Revised were in a range comparable with nonadopted children diagnosed with ASD. These children had limited social awareness of others, lacked social reciprocity, and showed limited empathy toward others. Similar to nonadopted children with ASD, they showed preoccupations with sensations (particularly touch or smell) and intensely circumscribed interests (eg, fascination with watches, intense interest in £10 notes). At the time of adoption, this group had more significant cognitive delays than the other adopted children. Similar findings were noted in Romanian children adopted by Dutch families, where the phenomenon was referred to as postinstitutional autistic syndrome (PIAS).[39] Unlike nonadopted children diagnosed with ASD, the symptoms of autism declined steadily in many Romanian adoptees with PIAS following adoption. Despite these improvements, abnormal attachment behaviors and problems with peer relationships persisted in most children.[40]

Differential Diagnosis of Reactive Attachment Disorder, Postinstitutional Autistic Syndrome, and Autism Spectrum Disorders

RAD, PIAS, and ASD are characterized by significant impairments in social interest and interaction, and cognitive and language delays. Stereotypic behaviors, such as rocking or flapping, may also be present in all three conditions.[41] Fixated interests and unusual sensory reactions are not seen in children with RAD, but are part of PIAS and ASD. RAD and PIAS are always associated with a history of severe emotional neglect or institutionalization, whereas ASD is not caused by inappropriate nurturing. Following adoption, children with PIAS often have a steady decline in symptoms associated with autism and increase in overall cognitive abilities.

INTELLECTUAL DISABILITY

Intellectual disability (ID) affects cognitive and adaptive functioning. Using scores derived from standardized tests, intellectual ability is categorized as mild, moderate, severe, and profound degrees of impairment. Adaptive functioning is reflected in conceptual (academic), social (relationship), and practical (personal) domains. Because there are discrepancies between intellectual and adaptive functioning, IQ measures alone are insufficient to diagnose ID. The overall population prevalence of ID is approximately 1%, of which approximately 85% have a mild disability. Etiologies are heterogeneous and ID is often associated with other disabilities, including ASD. A firm diagnosis of ID may be difficult to establish in preschool children, who may improve intellectual and adaptive functioning as a result of early intervention programs. It is generally accepted that intellectual abilities become stable once children enter primary school (6 years and older). However, intellectual functioning may deteriorate at any age in the presence of acquired diseases (trauma, infection, exposure to toxins), or progressive neurologic or metabolic disorders.

Distinguishing Autism Spectrum Disorders in Children with Intellectual Disability

Children with mild and moderate degrees of ID often have generalized delays in overall development of language, behavior, and social skills that are often consistent with their cognitive level. Among individuals with severe and profound ID (IQ <50), many never develop expressive language abilities.[42] Social impairment and self-absorbed behaviors are chronic problems in people with severe ID whether or not they also have ASD.[43,44] In one population study, nearly half of children less than 15 years of age with severe ID demonstrated social interactions that were appropriate for their mental level. Among the group with poor social skills, those with ASD were distinguished by the presence of elaborate repetitive routines, the use of idiosyncratic language and pronoun reversals, and the absence of symbolic play despite having a mental age of greater than 20 months.[45]

VISUAL AND HEARING IMPAIRMENT

Childhood blindness is one of the least prevalent developmental disabilities (0.13%) among US children.[46] Prevalence of ASD in blind/severely visually impaired children is estimated to be about 50%, and is higher (65%–70%) in children who are congenitally blind.[47] The symptoms of blindness and visual impairment are variable and derive from several disparate causes (congenital and acquired). A key feature in the association between blindness and ASD is the total lack of light perception, not the cause of the blindness.

Blind children typically have motor and social delays caused by social isolation, and blindness is associated with several autistic symptoms, especially in young children. These symptoms, referred to as "blindisms," include eye pressing (more common in severe ocular visual loss, especially retinal disorders), light gazing (more common in cortical visual impairment), flicking fingers in front of lights (noted to be common in children with congenital rubella), and motor stereotypies (eg, rocking, spinning, tapping, and twirling).[48,49] Other behaviors often associated with autism include exploration through touch and smell, and pronoun reversal.[50] In addition, visually impaired children, as a group, develop imaginative play at a later stage than sighted children.

Although diagnoses of ASD have been strongly associated with blindness, there are several reports of blind and visually impaired children with well-documented ASD who improved to the point of no longer meeting diagnostic criteria.[47,51–53] ASD has also been associated with delayed visual maturation, a less severe form of visual impairment. In the report by Hobson and Lee,[53] the greatest improvements were in measures of "bizarre relating to others," appropriate use of language, developmentally appropriate imaginative activity including play, and decrease in RRBIs. However, despite no longer meeting diagnostic criteria for ASD, the blind children continued to have difficulties making peer friendships, initiating and sustaining conversations, engaging in imaginative play, and continued to demonstrate postural oddities or motor stereotypes. A variable pattern of autistic withdrawal, in some cases reversible, was noted in a series of young children with severe visual impairment in the United Kingdom.[54] Approximately one-third of these children showed a "setback" in "social accessibility and behavior" between 16 and 27 months of age; almost all had minimal or no light perception from birth. Partial recovery occurred in some of these children, apparently in association with additional developmental support at home or in a school setting.

No diagnostic scales for ASD have been standardized with respect to severely visually impaired children. Most clinicians rely on untested modifications and adaptations of existing scales to diagnose ASD in this population. However, a recent study found that certain behaviors on the Autism Diagnostic Observation Schedule were helpful in discriminating visually impaired children with ASD from those without ASD, particularly after the age of 4 to 5 years.[49] They found that as blind children without ASD matured, they were able to demonstrate social engagement and social communication behaviors on the Autism Diagnostic Observation Schedule that distinguished them from children with ASD. They also noted that self-stimulatory and repetitive behaviors that were common in younger blind children also decreased. The authors cautioned that it is difficult to make a diagnosis of ASD in young severely visually impaired children.

Congenital hearing loss has a prevalence of 0.001% to 0.003% in newborns, but occurs at a rate much higher than expected in children with ASD (0.1%–0.2%).[55] However, the severity of autism does not correlate with the severity of hearing loss,[56] and cochlear implants in young children with ASD do not improve their oral communication and language ability.[57] Delayed language acquisition and comprehension, and deficits in social knowledge and theory of mind competence are common in deaf children with and without ASD. Because there are no instruments suitable for the assessment of ASD in hearing-impaired children, differential diagnosis depends on clinical judgment from experts familiar with the developmental profiles of deaf children.

NORMAL BEHAVIORAL VARIATIONS

Behaviors found in otherwise typically developing children that are not associated with any impairment in functioning are considered normal behavioral variations. For example, repetitive behaviors (RRBIs), a need to follow daily routines, intense interests, and toe-walking are common in typically developing infants and preschool age children.[58–64] Similar behaviors also occur in children with autism, ID, and severe deprivation.[41,65,66] In typically developing children, motor stereotypies often begin before age 3 years, are more common in boys, and may persist into adulthood. Symptoms range from simple to complex motor patterns and are associated with periods of excitement, stress, fatigue, or boredom.[67] These behaviors can sometimes be suppressed and they are absent during sleep. Although often associated with other comorbid conditions (tics/Tourette syndrome, attention-deficit/hyperactivity disorder, obsessive-compulsive disorder), the stereotypic movements do not cause the child to be distressed and do not interfere with the child's daily activities.[68–70]

Differentiating Normal Behavioral Variants from Autism Spectrum Disorders

The presence of RRBIs constitutes the second major criteria for ASD in DSM-5. Because these behaviors are nonspecific and common in typically developing children, it may be difficult to know when they indicate ASD, especially during infancy and preschool years. Although no specific behaviors are unique to ASD, RBBIs occur more often and at a greater level of intensity in children with ASD and ID when compared with typically developing children.[71,72] This distinction is reflected in the number of qualifiers stated in DSM-5 (eg, "*inflexible* adherence to routines," "*extreme* distress at small changes," "*highly* restricted, *fixated* interests that are *abnormal* in intensity or focus" [emphasis added]). In addition, such behaviors in typically developing children seem appropriate in context. More importantly, children without ASD demonstrate appropriate social communication and social interaction skills despite the presence of restricted and RRBIs.

SUMMARY

ASD is a behavioral and dimensional syndrome defined by a combination of symptoms, many of which overlap with other behaviorally defined conditions including normal behavioral variants. Preschool children present unique challenges because their symptoms must be interpreted in light of their chronologic age, their cognitive and communication abilities, and the context in which the behaviors occur. All of these factors may change significantly as children mature.

DSM-5 provides a clear definition of ASD. If an individual does not meet the necessary criteria, another explanation should be sought. The gold standard of developmental diagnosis is evaluation by a multidisciplinary team of professionals who can observe a child in a variety of circumstances and develop a profile of strengths and deficits. Recent evidence, however, suggests that many children receive single discipline evaluations, even at academic centers.[73] When there is any doubt, the careful clinician may choose to refrain from making a definitive diagnosis until the child has had the benefit of appropriate developmental and educational interventions.

Children with RAD, PIAS, and blindness may meet the full diagnostic criteria for ASD at some point in their development, but they can change in response to altered experiences and maturity. This may also occur in some children with ASD who do not have an obvious cause. Those who remain ASD presumably lack the potential to respond to intervention. It seems that, under certain circumstances, there may be different paths in and out of the ASD.

For clinicians, distinguishing among similar disorders is a central part of clinical practice. Use of the term "autistic-like" is imprecise and should be avoided when possible. The desire to identify and treat children with autism early should be balanced by concern to avoid misdiagnosing what could be a benign transitory problem, a normal developmental variation, or a different condition altogether.

REFERENCES

1. Baxter AJ, Brugha TS, Erskine HE, et al. The epidemiology and global burden of autism spectrum disorders. Psychol Med 2015;45:601–13.
2. Charman T, Pickles A, Chandler S, et al. Commentary: effects of diagnostic thresholds and research vs service and administrative diagnosis on autism prevalence. Int J Epidemiol 2009;38:1234–8.
3. Matson JL, Kozlowski AM. The increasing prevalence of autism spectrum disorders. Res Autism Spectr Disord 2011;5:418–25.
4. Laidler JR. US Department of Education data on "autism" are not reliable for tracking autism prevalence. Pediatrics 2005;116:e120–4.
5. Carrington SJ, Kent RG, Maljaars J, et al. DSM-5 autism spectrum disorder: in search of essential behaviours for diagnosis. Res Autism Spectr Disord 2014;8: 701–15.
6. Happé F, Ronald A, Plomin R. Time to give up on a single explanation for autism. Nat Neurosci 2006;9:1218–20.
7. Rogers S, Stackhouse T, Hepburn S, et al. Imitation performance in toddlers with autism and those with other developmental disorders. J Child Psychol Psychiatry 2003;44:763–81.
8. Rutherford MD, Young GS, Hepburn S, et al. A longitudinal study of pretend play in autism. J Autism Dev Disord 2007;37:1024–39.
9. Baron-Cohen S, Leslie AM, Frith U. Does the autistic child have a 'theory of mind'? Cognition 1985;21:37–46.
10. Stefanatos GA. Regression in autistic spectrum disorders. Neuropsychol Rev 2008;18:305–19.
11. Holmboe K, Rijsdijk FV, Hallett V, et al. Strong genetic influences on the stability of autistic traits in childhood. J Am Acad Child Adolesc Psychiatry 2014;53:221–30.

12. Frombonne E. Epidemiology of pervasive developmental disorders. Pediatr Res 2009;65:591–8.
13. Gotham K, Pickles A, Lord C. Trajectories of autism severity in children using standardized ADOS scores. Pediatrics 2012;130:e1278–84.
14. Fountain C, Winter AS, Bearman PS. Six developmental trajectories characterize children with autism. Pediatrics 2012;129:e1112–20.
15. Helt M, Kelley E, Kinsbourne M, et al. Can children with autism recover? If so, how? Neuropsychol Rev 2008;18:339–66.
16. Zappella M. Reversible autism and intellectual disability in children. Am J Med Genet C Semin Med Genet 2012;160C:111–7.
17. Simms MD. Language disorders in children: classification and clinical syndromes. Pediatr Clin North Am 2007;54:437–67.
18. Rapin I, Allen D. Developmental language disorders: nosologic considerations. In: Kirk U, editor. Neuropsychology of language, reading, and spelling. New York: Academic Press; 1983. p. 155–84.
19. Russell RL. Social communication impairments: pragmatics. Pediatr Clin North Am 2007;54:483–506.
20. Tager-Flusberg H, Joseph RM. Identifying neurocognitive phenotypes in autism. Philos Trans R Soc Lond B Biol Sci 2003;358:303–14.
21. Bishop DVM, Norbury CF. Exploring the borderlands of autistic disorder and specific language impairment: a study using standardized diagnostic instruments. J Child Psychol Psychiatry 2002;43:917–29.
22. Ketelaars MP, Cuperus J, Jansonius K, et al. Pragmatic language impairment and associated behavioural problems. Int J Lang Commun Disord 2010;45:204–14.
23. Gibson J, Adams C, Lockton E, et al. Social communication disorder outside autism? A diagnostic classification approach to delineating pragmatic language impairment, high functioning autism, and specific language impairment. J Child Psychol Psychiatry 2013;54:1186–97.
24. Staikova E, Gomes H, Tartter V, et al. Pragmatic deficits and social impairment in children with ADHD. J Child Psychol Psychiatry 2013;54:1275–83.
25. Simms MD, Jin XM. Autism, language disorder, and social (pragmatic) communication disorder: DSM-V and differential diagnoses. Pediatr Rev 2015;36:355–63.
26. Baird G, Norbury CF. Social (pragmatic) communication disorders and autism spectrum disorder. Arch Dis Child 2016;101:745–51. Available at: http://dx.doi.org/10.1136/archdischild-2014-306944. Accessed February 16, 2016.
27. Beesdo K, Knappe S, Pine DS. Anxiety and anxiety disorders in children and adolescents: developmental issues and implications for DSM-V. Psychiatr Clin North Am 2009;32:483–524.
28. Kagan J, Reznick JS, Snidman N. Biological bases of childhood shyness. Science 1988;240:167–71.
29. Hirshfeld-Becker DR, Rosenbaum JF, Biederman JF, et al. Stable behavioral inhibition and its association with anxiety disorder. J Am Acad Child Adolesc Psychiatry 1992;31:103–11.
30. Muris P, van Brackel AM, Arntz A, et al. Behavioral inhibition as a risk factor for the development of childhood anxiety disorders: a longitudinal study. J Child Fam Stud 2011;20:157–70.
31. Viana AG, Beidel DC, Rabian B. Selective mutism: a review and integration of the last 15 years. Clin Psychol Rev 2009;29:57–67.
32. Muris P, Ollendick TH. Children who are anxious in silence: a review on selective mutism, the new anxiety disorder in DSM-5. Clin Child Fam Psychol Rev 2015;18:151–69.

33. Simonoff E, Pickles A, Charman T, et al. Psychiatric disorders in children with autism spectrum disorders: prevalence, comorbidity, and associated factors in a population-derived sample. J Am Acad Child Adolesc Psychiatry 2008;47: 921–9.

34. Settipani CA, Puleo CM, Conner BT, et al. Characteristics and anxiety symptom presentation associated with autism spectrum traits in youth with anxiety disorders. J Anxiety Disord 2012;26:459–67.

35. Towbin KE, Pradella A, Gorrindo T, et al. Autism spectrum traits in children with mood and anxiety disorders. J Child Adolesc Psychopharmacol 2005;15:452–64.

36. Tyson KE, Cruess DG. Differentiating high-functioning autism and social phobia. J Autism Dev Disord 2012;42:1477–90.

37. Zeenah CH, Gleason MM. Annual research review: attachment disorder in early childhood – clinical presentation, causes, correlates, and treatment. J Child Psychol Psychiatry 2015;56:207–22.

38. Rutter M, Andersen-Wood L, Beckett C, et al. Quasi-autistic patterns following severe early global privation. J Child Psychol Psychiatry 1999;40:537–49.

39. Hoksbergen R, ter Laak J, Rijk K, et al. Post-institutional autistic syndrome in Romanian adoptees. J Autism Dev Disord 2005;35:615–23.

40. Rutter M, Kreppner J, Croft C, et al. Early adolescent outcomes of institutionally deprived and non-deprived adoptees. III. Quasi-autism. J Child Psychol Psychiatry 2007;48:1200–7.

41. Sweeney JK, Bascom BB. Motor development and self-stimulatory movement in Institutionalized Romanian children. Pediatr Phys Ther 1995;7:124–32.

42. Gould J. Language development and non-verbal skills in severely mentally retarded children: an epidemiological study. J Ment Defic Res 1976;2:129–46.

43. Beadle-Brown J, Murphy G, Wing L, et al. Changes in social impairment for people with intellectual disabilities: a follow-up of the Camberwell cohort. J Autism Dev Disord 2002;32:195–206.

44. Tonge B, Einfeld S. The trajectory of psychiatric disorders in young people with intellectual disabilities. Aust N Z J Psychiatry 2000;34:80–4.

45. Wing L, Gould J. Severe impairments of social interaction and associated abnormalities in children: epidemiology and classification. J Autism Dev Disord 1979;9: 11–29.

46. Boyle CA, Boulet S, Schieve LA, et al. Trends in the prevalence of developmental disabilities in US children, 1997-2008. Pediatrics 2011;127:1034–42.

47. Jure R, Pogonza R, Rapin I. Autism spectrum disorders (ASD) in blind children: very high prevalence, potentially better outlook. J Autism Dev Disord 2016;46: 749–59.

48. Carvill S. Sensory impairment, intellectual disability and psychiatry. J Intellect Disabil Res 2001;45:467–83.

49. Williams ME, Fink C, Zamora I, et al. Autism assessment in children with optic nerve hypoplasia and other vision impairments. Dev Med Child Neurol 2014;56: 66–72.

50. Brown R, Hobson RP, Lee A. Are there "autistic-like" features in congenitally blind children? J Child Psychol Psychiatry 1997;38:693–703.

51. Chess S. Follow-up report on autism in congenital rubella. J Autism Child Schizophr 1977;7:69–81.

52. Goodman R, Ashby L. Delayed visual maturation and autism. Dev Med Child Neurol 1990;32:814–9.

53. Hobson RP, Lee A. Reversible autism among congenitally blind children? A controlled follow-up study. J Child Psychol Psychiatry 2010;51:1235–41.

54. Cass HD, Sonksen PM, McConachie HR. Developmental setback in severe visual impairment. Arch Dis Child 1994;70:192–6.
55. Rosenhall U, Nordin V, Sandstrom M, et al. Autism and hearing loss. J Autism Dev Disord 1999;29:349–57.
56. Jure R, Rapin I, Tuchman R. Hearing impaired autistic children. Dev Med Child Neurol 1991;33:1062–72.
57. Edwards L. Children with cochlear implants and complex needs: a review of outcome research and psychological practice. J Deaf Stud Deaf Educ 2007; 12:258–68.
58. Thelen E. Rhythmical stereotypies in normal human infants. Anim Behav 1979;27: 699–715.
59. Werry JS, Carlielle J, Fitzpatrick J. Rhythmic motor activities (stereotypies) in children under five: etiology and prevalence. J Am Acad Child Psychiatry 1983;22: 329–36.
60. Evans DW, Leckman JF, Carter A, et al. Ritual, habit, and perfectionism: the prevalence and development of compulsive-like behavior in normal young children. Child Dev 1997;68:58–68.
61. DeLoache JS, Macari S, Simcock G. Planes, trains, automobiles and tea sets: extremely intense interest in very young children. Dev Psychol 2007;43:1579–86.
62. Leekam S, Tandos J, McConachie H, et al. Repetitive behaviours in typically developing 2-year-olds. J Child Psychol Psychiatry 2007;48:1131–8.
63. Arnott B, McConachie H, Meins E, et al. The frequency of restricted and repetitive behaviors in a community sample of 15-month-old infants. J Dev Behav Pediatr 2010;31:223–9.
64. Pernet J, Billiaux A, Auvin S, et al. Early onset toe-walking in toddlers: a cause for concern? J Pediatr 2010;157:496–8.
65. Bodfish JW, Symons FJ, Parker DE, et al. Varieties of repetitive behavior in autism: comparisons to mental retardation. J Autism Dev Disord 2000;30:237–43.
66. Berkson G, Tupa M, Sherman L. Early development of stereotyped and self-injurious behaviors: I. incidence. Am J Ment Retard 2001;106:539–47.
67. Singer HS. Motor stereotypies. Semin Pediatr Neurol 2009;16:77–81.
68. Harris KM, Mahone EM, Singer HS. Nonautistic motor stereotypies: clinical features and longitudinal follow-up. Pediatr Neurol 2008;38:267–72.
69. Freeman RD, Soltanifar A, Baer S. Stereotypic movement disorder: easily missed. Dev Med Child Neurol 2010;52:733–8.
70. Barry S, Baird G, Lascelles K, et al. Neurodevelopmental movement disorders-an update on childhood motor stereotypies. Dev Med Child Neurol 2011;53:979–85.
71. Goldman S, Wang C, Salgado M, et al. Motor stereotypies in children with autism and other developmental disorders. Dev Med Child Neurol 2009;51:30–8.
72. Hoch J, Spofford L, Dimian A, et al. A direct comparison of self-injurious and stereotyped motor behavior between preschool-aged children with and without developmental delays. J Pediatr Psychol 2016;41:566–72.
73. Hansen RL, Blum NJ, Graham A, et al. Diagnosis of autism spectrum disorder by developmental-behavioral pediatricians in academic centers: a DBPNet study. Pediatrics 2016;137(Suppl 2):S79–89.

Nonclassic Inflammatory Bowel Disease in Young Infants

Immune Dysregulation, Polyendocrinopathy, Enteropathy, X-Linked Syndrome, and Other Disorders

Shanmuganathan Chandrakasan, MD[a,b],
Suresh Venkateswaran, PhD[a,c], Subra Kugathasan, MD[a,d],*

KEYWORDS

- Very early onset IBD (VEO-IBD) • IPEX • IL-10 defects • Inflammasome
- Epithelial barrier defects • Neutrophil defects • T cell or B cell defects

KEY POINTS

- IBD in infant and children is rare. However, its incidence in this age group is increasing.
- Etiology of IBD in this age group is very diverse, a significant proportion of these patients have underlying primary immune defect. Many VEO-IBD have non-classical gut pathology, may not be categorized as Crohn's disease or ulcerative colitis.
- Earnest attempt need to be made to identify underlying genetic defect in a patient with VEO-IBD. Identification of genetic defects could facilitate the use of targeted therapy in this disease that could otherwise be resistant to usual first line therapy for IBD.
- In many VEO-IBD patients with underlying primary immune defect hematopoietic stem cell transplantation could result in definitive cure.

INTRODUCTION

From conception of an embryo in the womb to end of life, the human gastrointestinal (GI) tract interfaces dynamically with the microbial environment and the host immune system.[1–3] The GI system, which is the largest lymphoid and immune organ in infants

[a] Department of Pediatrics, Children's Health Care of Atlanta, Emory University School of Medicine, Atlanta, GA, USA; [b] Division of Hematology, Oncology and BMT, Emory University School of Medicine, Atlanta, GA, USA; [c] Division of Pediatric Gastroenterology, Emory University School of Medicine, Atlanta, GA, USA; [d] Division of Gastroenterology, Emory University School of Medicine, Atlanta, GA, USA
* Corresponding author. Division of Pediatric Gastroenterology, Emory Children's Center, Emory University School of Medicine, 2015 Uppergate Drive, Suite 248, Atlanta, GA 30322.
E-mail address: skugath@emory.edu

Pediatr Clin N Am 64 (2017) 139–160
http://dx.doi.org/10.1016/j.pcl.2016.08.010
0031-3955/17/© 2016 Elsevier Inc. All rights reserved.

and young children, is relatively sterile at birth and encounters a huge onslaught of antigens in the forms of diet and microbes during first few years of life. Robust GI tract barrier function, maturing immune function, and controlled immune tolerance are needed to maintain a healthy interface. This healthy GI mucosa is required to maintain a low-grade physiologic inflammation characterized by normal balance of immune cells, lymphocytes, and plasma cells.[4,5] Therefore, defects in either mucosal barrier or immune tolerance networks results in abnormal and inappropriate innate and adaptive responses, perhaps directed against intestinal microbes or diet, resulting in mucosal injury and GI inflammation.[5,6] The human GI system has limited ways to respond to insults and injury. The common form of mucosal injury is infiltration of the GI mucosa with immune cells, neutrophils, and epithelial or crypt architectural damage, which clinicians and pathologists classify under the umbrella term of inflammatory bowel disease (IBD).

The common form of IBD occurs in older children and young adults and comprises Crohn disease (CD) and ulcerative colitis, 2 distinct entities with characteristic clinical, endoscopic, and pathologic features. A subgroup of IBD occurs very early in life and is thus called very early onset IBD (VEO-IBD).[7,8] Historically, the incidence of VEO-IBD in infants and children has been very low. However, due to still not well-understood reasons, the occurrence of IBD and other autoimmune disease such as type 1 diabetes mellitus has been increasing in alarming rates over the last couple of decades.[9–11] The incidence of IBD in children younger than 5 years of age has grown by more than 50% over the last 10 years, hypothesized to be due to changing environmental or diet interaction with microbes and genes.[11,12] Though VEO-IBD contribute to a small percentage to the overall prevalence of IBD, for proper evaluation and management it is important to recognize the salient difference between VEO-IBD and IBD presenting at the older age group. Some of these cardinal features are listed in **Table 1**.[7,13–16]

Immune dysregulation, polyendocrinopathy, enteropathy, X-linked (IPEX) syndrome, a disorder of T-cell immune tolerance, a well recognized entity in this group was first reported decades ago.[17] It presents with multiple autoimmune manifestations, with VEO-IBD being among the most prominent clinical presentation, leading to significant diarrhea and failure to thrive.[18] Over the last decade, multiple other defects, most importantly interleukin (IL)-10 receptor (10R) and IL-10 defects, and other monogenetic disorders and variants in the immune pathway and intestinal barrier function have been associated with VEO-IBD.[19–23]

Early evaluation of these patients is important because identification of underlying immune defects would facilitate the use of better-targeted therapy for the specific genetic defect. Moreover, in a subset of carefully identified patients presenting with VEO-IBD, hematopoietic stem cell transplant (HSCT) could be curative.[24–26] With more than 50 monogenetic defects that can present with VEO-IBD, evaluation and management

Table 1 Cardinal clinical features of very early onset inflammatory bowel disease	
Features	References
Chronic intestinal inflammation often tend to involve colon	7,13,14
In a significant percentage of these patients, IBD is the presenting manifestation of underlying primary immune deficiency	13–15
The pathologic features might be unclassifiable, patients have IBD-like inflammation without classic CD or ulcerative colitis pathologic features	13,14
Severe course with poor response to multiple immunosuppressive medications	7

A   B

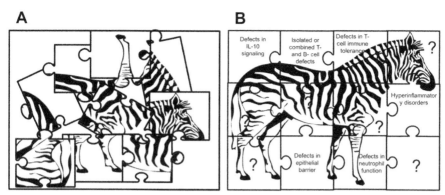

Fig. 1. The unsolved and solved jigsaw puzzle of zebra. (*A*) Jigsaw puzzle pieces represent different categories of research progress to resolve the IBD in young infants, especially in IPEX and other related disorders in the past 10 years. (*B*) Solved jigsaw Zebra represents the solved areas of IBD in young infants, IPEX, and other related disorders.

of this condition could be challenging and time-consuming. This article presents IBD in infants and very young children as an unsolved jigsaw puzzle (**Fig. 1**) and then describes at least 6 broad categories to partially resolve the puzzle, leaving some of the pieces yet to be filled with future discoveries.

CLINICAL PRESENTATION AND CASE DISCUSSION BASED ON PATHOPHYSIOLOGICAL SUBTYPES

Depending on the extent and severity of inflammation of GI tract, infants with IBD can have varied clinical manifestations. Infantile colitis can have an insidious course, with frequent small volume diarrhea with blood and mucus. Because of this insidious onset with symptoms of mild colitis, these infants invariably undergo initial evaluation for allergic colitis and infectious colitis. Many are treated with antibiotics despite negative infectious workup and undergo multiple formula changes for presumed allergic colitis. Clinical presentation of severe enterocolitis in infants is usually much more dramatic. There is usually explosive large volume watery diarrhea and many of these patients have manifestations similar to severe acute graft-versus-host disease (GVHD) of the gut.[27] This presentation is common in infants with IPEX and IPEX-like disorders. Pathologic findings show villous atrophy and apoptotic enterocolitis.[27] Overlapping presentation of large volume diarrhea with blood and mucus is also common. Transmural inflammation resulting in fistulating intestinal disease can be seen in patients with defects in IL-10 signaling,[19] X-linked inhibitor of apoptosis protein (XIAP),[28] and nicotinamide adenine dinucleotide phosphate (NADPH) oxidase leading to chronic granulomatous disease (CGD).[29] Infants with IBD can also present with other clinical manifestations of autoimmunity from broader immune dysregulation. Autoimmune endocrinopathy and autoimmune cytopenia are some of the common autoimmune manifestation seen in patients with IPEX and IPEX-like disorders presenting with VEO-IBD.

Serious and opportunistic infections can also be another associated manifestation because many monogenic primary immune deficiency disorders present with IBD.[29] Recognizing the underlying immune defect could help in identifying the cause of infantile-onset IBD (eg, a *Serratia marcescens* abscess on the scalp of an infant with IBD would lead us to the diagnosis of CGD). There are also nonimmune somatic defects in many of the disorders that present with IBD in infants. Knowing these finding could be of immense help in the diagnosis of the underlying genetic condition. For example, infants with nuclear factor-kappa B (NF-κB) essential modulator (NEMO) deficiency usually have a varying degree of ectodermal dysplasia, sparse and brittle hair, and conical teeth, along with IBD.[30]

Defects in every aspect of the immune system, such as neutrophils, T-cell and B-cell lymphocytes, and macrophages, are associated with IBD in infants. Also, nonlympho-hematopoietic defects with primary defects in enterocytes can also lead to IBD-like manifestations. Based on the pathophysiology, VEO-IBD can be categorized as

1. Defects in T-cell immune tolerance (IPEX and IPEX-like disorders)
2. Defects in IL-10 signaling
3. Hyperinflammatory disorders (defect in T-cell cytotoxicity or inflammasome)
4. Defects in neutrophil function
5. Defects in epithelial barrier function
6. Isolated or combined T-cell and B-cell defects.

DEFECTS IN T-CELL IMMUNE TOLERANCE

CLINICAL VIGNETTE

A 2-week-old breastfed infant presented with acute onset large volume watery diarrhea requiring hospitalization and intravenous fluid resuscitation. Over the next 2 weeks he became significantly malnourished and had multiple bouts of significant dehydration from large-volume diarrhea. At 1 month of age, he was also diagnosed to have type 1 diabetes mellitus. He was also noted to have eczematous dermatitis, elevated immunoglobulin (Ig)-E, and periph-eral eosinophilia. Laboratory screen for autoantibodies revealed features of autoimmune thyroiditis with high antithyroglobulin antibodies and elevation of IgG tissue transglutaminase antibodies. His duodenal biopsy showed total villous atrophy with mucosal lymphocytic and eosinophil infiltration with apoptosis of epithelial cells and significant depletion of goblet cells mimicking GVHD-like pathologic findings. Based on these findings, a diagnosis of IPEX was sus-pected. Further work-up revealed marked decrease in T-regulatory (Treg) cells and mutational analysis revealed known mutations in the FOXP3 gene. He received pulse steroids followed by sirolimus with significant improvement in watery diarrhea. He underwent a reduced-intensity HSCT from an unaffected matched sibling. He is currently doing well with resolution of GI symp-toms and no new autoimmune manifestations.

Mutations in *FOXP3* result in either absent or decreased Treg cell numbers or a qual-itative defect in Treg cells, resulting in reduced Treg cell suppressive activity (**Fig. 2**).[31] This defect results in broader immune dysregulation, resulting in multisystem autoim-munity with autoimmune endocrinopathy, autoimmune cytopenia, autoimmune hepa-titis, and severe eczema.[32] Though classic IPEX presents in infancy, depending on the residual protein function, IPEX can present with varying severity of GI involvement. The varying presentation and variable age of onset resulting in disease heterogeneity and phenotype is attributed to the location of the mutation within the FOXP3 gene.[32–34] The FOXP3 gene is located in the X chromosome, hence male infants are affected but fe-male infants with 1 copy of the gene also exhibit IPEX-like disorders albeit mild disease phenotype.[34] There are many IPEX-like disorders resulting from mutations directly affecting Treg cell development, such as mutation in CD25[35] and signal transducer and activator of transcription (STAT)-5b[36]. However, a qualitative defect in Treg cell numbers and function resulting in VEO-IBD have also been reported in other immune dysregulation disorders such as STAT-1 gain-of-function (GOF) mutation,[37] STAT-3 GOF mutation,[38,39] lipopolysaccharide responsive beige-like anchor protein (LRBA) deficiency,[40,41] and cytotoxic T-lymphocyte-associated protein (CTLA)-4 haploinsufficiency.[42,43]

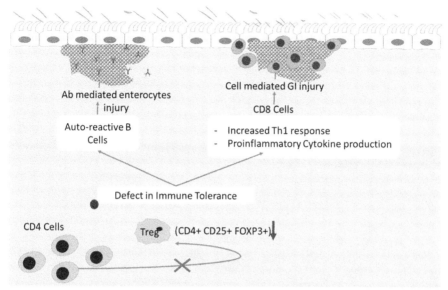

Fig. 2. Defects in T-cell immune tolerance (IPEX and IPEX-like disorders). Quantitative and qualitative defects in Treg cells lead to defective immune tolerance, leading to T-cell and B-cell immune dysregulation. This results in both antibody and cell-mediated GI injury and inflammation. Other diseases included in this group are CD25 and STAT5b defects. Additionally, varying degrees of Treg dysfunction leading to IBD can also be noted in defects such as LRBA deficiency, CTLA4-haploinsufficiency, STAT1 GOF, and STAT3 GOF.

DEFECTS IN INTERLEUKIN-10 SIGNALING

CLINICAL VIGNETTE

An 8-week-old female infant presented with the history of bloody diarrhea and failure to thrive. She had 1 hospital admission for documented bacterial sepsis. She had developed perianal enterocutaneous fistula and an abscess needing surgical drainage and antibiotics. Colonoscopy revealed severe discontinuous colitis with deep ulceration. Histology showed nonspecific acute colitis with dense neutrophilic infiltrates. The systemic examination is significant for deep oral aphthous ulcers and folliculitis. The immune evaluation showed normal T, B, and natural killer (NK) cells with normal proliferative response to mitogens. She had elevated IgA and IgG, and normal IgM, and a neutrophil oxidative burst test was normal. Based on the severe fistulating colitis, a STAT3 phosphorylation study was done that showed normal phosphorylation to IL-6 and no STAT3 phosphorylation to IL-10, suggestive of IL-10R defect. Further, genetic testing (mutation testing) confirmed the presence of the mutation in IL-10R-α. She later underwent allogeneic HSCT with complete resolution of colitis and resolution of perianal enterocutaneous fistula.

A few dozen cases are reported in the literature in IL-10 or IL-10R defects resulting in severe infantile colitis mimicking IBD (**Fig. 3**).[19,20,44] In addition to colitis and fistulating perianal disease, additional clinical manifestations include recurrent infections, folliculitis, and arthritis.[19,44] A high degree of consanguinity is reported because both copies of IL-10 and IL-10R need to be mutated for this autosomal recessive condition

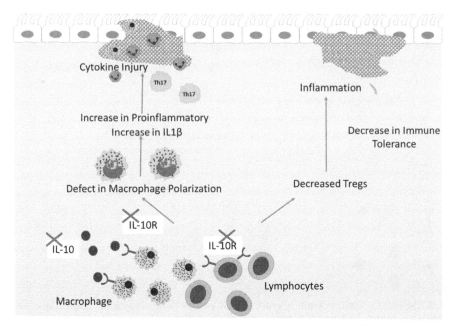

Fig. 3. Defects in IL-10 signaling. Defects in IL-10 and IL-10R lead to proinflammatory macrophage polarization and cytokine cell-mediated tissue injury. In addition, it results in decreased Treg cells, leading to defective mucosal immune tolerance.

to occur. IL-10 is an important immunomodulatory cytokine.[45] Through its effects on the innate and adaptive immune systems, it maintains mucosal immune tolerance in the GI tract. Its immune modulatory effects are, in part, mediated by promoting Treg cell function and by modulating macrophage to a more antiinflammatory phenotype.[20] Hence, deleterious mutations in IL-10 or its receptor results in the breakdown of immune tolerance and skewed proinflammatory macrophage phenotype with excess IL-1β production, leading to inflammation in GI tract. Patients with IL-10, IL-10RA, and IL-10RB have similar disease phenotype.[20] Recently, increased risk of non-Hodgkin lymphoma is also recognized in these patients.[46,47]

HYPERINFLAMMATORY DISORDERS (DEFECT IN T-CELL CYTOTOXICITY OR INFLAMMASOME)

CLINICAL VIGNETTE

A 12-month-old male infant presented with history of diarrhea, weight loss, and perianal abscess. The abscess failed to heal despite surgical drainage and several courses of antibiotics. His clinical history is also significant for several episodes of self-limiting high-grade fever, variable cytopenia, and mild-to-moderate elevation of liver enzymes. His growth was significantly stunted and he was malnourished (all growth parameters were less than third centile). Further evaluation revealed perianal fistulae with additional deep fissures. Endoscopy showed features of active colitis. Colonoscopic or histologic findings from biopsies were similar to CD pathologic findings with skip lesions, deep linear ulcerations, and chronic inflammation with crypt architectural changes but without granulomas. Despite multiple immunosuppressive and biologic medications for 6 months he had no improvement in IBD. He eventually underwent total *abdominal colectomy and end ileostomy. He had extensive immune evaluation, which showed normal neutrophil oxidative burst, lymphopenia with inverted CD4/CD8 ratio, normal percentage of naïve T cells, and decreased NK cell cytotoxicity. His ferritin was elevated at 7286 ng/mL (normal <79 ng/mL) and serum IL-18 was elevated. Flow cytometry-based XIAP protein expression was markedly decreased. Follow-up mutation testing showed he has a known mutation in baculovirus inhibitor of apoptosis repeat containing protein 4 (BIRC4) gene-encoding XIAP protein, leading to markedly decreased XIAP protein expression.*

Hyperinflammation could either result from a defect in inflammasome pathway or a defect in T-cell and NK-cell cytotoxicity (**Fig. 4**). Mutation in BIRC4 results in XIAP deficiency. It is increasingly considered as an inflammasome disorder. In the physiologic state, normal XIAP protects from toll-like receptor and tumor necrosis factor (TNF)-driven inflammasome formation and cell death. Defects in XIAP lead to exaggerated IL-1β and IL-18 secretion, and cell death.[48] A significant percentage of these patients present with recurrent fever and enteropathy, progressing to fistulating VEO-IBD.[28] Recently, GOF mutation in an important inflammasome protein NOD-Like Receptor C4 (NLRC4) is reported to be associated with neonatal-onset enterocolitis, periodic fever, and fatal or near-fatal episodes of autoinflammation.[49,50] Recurrent fever and colitis can also been seen in other autoinflammatory periodic fever syndromes, such with mevalonate kinase deficiency.[51]

Usually, defects in T-cell and NK-cell cytotoxicity lead to primary hemophagocytic lymphohistiocytosis (HLH). Primary HLH from defects in syntaxin-binding protein 2 (STXBP2) are known to present with significant colitis and diarrhea.[52] In some cases,

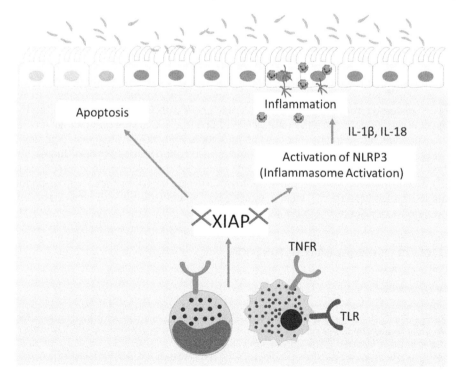

Fig. 4. Hyperinflammatory disorders (defect in T-cell cytotoxicity or inflammasome). Defects in XIAP lead to increased inflammasome activation, resulting in hyperinflammation and inflammation-driven apoptosis.

the onset of diarrhea could precede the development of HLH. In many cases, the control of hyperinflammation usually controls to diarrhea. A similar presentation can also be seen in Hermansky-Pudlak syndrome, which is an extremely rare autosomal recessive disorder resulting in oculocutaneous albinism (decreased pigmentation) and bleeding problems due to a platelet abnormality (platelet storage pool defect).[53,54]

DEFECTS IN NEUTROPHIL FUNCTION

CLINICAL VIGNETTE

An 8-month-old male infant presented with complaints of blood in stool since 1 week of age and new left inguinal lymphadenopathy for the last 2 weeks. Given his bright red blood in stool and diarrhea, he has had multiple formula changes. Diarrhea slightly improved on soy-based formula. However, he continued to have blood and mucus stools 7 times a day. Stool calprotectin was 1479 μg/gm (normal <100). Immunoglobulin profile showed elevation in IgA and IgG. The left inguinal budging was later diagnosed as cold abscess from Staphylococcus aureus. Because the abscess caused by commensal skin bacteria, along with IBD-like symptoms, CGD as a diagnosis was considered. Dihydrorhodamine (DHR) testing showed absent neutrophil oxidative burst suggestive of X-linked CGD. Genetic testing showed mutations in Cytochrome B(558) Alpha(CYBA) gene consistent with the molecular diagnosis for CGD.

CGD is a result of defective phagocytosis, specifically in the granulocytes responsible for bacterial killing and clearance (**Fig. 5**). The NADPH oxidase complex that is responsible for killing ingested bacteria through the production of respiratory burst. Mutation involving NADPH complex (CYBA, CYBB, neutrophil cytosolic factor [NCF]-1, NCF2, NCF4) present with CGD and intestinal inflammation similar to VEO-IBD can be seen up to 40%.[55,56] Recently, even missense variant in the NCF2 gene and NADPH oxidases are associated with VEO-IBD.[57–59] Patients with CGD often present during infancy with colitis, severe perianal disease, hepatosplenomegaly, abscesses, and fistulas.[56] Histology from intestinal biopsies may show well-formed granulomas but the main clue with CGD that differentiates it from CD is that in CGD the granulomas are not associated with surrounding mucosal inflammation. Early diagnosis showing absence or very low oxidative burst with DHR tests is essential because some of the established IBD therapies, such as anti-TNF, may increase the risk of serious infections in CGD. Colitis resulting from defective neutrophils is also seen in patients with glycogen storage disease type 1b,[60,61] leukocyte adhesion defect type 1,[62] and other less common defects highlighted in **Table 2**.

DEFECTS IN EPITHELIAL BARRIER FUNCTION

CLINICAL VIGNETTE

A 7-day-old male infant presented with a history of bloody diarrhea since birth. Colonoscopy revealed severe friability and mucosal exfoliative changes. Colonic biopsy showed glandular dropout, enterocyte and crypt apoptosis, and focal areas of scarring mimicking acute GVHD of the gut. He was also noted to have multiple intestinal atresias. Also, he had profound T-cell lymphopenia. Based on these findings, TTC7a defect was considered. Targeted sequencing revealed a biallelic mutation in TTC7a. He was total parenteral nutrition (TPN)-dependent and had a poor response to systemic steroids. He eventually succumbed to Klebsiella pneumonia and associated septicemia at 4 months of age.

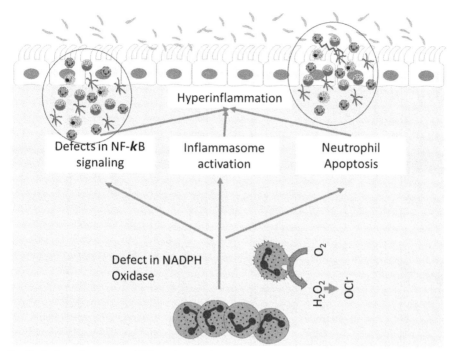

Fig. 5. Defects in neutrophil function. Defective oxidative burst in CGD results in hyperinflammation and IBD through the mechanisms shown.

Intact epithelial integrity and function are critical for barrier function and modulation, and adaptive and innate immune response to commensal bacteria. Breakdown or defective barrier function could lead to loss of intestinal immune tolerance and result in a proinflammatory intestinal milieu, resulting in IBD (**Fig. 6**). In addition to TTC7a, several other disorders affect intestinal epithelial barrier function. Deficiency in the NEMO from mutations in the Inhibitor of Kappa Light Polypeptide Gene Enhancer in B cell Kinase Gamma (*IKBKG*) gene.[63] NEMO-deficient intestinal epithelial cells lack the ability to activate NF-κB and are sensitive to proinflammatory cytokine-mediated apoptosis[63,64] and have compromised epithelial barrier thereby facilitating bacterial translocation and inflammation.[64] A disintegrin and metalloproteinase domain 17 (ADAM17) deficiency from biallelic loss of function in *ADAM17* gene can also lead to colitis and VEO-IBD–like inflammation.[65] Colitis and innate immune deficiency in infants has been increasingly recognized as a presentation of telomere biology defects, such as dyskeratosis congenita (DKC).[66,67] Defects in *DKC-1*[66] and regulator of telomere elongation helicase 1 (*RTEL1*)[67] are known to present with varying immune deficiency and enterocolitis, even before the development of apparent bone marrow failure. Other less common disorders and associated clinical manifestations are highlighted in **Table 2**.

Table 2
Known defects associated with very early onset inflammatory bowel disease and its associated extraintestinal manifestations and laboratory findings

Defects	Gene Defect	Extra Intestinal Immune, Hematologic, or Somatic Manifestations	Laboratory Findings and Functional Evaluation
IPEX and IPEX-like disorders			
IPEX	FOXP3	Autoimmune endocrinopathy, cytopenia, hepatitis and kidney disease, eczema, food allergy, eosinophilia	Decrease in Treg cells number and function Decreased Foxp3 expression
CD25 deficiency	CD25	Autoimmune endocrinopathy, cytopenia, eczema, gingivitis, alopecia universalis, bullous pemphigoid, CMV, EBV disease	Absent CD25 expression
STAT5b deficiency	STAT5B	Autoimmune endocrinopathy, eczema, short stature, interstitial pneumonitis, alopecia universalis, bullous pemphigoid, varicella and herpes zoster infections	Variable immune abnormality Normal to low T, B, and NK cells
STAT1 GOF mutation	STAT1	Mucocutaneous candidiasis, short stature, eczema, autoimmune endocrinopathy, sinopulmonary infection, hypertension, aneurysm	Most have normal Treg cell number and Foxp3 expression, abnormal STAT1 phosphorylation studies
STAT3 GOF mutation	STAT3	Multisystem autoimmunity, variable short stature, lymphoproliferation	Hypogammaglobulinemia Decreased class switched memory B cells
LRBA deficiency	LRBA	Multisystem autoimmunity, cytopenia, arthritis, recurrent sinopulmonary infection, granuloma, hypogammaglobulinemia	Hypogammaglobulinemia Decreased class switched memory B cells
CTLA4 haploinsufficiency	CTLA4	Diarrhea, enteropathy, hypogammaglobulinemia, granulomatous lymphocytic interstitial lung disease, multisystem autoimmunity	Hypogammaglobulinemia Decreased class switched memory B cells
Defects in IL-10 signaling			
Defects in IL-10 and IL-10R	IL-10RA IL-10RB IL-10	Perianal fistula, folliculitis, arthritis, abscess, lymphoma	STAT3 phosphorylation by IL-6 and IL-10 studies[a]
Defects in neutrophil function			
CGD	CYBB CYBA NCF1 NCF2 NCF4	Perianal fistula, recurrent cold abscess from catalase positive organisms,[b] gastric outlet obstruction	Decreased neutrophil oxidative burst study Elevated IgG

Disease	Gene	Clinical features	Immune/laboratory findings
Glycogen storage disease 1b	SLC37A4	Recurrent bacterial infections, hypoglycemia, hepatomegaly	Neutropenia, hypoglycemia, hyperuricemia, hyperlipidemia
Leukocyte adhesion defect	ITGB2	Neutrophilia, recurrent bacterial infections, delayed separation of umbilical cord, poor wound healing	Leukocytosis, Absent CD18 expression
Congenital neutropenia	G6PC3	Cutaneous vascular malformation and cardiac defect	Severe neutropenia
Hyperinflammatory disorders			
XIAP	BIRC4	Perianal fistula, recurrent HLH, EBV, and CMV infections, hypogammaglobinemia	Markedly elevated IL-18, Decreased or absent XIAP protein expression by flow
NLRC4 GOF mutation	NLRC4	Recurrent macrophage activation, rash	Markedly elevated IL-18
Mevalonate kinase deficiency	MVK	Recurrent fever, rash, abdominal pain and emesis	Elevated inflammatory markers, Elevated IgD, Elevated urine mevalonate
Familial Mediterranean fever	MEFV	Recurrent fever, abdominal pain, arthralgia, peritonitis	Elevated inflammatory markers
Familial HLH type 5	STXBP2	HLH, hypogammaglobinemia, sensorineural hearing loss	Marked elevated ferritin and sIL-2R, Decreased CD107a degranulation
Hermansky-Pudlak syndrome	HPS1 HPS4 HPS6	Partial albinism, bleeding tendency, recurrent infection and immunodeficiency	Decreased CD107a degranulation
Defects in epithelial barrier function			
TTC7A deficiency	TTC7A	Varying degree of intestinal atresia, T-cell immune defect and recurrent infections	Mild to severe T-cell immune deficiency, Hypogammaglobinemia
X-linked ectodermal immunodeficiency (NEMO deficiency)	IKBKG	Varying degree of ectodermal dysplasia, conical teeth, space and brittle hair, recurrent bacterial, viral and mycobacterial infections	Hypogammaglobinemia, Decreased class switched memory B cells
ADAM17 deficiency	ADAM17	Neonatal inflammatory skin and bowel disease, generalized pustular rash	Normal T-cell and B-cell numbers
Dystrophic epidermolysis bullosa	COL7A1	Blistering disorder primarily affect the hands, feet, knees, and elbows	Unremarkable immune findings

(continued on next page)

Table 2
(continued)

Defects	Gene Defect	Extra Intestinal Immune, Hematologic, or Somatic Manifestations	Laboratory Findings and Functional Evaluation
Kindler syndrome	*FERMT1*	Acral skin blistering, photosensitivity, progressive poikiloderma, and diffuse cutaneous atrophy	Eosinophilia
Isolated or combined T-cell and B-cell immune defects			
X-Linked agammaglobulinemia	*BTK*	Recurrent sinopulmonary infection	Absent B cells in peripheral blood Absent plasma cells in tissue Decreased class switched memory B cells
Common variable immune defect (CVID)		Heterogeneous group of defects with sinopulmonary infections, autoimmunity, lymphoproliferation, and variable T cell immune defect	Hypogammaglobinemia Variable T-cell lymphopenia
X-linked hyper IgM (CD40L)	*CD40L*	Sclerosing cholangitis, cryptosporidium diarrhea and pneumocystis infection	Elevated or normal IgM, neutropenia Absent class switched memory B cells
Wiskott-Aldrich syndrome	*WAS*	Eczema, recurrent infection, autoimmunity, vasculitis	Microthrombocytopenia Variable lymphopenia, low IgM Decreased WAS protein
Leaky SCID or Omenn	*RAG1, RAG2* *IL-7Ra* *IL-2RG*	Generalized erythroderma, hepatosplenomegaly, lymphadenopathy	Eosinophilia T-cell lymphopenia Decreased naïve T cells

[a] STAT3 signaling following IL-6 and IL-10 will only identify IL-10R A and B defects, it will not identify IL-10 deficiency.
[b] *Staphylococcus aureus, Serratia marcescens, Burkholderia cepacia, Aspergillus,* and *Candida.*

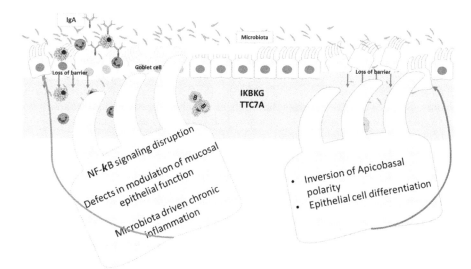

Fig. 6. Defects in epithelial barrier function. Figure shows 2 epithelial barrier mucosal defects: defects in NFκB signaling lead to defects in modulation of mucosal epithelial function, thereby resulting in intestinal microbiota-driven chronic intestinal inflammation; and defects in TTC7A lead to inversion of apicobasal polarity and defective epithelial cell differentiation and poor mucosal barrier function.

ISOLATED OR COMBINED T-CELL AND B-CELL DEFECTS

CLINICAL VIGNETTE

A 14-day-old infant presented with 15 loose bowel movements a day. Over the next few days he developed diffuse popular scaly rash in his extremities that spread quickly to involve his entire body. He was also noted to have purulent conjunctivitis. Generalized lymphadenopathy and hepatosplenomegaly was noted on physical examination. He was noted to have oral thrush and his blood culture grew Candida albicans. Complete blood count (CBC) reveled a hemoglobin of 7.8gm/dL (low) and platelets of 596,000 (elevated). White blood count was 6800μl-1, of which 48% were eosinophils, 28% neutrophils, 20% monocytes, and 8% lymphocytes (normal 55%). Skin and GI biopsy showed marked infiltration with eosinophils, monocytes, and lymphocytes. Based on candida infection and profound lymphopenia, an immune evaluation was done. There was profound T-cell and B-cell lymphopenia, and most of the T cells were of memory phenotype (98% CD3+ CD8+ CD45RO+) with near complete absence of naïve T cells. Functional T-cell evaluation showed poor T-cell proliferation to mitogen phytohemagglutinin, and analysis of T-cell repertoire showed oligoclonal population. Further genetic evaluation showed hypomorphic mutation in recombination-activating gene (RAG)-1. Based on these, a diagnosis of Omenn syndrome from hypomorphic RAG-1 defect was made.

Several known and unknown (yet to be characterized) entities belong in this category of disorders. Defects that affect the development of or function of either T cells or B cells can present with VEO-IBD. Infants and children with leaky severe combined immune deficiency (SCID) from hypomorphic mutations are known to present with IBD-like pathologic features. Unlike classic SCID, patients with leaky SCID have some residual T cells. However, the T cells are dysregulated, autoreactive, and oligoclonal in nature. In some patients, this dysregulated immune compartment manifests as Omenn syndrome,[68,69] characterized by generalized rash (erythroderma), protracted diarrhea, enlarged liver, spleen and lymph node, and eosinophilia. Mutations in RAG1 or RAG2, IL-7Rα, and IL-2Rγ are common causes of Omenn syndrome.[68,69] Another well-known entity that presents with VEO-IBD is Wiskott-Aldrich syndrome (WAS).[29] It is a rare, inherited, X-linked, recessive disease characterized by immune dysregulation that results from a defective WAS protein (mutations in the WAS gene). Infants and children with this disorder present with thrombocytopenia, severe eczema, chronic ear infections, and VEO-IBD. In addition to T-cell immune defects, patients with primary B-cell defects, such as X-linked agammaglobulinemia (XLA from Bruton tyrosine kinase [BTK] mutation) and common variable immunodeficiency (CVID) from diverse genetic causes can also present with VEO-IBD.[39,70,71]

EVALUATION AND DIAGNOSTIC APPROACH

More than 50 monogenetic defects in innate and adaptive immune system are associated with VEO-IBD and this list is likely to grow in the coming years when advances in genome sequencing become widely available along with molecular diagnostic technologies.[7] Nevertheless, these are still rare disorders and pediatricians and subspecialists are only expected to see these cases a few times in their lives. Initial immune evaluation should aim to identify common immune deficiency disorders that present with VEO-IBD. In the absence of specific diagnostic clue from clinical findings, for most patients initial immune evaluation should include a CBC, peripheral smear evaluation, lymphocyte subsets with T-cell, B-cell and NK-cell enumeration, CD45RA/RO enumeration and B-cell panel for class-switched memory B cells, neutrophil oxidative burst, and T regulatory cell (CD4+CD25+FOXP3+) cell enumeration. Additional studies, such as IL-10R signaling, IL-18 levels, CD107a degranulation, and telomere length, could be considered based on the clinical evaluation. **Table 3** highlights the utility of immune evaluation in a setting of VEO-IBD. Later, targeted immune evaluation based on initial immune phenotype or functional immune studies to validate genetic findings from VEO-IBD diagnostic panels based on next-generation sequencing or whole exome-based testing should be considered.

GENETIC TESTING IN VERY EARLY ONSET INFLAMMATORY BOWEL DISEASE

Traditional and individual single gene testing can be cumbersome and expensive for clinical use. Although gene panel testing is widely available for many diseases or disorders, few organizations or laboratories offer commercially available VEO-IBD gene panels. Any commercial testing that is covered by insurance for patients living in the United States and certified by Clinical Laboratory Improvement Amendments (CLIA) and/or College of American Pathologists (CAP) is necessary because the costs of sequencing can be significant for a family. The diagnostic laboratory at the authors' institution offer such a CLIA/CAP certified genetic test (http://geneticslab.emory. edu/tests/MM160) for VEO-IBD in which a 26-gene panel (AICDA, BTK, CD40LG, CYBA, CYBB, DCLRE1C, FOXP3, HPS1, HPS4, HPS6, ICOS, IL-10RA, IL-2RA, LRBA, MEFV, MVK, NCF2, NCF4, PTEN, RET, SH2D1A, SLC37A4, STXBP2, TTC37, WAS, XIAP) is included. Such testing provides targeted full gene sequencing for 26 genes implicated with VEO-IBD and provides comprehensive interpretation of the results. If the test yields no known mutations within the panel, testing is offered that is scalable to full exome genome sequencing in patients with initial negative results; full exome sequencing needs to be requested separately after the first round of results. The genetic testing for IBD not only establishes the molecular diagnosis with the basis of pathogenesis, it also allows rationale for patient-specific early intervention with emerging or experimental therapeutics and cell-based approaches, as well as the opportunity to screen family members for carrier detection and genetic counseling.

Table 3
Immune abnormalities in patients with very early onset inflammatory bowel disease

Immune Studies	Findings	Diagnostic Implications and Genetic Defects
CBC	Lymphopenia	T-cell immune defects
	Neutropenia	X-linked hyper IgM, XLA, HLH, autoimmune neutropenia, DKC, G6PC3 deficiency, and other severe congenital neutropenia
	Thrombocytopenia	WAS or immune thrombocytopenia
T, B, NK cell enumeration	T-cell lymphopenia	SCID or combined immune defects
	B-cell lymphopenia	XLA, combined immune defects
IgG, IgA, IgM	Low IgA	Common in infants, isolated low IgA should not warrant an extensive immune evaluation
	Decreased IgG, IgM	XLA, SCID/CID, CVID
	Elevated IgG	Marker of chronic inflammation in setting of IBD
Neutrophil oxidative burst	Decreased oxidative burst	CGD, RAC2
CD45RA/RO	Markedly skewed memory	SCID
	Mild to moderate skewing	Immune dysregulation PIK3CD defect, LRBA deficiency, STAT1 GOF, STAT3GOF, CTLA4 haploinsufficiency
Class switched B cells	Decreased CD27+,IgD- IgM- B cells	X-linked hyper IgM, CVID
FOXP3+Tregs cells	Decreased	IPEX, deficiency in CD25 and STAT5b
	Variable	Deficiency in LRBA, CTLA4, IL-10R
IL-10R signaling	Decreased STAT3 phosphorylation to IL-10	IL-10R defects
IL-18 levels	Elevated IL-18	XIAP and NLRC4 defect
CD107a	Decreased NK degranulation	HLH
Disease-specific flow	Decreased or absent expression of CD40L, WAS, XIAP, and BTK	Defects in CD40L, WAS, XIAP, and BTK
IKBα degradation	Abnormal degradation	NEMO/IKBα pathway defects
Telomere length	Decreased in T cells	Immune dysregulation disorders characterized by increased in T-cell memory phenotype
	Decreased in all cell types, especially in naive T cells and B cells	DKC

MANAGEMENT
Targeted Therapy

Apart from conventional management, understanding the specific defects and under-lying drivers of inflammation enables pathophysiology-based targeted treatment of patients with VEO-IBD. In general, these infants and young children do not respond to commonly used immunosuppressive IBD therapies and biologics, IL-1β antagonist anakinra has been shown to be effective in the management of colitis in patients with CGD.[72] This improvement with anakinra is thought to be due to improvement in auto-phagy and decrease in inflammasome activation. However, a recent report showed a more variable and unsustained response of colitis with anakinra treatment in patients with CGD.[73] Based on these reports, it seems that anakinra might be effective in sub-set of patients with CGD-associated colitis. Because the infectious complication is less with anakinra when compared with anti-TNF blocking biologic agents, anakinra could potentially be tried early in management CGD-associated colitis. Additionally, IL-1β blocking strategy has been shown to be effective in experimental mouse models of IL-10R associated colitis.[74]

In patients with LRBA deficiency and CTLA4 haploinsufficiency presenting with en-teropathy, abatacept, a CTLA4-immunoglobulin fusion drug that blocks T-cell costi-mulation has shown excellent response and long-term disease control.[75] Similarly, tocilizumab, an IL-6 receptor blocking antibody, has been reported to be effective in management of enteropathy associated with STAT3 GOF mutation.[39] Sirolimus has been reported to improve the number and function of Treg in experimental studies.[76,77] Based on these observations, sirolimus has been used in IPEX and IPEX-like conditions with significant improvement in enteropathy.[78,79] Despite these recent advances and observations, these infants and children respond poorly to med-ical therapy, Hence, medically refractory patients often undergo colectomies and are considered for HSCT.

Bone Marrow Transplant (Hematopoietic Stem Cell Transplant)

VEO-IBD caused by immune dysregulation could potentially be corrected by bone marrow transplant (BMT), or HSCT. Many of these diseases, such as CGD, IL-10 signaling defects, and SCID, have underlying significant immune deficiency predis-posing to multiple infections. Continuing long-term immune suppression for manage-ment of IBD in patients with underlying primary immune deficiency becomes challenging. In addition to the risk of recurrent and opportunistic infections, there is increased risk of lymphoma (in IL-10R), HLH (in XIAP and STXBP2), bone marrow fail-ure (in DKC), and progression of multisystem autoimmunity (in IPEX, LRBA deficiency, and IPEX-like disorders). HSCT will not only correct underlying immune dysregulation but also correct the underlying immune deficiency. Hence, adequate immune recon-stitution following HSCT could not only ameliorate IBD and other autoimmune mani-festations but also correct the predisposition to opportunistic infections.

HSCT for IPEX[24,25,80] and IL-10 signaling defects[20,26] has resulted in dramatic improvement in enterocolitis, healing of perianal disease, and fistula. Because HSCT only corrects defects in the immune compartment, IBD from primary epithe-lial defects are less likely to improve following HSCT. On the contrary, there are re-ports to suggest the IBD could potentially worsen following HSCT. For diseases such as NEMO and TTC7a deficiency (and potentially other epithelial barrier de-fects) there is a concern for unresolved or worsening colitis after HSCT.[22,81-83] Because many of the defects associated with VEO-IBD were identified in last decade, there are limited data to determine the role of HSCT in these disorders.[84]

Table 4
Role of bone marrow transplant (hematopoietic stem cell transplant) in very early onset inflammatory bowel disease

Role of BMT (HSCT[a])	Disease/Genetic Defect
Definitive Standard of care with overall good outcome	IL-10R, IL-10, IPEX, CGD, SCID, WAS, CD40L
Probable Based on the current understanding of the disease, HSCT is likely to work; however, there are currently not enough HSCT data to support BMT as the standard of care	STAT3 GOF, LRBA, CTLA4
Variable HSCT has resulted in variable outcome precluding defective recommendation	NEMO,[c] XIAP,[b] STAT1 GOF,[b] DKC
Not indicated HSCT not likely to help, could cause more harm than good	TTC7a[d] and other epithelial barrier defects

[a] The role of HSCT decided based on standard matched sibling and matched unrelated HSCT outcomes.
[b] High mortality with myeloablative conditioning.
[c] Experimental models and some case reports suggest there could be worsening of colitis after HSCT; however, there are reports of patients with complete immune reconstitution and no worsening of colitis after HSCT.
[d] HSCT has been done in some patients to correct underlying severe immune deficiency.

Nevertheless, based on the limited data and understanding of the disease processes, **Table 4** is intended to highlight the role of HSCT in various VEO-IBD disorders.[85–92]

HSCT should be entertained if there are good donor options (HLA-matched unaffected sibling, matched unrelated donor). When related donors are used for HSCT, every attempt should be made (both genetic and immune evaluation) to avoid apparently asymptomatic sibling harboring the same genetic defect. Though HSCT offers a potential opportunity for a long-term cure for patients with VEO-IBD, there are still significant short-term and long-term complications associated with HSCT. The authors recommend that HSCT evaluation should be done in centers where there is significant medical expertise in managing these complicated patients. In general, transplants outcomes are better when HSCT is offered early in life.[87] Early preclinical and clinical data on FOXp3 gene therapy for IPEX and other monogenetic immune defects are very promising and could potentially be a very attractive treatment option for these disorders in the future.[93–95]

REFERENCES

1. Strober W. The multifaceted influence of the mucosal microflora on mucosal dendritic cell responses. Immunity 2009;31(3):377–88.
2. Chu H, Mazmanian SK. Innate immune recognition of the microbiota promotes host-microbial symbiosis. Nat Immunol 2013;14(7):668–75.
3. Chistiakov DA, Bobryshev YV, Kozarov E, et al. Intestinal mucosal tolerance and impact of gut microbiota to mucosal tolerance. Front Microbiol 2014;5:781.
4. Tourneur E, Chassin C. Neonatal immune adaptation of the gut and its role during infections. Clin Dev Immunol 2013;2013:270301.

5. Kamada N, Seo SU, Chen GY, et al. Role of the gut microbiota in immunity and inflammatory disease. Nat Rev Immunol 2013;13(5):321–35.

6. de Souza HS, Fiocchi C. Immunopathogenesis of IBD: current state of the art. Nat Rev Gastroenterol Hepatol 2016;13(1):13–27.

7. Uhlig HH, Schwerd T, Koletzko S, et al. The diagnostic approach to monogenic very early onset inflammatory bowel disease. Gastroenterology 2014;147(5): 990–1007.e3.

8. Moran CJ, Klein C, Muise AM, et al. Very early-onset inflammatory bowel disease: gaining insight through focused discovery. Inflamm Bowel Dis 2015;21(5):1166–75.

9. Malmborg P, Hildebrand H. The emerging global epidemic of paediatric inflammatory bowel disease - causes and consequences. J Intern Med 2016;279(3):241–58.

10. Bendas A, Rothe U, Kiess W, et al. Trends in incidence rates during 1999-2008 and prevalence in 2008 of childhood type 1 diabetes mellitus in Germany–model-based national estimates. PLoS One 2015;10(7):e0132716.

11. Benchimol EI, Guttmann A, Griffiths AM, et al. Increasing incidence of paediatric inflammatory bowel disease in Ontario, Canada: evidence from health administrative data. Gut 2009;58(11):1490–7.

12. Benchimol EI, Mack DR, Nguyen GC, et al. Incidence, outcomes, and health services burden of very early onset inflammatory bowel disease. Gastroenterology 2014;147(4):803–13.e7 [quiz: e814–5].

13. Oliva-Hemker M, Hutfless S, Al Kazzi ES, et al. Clinical presentation and five-year therapeutic management of very early-onset inflammatory bowel disease in a large North American Cohort. J Pediatr 2015;167(3):527–32.e1–3.

14. Kelsen JR, Baldassano RN, Artis D, et al. Maintaining intestinal health: the genetics and immunology of very early onset inflammatory bowel disease. Cell Mol Gastroenterol Hepatol 2015;1(5):462–76.

15. Kelsen JR, Dawany N, Moran CJ, et al. Exome sequencing analysis reveals variants in primary immunodeficiency genes in patients with very early onset inflammatory bowel disease. Gastroenterology 2015;149(6):1415–24.

16. Al-Hussaini A, El Mouzan M, Hasosah M, et al. Clinical pattern of early-onset inflammatory bowel disease in Saudi Arabia: a multicenter national study. Inflamm Bowel Dis 2016;22(8):1961–70.

17. Bennett CL, Yoshioka R, Kiyosawa H, et al. X-Linked syndrome of polyendocrinopathy, immune dysfunction, and diarrhea maps to Xp11.23-Xq13.3. Am J Hum Genet 2000;66(2):461–8.

18. Barzaghi F, Passerini L, Bacchetta R. Immune dysregulation, polyendocrinopathy, enteropathy, x-linked syndrome: a paradigm of immunodeficiency with autoimmunity. Front Immunol 2012;3:211.

19. Glocker EO, Kotlarz D, Boztug K, et al. Inflammatory bowel disease and mutations affecting the interleukin-10 receptor. N Engl J Med 2009;361(21):2033–45.

20. Kotlarz D, Beier R, Murugan D, et al. Loss of interleukin-10 signaling and infantile inflammatory bowel disease: implications for diagnosis and therapy. Gastroenterology 2012;143(2):347–55.

21. Moran CJ, Walters TD, Guo CH, et al. IL-10R polymorphisms are associated with very-early-onset ulcerative colitis. Inflamm Bowel Dis 2013;19(1):115–23.

22. Chen R, Giliani S, Lanzi G, et al. Whole-exome sequencing identifies tetratricopeptide repeat domain 7A (TTC7A) mutations for combined immunodeficiency with intestinal atresias. J Allergy Clin Immunol 2013;132(3):656–64.e17.

23. Lemoine R, Pachlopnik-Schmid J, Farin HF, et al. Immune deficiency-related enteropathy-lymphocytopenia-alopecia syndrome results from tetratricopeptide repeat domain 7A deficiency. J Allergy Clin Immunol 2014;134(6):1354–64.e6.

24. Burroughs LM, Torgerson TR, Storb R, et al. Stable hematopoietic cell engraftment after low-intensity nonmyeloablative conditioning in patients with immune dysregulation, polyendocrinopathy, enteropathy, X-linked syndrome. J Allergy Clin Immunol 2010;126(5):1000–5.

25. Rao A, Kamani N, Filipovich A, et al. Successful bone marrow transplantation for IPEX syndrome after reduced-intensity conditioning. Blood 2007;109(1):383–5.

26. Engelhardt KR, Shah N, Faizura-Yeop I, et al. Clinical outcome in IL-10- and IL-10 receptor-deficient patients with or without hematopoietic stem cell transplantation. J Allergy Clin Immunol 2013;131(3):825–30.

27. Patey-Mariaud de Serre N, Canioni D, Ganousse S, et al. Digestive histopathological presentation of IPEX syndrome. Mod Pathol 2009;22(1):95–102.

28. Worthey EA, Mayer AN, Syverson GD, et al. Making a definitive diagnosis: successful clinical application of whole exome sequencing in a child with intractable inflammatory bowel disease. Genet Med 2011;13(3):255–62.

29. Cannioto Z, Berti I, Martelossi S, et al. IBD and IBD mimicking enterocolitis in children younger than 2 years of age. Eur J Pediatr 2009;168(2):149–55.

30. Hanson EP, Monaco-Shawver L, Solt LA, et al. Hypomorphic nuclear factor-kappaB essential modulator mutation database and reconstitution system identifies phenotypic and immunologic diversity. J Allergy Clin Immunol 2008; 122(6):1169–77.e16.

31. Le Bras S, Geha RS. IPEX and the role of Foxp3 in the development and function of human Tregs. J Clin Invest 2006;116(6):1473–5.

32. Bacchetta R, Barzaghi F, Roncarolo MG. From IPEX syndrome to FOXP3 mutation: a lesson on immune dysregulation. Ann N Y Acad Sci 2016. [Epub ahead of print].

33. Zama D, Cocchi I, Masetti R, et al. Late-onset of immunodysregulation, polyendocrinopathy, enteropathy, x-linked syndrome (IPEX) with intractable diarrhea. Ital J Pediatr 2014;40:68.

34. Okou DT, Mondal K, Faubion WA, et al. Exome sequencing identifies a novel FOXP3 mutation in a 2-generation family with inflammatory bowel disease. J Pediatr Gastroenterol Nutr 2014;58(5):561–8.

35. Sharfe N, Dadi HK, Shahar M, et al. Human immune disorder arising from mutation of the alpha chain of the interleukin-2 receptor. Proc Natl Acad Sci U S A 1997;94(7):3168–71.

36. Bernasconi A, Marino R, Ribas A, et al. Characterization of immunodeficiency in a patient with growth hormone insensitivity secondary to a novel STAT5b gene mutation. Pediatrics 2006;118(5):e1584–92.

37. Uzel G, Sampaio EP, Lawrence MG, et al. Dominant gain-of-function STAT1 mutations in FOXP3 wild-type immune dysregulation-polyendocrinopathy-enteropathy-X-linked-like syndrome. J Allergy Clin Immunol 2013;131(6): 1611–23.

38. Flanagan SE, Haapaniemi E, Russell MA, et al. Activating germline mutations in STAT3 cause early-onset multi-organ autoimmune disease. Nat Genet 2014; 46(8):812–4.

39. Milner JD, Vogel TP, Forbes L, et al. Early-onset lymphoproliferation and autoimmunity caused by germline STAT3 gain-of-function mutations. Blood 2015;125(4):591–9.

40. Lopez-Herrera G, Tampella G, Pan-Hammarstrom Q, et al. Deleterious mutations in LRBA are associated with a syndrome of immune deficiency and autoimmunity. Am J Hum Genet 2012;90(6):986–1001.

41. Charbonnier LM, Janssen E, Chou J, et al. Regulatory T-cell deficiency and immune dysregulation, polyendocrinopathy, enteropathy, X-linked-like disorder

caused by loss-of-function mutations in LRBA. J Allergy Clin Immunol 2015; 135(1):217–27.

42. Kuehn HS, Ouyang W, Lo B, et al. Immune dysregulation in human subjects with heterozygous germline mutations in CTLA4. Science 2014;345(6204):1623–7.

43. Schubert D, Bode C, Kenefeck R, et al. Autosomal dominant immune dysregulation syndrome in humans with CTLA4 mutations. Nat Med 2014;20(12):1410–6.

44. Beser OF, Conde CD, Serwas NK, et al. Clinical features of interleukin 10 receptor gene mutations in children with very early-onset inflammatory bowel disease. J Pediatr Gastroenterol Nutr 2015;60(3):332–8.

45. Couper KN, Blount DG, Riley EM. IL-10: the master regulator of immunity to infection. J Immunol 2008;180(9):5771–7.

46. Shouval DS, Ebens CL, Murchie R, et al. Large B-cell lymphoma in an adolescent patient with interleukin-10 receptor deficiency and history of infantile inflammatory bowel disease. J Pediatr Gastroenterol Nutr 2016;63(1):e15–7.

47. Neven B, Mamessier E, Bruneau J, et al. A Mendelian predisposition to B-cell lymphoma caused by IL-10R deficiency. Blood 2013;122(23):3713–22.

48. Yabal M, Muller N, Adler H, et al. XIAP restricts TNF- and RIP3-dependent cell death and inflammasome activation. Cell Rep 2014;7(6):1796–808.

49. Romberg N, Al Moussawi K, Nelson-Williams C, et al. Mutation of NLRC4 causes a syndrome of enterocolitis and autoinflammation. Nat Genet 2014;46(10): 1135–9.

50. Canna SW, de Jesus AA, Gouni S, et al. An activating NLRC4 inflammasome mutation causes autoinflammation with recurrent macrophage activation syndrome. Nat Genet 2014;46(10):1140–6.

51. Bader-Meunier B, Florkin B, Sibilia J, et al. Mevalonate kinase deficiency: a survey of 50 patients. Pediatrics 2011;128(1):e152–9.

52. Pagel J, Beutel K, Lehmberg K, et al. Distinct mutations in STXBP2 are associated with variable clinical presentations in patients with familial hemophagocytic lymphohistiocytosis type 5 (FHL5). Blood 2012;119(25):6016–24.

53. Hazzan D, Seward S, Stock H, et al. Crohn's-like colitis, enterocolitis and perianal disease in Hermansky-Pudlak syndrome. Colorectal Dis 2006;8(7):539–43.

54. Yoshiyama S, Miki C, Araki T, et al. Complicated granulomatous colitis in a Japanese patient with Hermansky-Pudlak syndrome, successfully treated with infliximab. Clin J Gastroenterol 2009;2(1):51–4.

55. Schappi MG, Smith VV, Goldblatt D, et al. Colitis in chronic granulomatous disease. Arch Dis Child 2001;84(2):147–51.

56. Kawai T, Arai K, Harayama S, et al. Severe and rapid progression in very early-onset chronic granulomatous disease-associated colitis. J Clin Immunol 2015; 35(6):583–8.

57. Muise AM, Xu W, Guo CH, et al. NADPH oxidase complex and IBD candidate gene studies: identification of a rare variant in NCF2 that results in reduced binding to RAC2. Gut 2012;61(7):1028–35.

58. Dhillon SS, Fattouh R, Elkadri A, et al. Variants in nicotinamide adenine dinucleotide phosphate oxidase complex components determine susceptibility to very early onset inflammatory bowel disease. Gastroenterology 2014;147(3):680–9.e2.

59. Hayes P, Dhillon S, O'Neill K, et al. Defects in NADPH oxidase genes and in very early onset inflammatory bowel disease. Cell Mol Gastroenterol Hepatol 2015; 1(5):489–502.

60. Yamaguchi T, Ihara K, Matsumoto T, et al. Inflammatory bowel disease-like colitis in glycogen storage disease type 1b. Inflamm Bowel Dis 2001;7(2):128–32.

61. Visser G, Rake JP, Fernandes J, et al. Neutropenia, neutrophil dysfunction, and inflammatory bowel disease in glycogen storage disease type Ib: results of the European Study on glycogen storage disease type I. J Pediatr 2000;137(2): 187–91.

62. D'Agata ID, Paradis K, Chad Z, et al. Leucocyte adhesion deficiency presenting as a chronic ileocolitis. Gut 1996;39(4):605–8.

63. Schmidt-Supprian M, Bloch W, Courtois G, et al. NEMO/IKK gamma-deficient mice model incontinentia pigmenti. Mol Cell 2000;5(6):981–92.

64. Nenci A, Becker C, Wullaert A, et al. Epithelial NEMO links innate immunity to chronic intestinal inflammation. Nature 2007;446(7135):557–61.

65. Blaydon DC, Biancheri P, Di WL, et al. Inflammatory skin and bowel disease linked to ADAM17 deletion. N Engl J Med 2011;365(16):1502–8.

66. Jyonouchi S, Forbes L, Ruchelli E, et al. Dyskeratosis congenita: a combined immunodeficiency with broad clinical spectrum–a single-center pediatric experience. Pediatr Allergy Immunol 2011;22(3):313–9.

67. Ballew BJ, Joseph V, De S, et al. A recessive founder mutation in regulator of telomere elongation helicase 1, RTEL1, underlies severe immunodeficiency and features of Hoyeraal Hreidarsson syndrome. PLoS Genet 2013;9(8):e1003695.

68. Villa A, Notarangelo LD, Roifman CM. Omenn syndrome: inflammation in leaky severe combined immunodeficiency. J Allergy Clin Immunol 2008;122(6):1082–6.

69. Marrella V, Maina V, Villa A. Omenn syndrome does not live by V(D)J recombination alone. Curr Opin Allergy Clin Immunol 2011;11(6):525–31.

70. Washington K, Stenzel TT, Buckley RH, et al. Gastrointestinal pathology in patients with common variable immunodeficiency and X-linked agammaglobulinemia. Am J Surg Pathol 1996;20(10):1240–52.

71. Serwas NK, Kansu A, Santos-Valente E, et al. Atypical manifestation of LRBA deficiency with predominant IBD-like phenotype. Inflamm Bowel Dis 2015; 21(1):40–7.

72. de Luca A, Smeekens SP, Casagrande A, et al. IL-1 receptor blockade restores autophagy and reduces inflammation in chronic granulomatous disease in mice and in humans. Proc Natl Acad Sci U S A 2014;111(9):3526–31.

73. Hahn KJ, Ho N, Yockey L, et al. Treatment with anakinra, a recombinant IL-1 receptor antagonist, unlikely to induce lasting remission in patients with CGD colitis. Am J Gastroenterol 2015;110(6):938–9.

74. Shouval DS, Biswas A, Goettel JA, et al. Interleukin-10 receptor signaling in innate immune cells regulates mucosal immune tolerance and anti-inflammatory macrophage function. Immunity 2014;40(5):706–19.

75. Lo B, Zhang K, Lu W, et al. AUTOIMMUNE DISEASE. Patients with LRBA deficiency show CTLA4 loss and immune dysregulation responsive to abatacept therapy. Science 2015;349(6246):436–40.

76. Battaglia M, Stabilini A, Tresoldi E. Expanding human T regulatory cells with the mTOR-inhibitor rapamycin. Methods Mol Biol 2012;821:279–93.

77. Ogino H, Nakamura K, Iwasa T, et al. Regulatory T cells expanded by rapamycin in vitro suppress colitis in an experimental mouse model. J Gastroenterol 2012; 47(4):366–76.

78. Bindl L, Torgerson T, Perroni L, et al. Successful use of the new immunesuppressor sirolimus in IPEX (immune dysregulation, polyendocrinopathy, enteropathy, X-linked syndrome). J Pediatr 2005;147(2):256–9.

79. Yong PL, Russo P, Sullivan KE. Use of sirolimus in IPEX and IPEX-like children. J Clin Immunol 2008;28(5):581–7.

80. Kucuk ZY, Bleesing JJ, Marsh R, et al. A challenging undertaking: stem cell transplantation for immune dysregulation, polyendocrinopathy, enteropathy, X-linked (IPEX) syndrome. J Allergy Clin Immunol 2016;137(3):953–5.e4.
81. Klemann C, Pannicke U, Morris-Rosendahl DJ, et al. Transplantation from a symptomatic carrier sister restores host defenses but does not prevent colitis in NEMO deficiency. Clin Immunol 2016;164:52–6.
82. Fish JD, Duerst RE, Gelfand EW, et al. Challenges in the use of allogeneic hematopoietic SCT for ectodermal dysplasia with immune deficiency. Bone Marrow Transplant 2009;43(3):217–21.
83. Samuels ME, Majewski J, Alirezaie N, et al. Exome sequencing identifies mutations in the gene TTC7A in French-Canadian cases with hereditary multiple intestinal atresia. J Med Genet 2013;50(5):324–9.
84. Marsh RA, Rao K, Satwani P, et al. Allogeneic hematopoietic cell transplantation for XIAP deficiency: an international survey reveals poor outcomes. Blood 2013; 121(6):877–83.
85. Morillo-Gutierrez B, Beier R, Rao K, et al. Treosulfan based conditioning for allogeneic HSCT in children with chronic granulomatous disease: a multicentre experience. Blood 2016;128(3):440–8.
86. Gungor T, Teira P, Slatter M, et al. Reduced-intensity conditioning and HLA-matched haemopoietic stem-cell transplantation in patients with chronic granulomatous disease: a prospective multicentre study. Lancet 2014;383(9915): 436–48.
87. Pai SY, Cowan MJ. Stem cell transplantation for primary immunodeficiency diseases: the North American experience. Curr Opin Allergy Clin Immunol 2014; 14(6):521–6.
88. Moratto D, Giliani S, Bonfim C, et al. Long-term outcome and lineage-specific chimerism in 194 patients with Wiskott-Aldrich syndrome treated by hematopoietic cell transplantation in the period 1980-2009: an international collaborative study. Blood 2011;118(6):1675–84.
89. Pai SY, Logan BR, Griffith LM, et al. Transplantation outcomes for severe combined immunodeficiency, 2000-2009. N Engl J Med 2014;371(5):434–46.
90. Tesi B, Priftakis P, Lindgren F, et al. Successful hematopoietic stem cell transplantation in a patient with LPS-Responsive Beige-Like Anchor (LRBA) gene mutation. J Clin Immunol 2016;36(5):480–9.
91. Seidel MG, Hirschmugl T, Gamez-Diaz L, et al. Long-term remission after allogeneic hematopoietic stem cell transplantation in LPS-responsive beige-like anchor (LRBA) deficiency. J Allergy Clin Immunol 2015;135(5):1384–90.e1–8.
92. Aldave JC, Cachay E, Nunez L, et al. A 1-year-old girl with a gain-of-function STAT1 mutation treated with hematopoietic stem cell transplantation. J Clin Immunol 2013;33(8):1273–5.
93. Passerini L, Rossi Mel E, Sartirana C, et al. CD4(+) T cells from IPEX patients convert into functional and stable regulatory T cells by FOXP3 gene transfer. Sci Transl Med 2013;5(215):215ra174.
94. Hacein-Bey-Abina S, Pai SY, Gaspar HB, et al. A modified gamma-retrovirus vector for X-linked severe combined immunodeficiency. N Engl J Med 2014;371(15): 1407–17.
95. Hacein-Bey Abina S, Gaspar HB, Blondeau J, et al. Outcomes following gene therapy in patients with severe Wiskott-Aldrich syndrome. JAMA 2015;313(15): 1550–63.

Presentation and Diagnostic Evaluation of Mitochondrial Disease

David P. Dimmock, MD[a,b], Michael W. Lawlor, MD, PhD[c],*

KEYWORDS

- Mitochondrial • Myopathy • Metabolic • Electron transport chain • mtDNA
- Diagnosis

KEY POINTS

- Mitochondrial diseases (MD) are a heterogeneous group of disorders with symptoms of organ dysfunction across multiple body systems.
- The unifying feature in MD is the dysfunction of mitochondrial respiratory chain complex function caused by genetic mutations.
- Diagnosis of MD is complicated by the lack of gold standard diagnostic testing strategies and the potential for false-negative test results caused by sampling issues.
- By integrating data obtained from clinical, imaging, pathologic, molecular, and enzymatic assessments, it is often possible to identify MD despite these issues.

FEATURES OF MITOCHONDRIAL DISEASE

Mitochondrial disease (MD) occurs when alteration of mitochondrial respiratory chain (RC) complex function caused by genetic mutation produces a detectable disease state. Activities of complexes I to V can be altered (**Fig. 1**), and physiologic consequences of

Disclosure Statement: Dr D.P. Dimmock is a member of advisory boards for Audentes Therapeutics and Biomarin. He has been funded for work performed for Biomarin, Shire, Alexion, Genzyme/Sanofi, and Cytonet. He has worked as a paid consultant for Illumina and Complete Genomics. He has also participated in a sponsored research agreement with Demeter Therapeutics. Dr M.W. Lawlor is a member of advisory boards for Audentes Therapeutics, and has been supported by sponsored research agreements by Audentes Therapeutics and Solid Biosciences. He is a scientific collaborator with Acceleron Pharma and Pfizer. He has recently been a consultant for Sarepta Therapeutics.
[a] Rady Children's Institute for Genomic Medicine, 3020 Children's Way MC 5129, San Diego, CA 92123, USA; [b] Division of Genetics, Department of Pediatrics, Human Molecular Genetics Center, Medical College of Wisconsin, Milwaukee, WI 53226, USA; [c] Division of Pediatric Pathology, Department of Pathology and Laboratory Medicine, Neuroscience Research Center, Medical College of Wisconsin, 8701 Watertown Plank Road, TBRC Building, Room C4490, Milwaukee, WI 53226, USA
* Corresponding author. 8701 Watertown Plank Road, TBRC Building, Room C4490, Milwaukee, WI 53226.
E-mail address: mlawlor@mcw.edu

Pediatr Clin N Am 64 (2017) 161–171
http://dx.doi.org/10.1016/j.pcl.2016.08.011
0031-3955/17/© 2016 Elsevier Inc. All rights reserved.

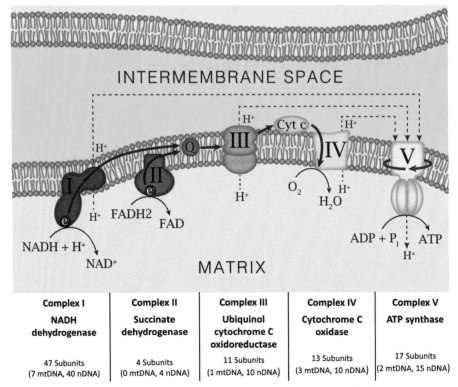

Fig. 1. Diagram of mitochondrial RC components. Each mitochondrial RC complex is depicted and named, as are the critical cofactors, coenzyme Q (CoQ) and cytochrome c (Cyt C). For each complex, the proportion of subunits encoded by the mtDNA and nDNA are shown. The flow of electrons (*solid red lines/arrows*) and protons (*dashed red lines/arrows*) in the RC are also displayed. The solid line encircling complex V depicts its rotation as it produces ATP. NADH, nicotinamide adenine dinucleotide.

mitochondrial RC defects include reduced metabolic capacity, reduced ATP synthesis, and increased oxidative and nitrosative stress.[1,2] Mutations in nuclear DNA (nDNA) or mitochondrial DNA (mtDNA) can lead to defects in the complexes essential for RC function or for the transport and assembly of mitochondrial proteins (**Box 1**). Additionally, because mtDNA mutations can impair mitochondrial function, mutations that affect

---

Box 1
Nuclear and mitochondrial genomes in mitochondrial disease

- The mitochondrial genome encodes 37 genes, encoding two ribosomal RNAs, 22 transfer RNAs, and 13 subunits of RCs.

- There are at least 1000 nuclear genes associated with mitochondrial function.

- Some pathologic patterns (cytochrome oxidase–negative/succinate dehydrogenase–overexpressing fibers) specifically suggest mutations in the mitochondrial genome.

- Gene diagnostic panels are available for disease subsets, along with sequencing of the mitochondrial and nuclear genomes separately.

the complement of factors that facilitate the recycling, synthesis, and import of nucleotides to the mitochondrial genome can also produce MD.

Because MD can present with an extraordinary range of clinical symptoms and testing abnormalities, it is often in the clinical differential diagnosis of patients with diseases involving the brain, muscle, or liver. Symptoms of MD are manifold and include abnormalities of the motor, sensory, gastrointestinal, endocrine, and cardiovascular systems; intolerance of some general anesthetics and antiepileptic drugs; increased susceptibility to infection; and pregnancy loss.[1,2] The exceptional variation seen in the MD phenotype can be caused by variations in the amount and distribution of dysfunctional mitochondria throughout the body. Dramatic differences in clinical phenotype are seen in different patients with the same mutation, particularly when that mutation is present in the mitochondrial genome. For MD caused by mtDNA mutation, the clinical phenotype depends on (1) the specific tissues that contain abnormal mitochondria, (2) the proportion of abnormal mitochondria within these tissues, and (3) the number of copies of mutant mtDNA within the tissue. For nuclear-encoded defects, the phenotype is driven by the dependence of that tissue on mitochondrial respiration, and the tissue-specific expression of the protein and of other potentially compensatory proteins. Several distinct MD syndromes have been described (**Box 2**), but it should be noted that these constitute particularly striking clinical phenotypes rather than the most common presentations of MD. In clinical practice, the most common presentation of MD is nonspecific, and may include the following issues:

- Unexplained combination of neuromuscular and nonneuromuscular symptoms
- Progressive course
- Involvement of an increasing number of seemingly unrelated organs
- Fluctuating symptomatology
- Exercise intolerance caused by premature fatigue after even mild activities (usually disproportionately severe compared with weakness)

Box 2
Examples of well-described mitochondrial syndromes

Mitochondrial encephalomyopathy, lactic acidosis stroke-like episodes
  Presentation includes weakness, headaches, followed by episodes of seizures and transient hemiparesis and cortical blindness.

Myoclonic epilepsy with ragged red fibers
  Presentation includes myoclonus (often the first symptom) followed by generalized epilepsy, ataxia, weakness, and dementia.

Progressive external ophthalmoplegia plus
  Presentation includes ptosis followed by ophthalmoplegia, and this may be associated with weakness of the upper limbs and exercise intolerance.

Alpers syndrome
  Presentation includes severe encephalopathy with intractable epilepsy and hepatic failure.

Navajo neurohepatopathy
  Presentation includes hepatopathy, peripheral neuropathy, corneal anesthesia and scarring, acral mutilation, cerebral leukoencephalopathy, failure to thrive, and recurrent metabolic acidosis with intercurrent infections

Leigh disease
  Presentation includes clinical evidence of brainstem/basal ganglia disease (including stepwise psychomotor retardation or regression), elevated blood or cerebrospinal fluid lactate levels, and imaging abnormalities in the brainstem and basal ganglia.

- Muscle cramps, stiffness, or the "second wind phenomenon" that is often seen in glycogenoses
- Elevated lactate levels at rest

Diagnostic approaches for MD are currently nonstandard and better diagnostic tools for MD are needed.[2] The clinical heterogeneity of MD complicates diagnosis because it can symptomatically overlap with a broad range of diseases, and testing abnormalities among the MDs are not uniform. MD is often suspected in early childhood, and traditional diagnostic methods for MD include assessment of clinical presentation, family history, pathology, metabolic profiling, enzyme activity levels, electrophysiology, MRI, magnetic resonance spectroscopy, and mtDNA analysis. Despite this arsenal of methods, the diagnostic work-up for the identification of MD is not standard across providers or institutions. Diagnostic algorithms have been used to predict the likelihood of MD.[2] Nevertheless, there is no clear consensus on when MD can be excluded, or where follow-up confirmatory testing should be performed.[2]

MD is likely vastly underdiagnosed at a level of 5 in 100,000 children,[1] whereas its suspected prevalence may be 1 in 5000 adults.[3] Conversely, a subset of patients with other causes of their symptoms may be incorrectly identified as having an MD because of secondary metabolic effects of their disease state. The determination of whether MD is present or can be excluded in a given patient is extremely complex, given the following:

- Mitochondrial function can be secondarily affected because of the disease processes in non-MDs.
- There is no specific or sensitive biomarker that identifies all or even most individuals with MD.
- There is extensive variability in the distribution of abnormal mitochondria within an individual patient, allowing a false-negative testing profile to occur when tissues used for diagnosis do not contain the abnormal mitochondria.
- There are no uniform, clear-cut pathologic abnormalities to distinguish all patients with MD from patients with other disorders, to the extent that some biopsy specimens from MD look structurally normal.

Unfortunately, the lack of standard strategies to identify true MD cases (especially less severe cases that do not have specific pathology) poses a substantial limitation on improving MD diagnosis. In our center, we have adopted a three-strike practice to identify whether genetic testing of the nuclear or mitochondrial genome is likely to be useful (**Box 3**), which has led to the identification of patients with pathogenic

---

Box 3
Integrating test abnormalities to diagnose MD: a three-strike approach

- Follow-up genetic testing is performed in cases with significant abnormalities in any three of the following categories
  - Clinical history
  - Light microscopy
  - Electron microscopy
  - Electron transport chain activity testing
  - mtDNA content
- Recognizing there may be rare false-negatives, we generally do not go forward with genetic testing for mitochondrial disease on cases without abnormalities in at least three of the categories listed previously.

mutations despite underwhelming test abnormalities on some of the other testing modalities. The remainder of this article provides descriptions of the diagnostic testing modalities that are useful in the diagnosis of MD.

DIAGNOSTIC TEST INTERPRETATION IN MITOCHONDRIAL DISEASE
Biochemical Screening Tests

Plasma lactate
Elevated lactate levels have long been associated with MD, although the finding is not a prerequisite for diagnosis. Plasma lactate can be normal or only mildly increased in many conditions, including mtDNA depletion syndromes. False-positive elevations in lactate may be seen in status of poor tissue perfusion/oxygenation or when samples are improperly collected or handled. Lactate levels are also often increased after feeding.[4]

Cerebrospinal fluid lactate
In Leigh disease, lactate elevation in the cerebrospinal fluid is more consistent than elevations in blood. Cerebrospinal fluid elevations in lactate, however, may also been seen after seizures of any cause.

Amino acid levels
Measurement of amino acids in plasma from patients with MD may demonstrate elevated alanine. This is formed from the transamination of pyruvate and reflects a persistent elevation of lactate but it may also be seen in other metabolic disorders.

Urine organic acids
Lactic aciduria is often seen in MD and urine analysis should be performed to exclude other organic acidurias. More specific biomarkers of mitochondrial dysfunction, such as 3-methylglutaconic acid, may be useful (although other genetic disorders including glycogen storage disease may also cause this). Elevations in tricarboxylic acid cycle intermediates may suggest MD but may also be seen in hepatic disease and starvation. Another common finding in MD is elevated urine amino acids that are suggestive of renal Fanconi syndrome.[5]

Cardiac Testing

Electrocardiogram
Cardiomyopathy, pre-excitation, or incomplete heart block are well described in mitochondrial encephalomyopathy, lactic acidosis stroke-like episodes (MELAS). Atrioventricular conduction defects are a specific concern in cases of Kearns-Sayre syndrome.

Echocardiogram
Cardiomyopathy is more common in MDs that also cause skeletal muscle myopathy. Systolic dysfunction is a frequent finding in MD, but the structural phenotype may vary. In MELAS, concentric left ventricular hypertrophy is common, whereas dilated cardiomyopathy is typical of Barth syndrome. Historically, mitochondrial mutations were thought to be the typical cause of left ventricular myocardial noncompaction (also known as left ventricular hypertrabeculation), but many other genetic syndromes can also lead to this cardiac phenotype.[6]

MRI of the Brain

MDs produce variable imaging abnormalities, and some patterns are helpful in diagnosis (**Fig. 2**). Cerebral and cerebellar atrophy are frequently observed across a broad

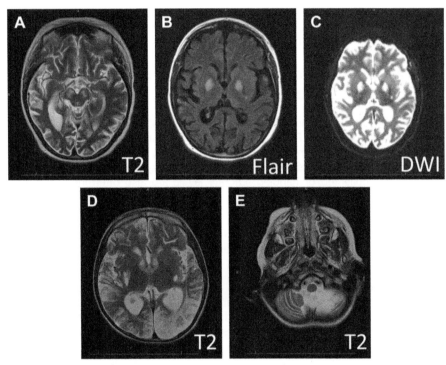

Fig. 2. Brain imaging findings in MD. MRI from two patients with MELAS are shown to illustrate the imaging findings in severe MD. Scans from the first patient (*A–C*) displayed patchy areas of restricted diffusion and long TR signal hyperintensity involving the parietal lobes, temporal lobes, and basal ganglia bilaterally. In the second patient (*D, E*), similar abnormalities were seen in the occipital lobes (*D*), and marked cerebellar atrophy was also noted (*E*). DWI, diffusion weighted sequence; Flair, fluid-attenuated inversion recovery sequence; T2, T2-weighted image sequence.

range of MDs. Additionally, metabolic impairment may produce stroke-like lesions of ischemia or infarction that may not correspond to specific vascular territories. In MELAS, increased T2 signal can be present, most frequently in the occipital areas. Slow spreading of these lesions is noted in the weeks following the initial event. The stroke-like lesions of MELAS show increased apparent diffusion coefficient, in contrast to the reduction seen in ischemic strokes. These stroke-like lesions may be confused with posterior reversible encephalopathy syndrome, and it is possible that both disease states have a similar cause related to endothelial dysfunction, ischemia, and subsequent vasogenic edema. The imaging abnormalities seen in Leigh disease are typically different from those of MELAS, including bilateral symmetric hyperintense signal abnormalities in the brainstem and/or basal ganglia on T2-weighted MRI.

Skeletal Muscle Biopsy

Light microscopy

Although muscle biopsy is extremely useful in the diagnosis of muscle disease, the degree of histopathology observed in most cases of MD is underwhelming. Structural characteristics consistent with MD include abnormalities of mitochondrial size, shape, location, number, and internal architecture. In some instances, these abnormalities are sufficiently severe to produce ragged red fibers that show mitochondrial aggregates at the light microscopic level (**Fig. 3**). In some cases, specific histochemical stains are useful in identifying mitochondrial abnormalities. Stains for reduced nicotinamide adenine dinucleotide, cytochrome oxidase (COX), and succinate dehydrogenase (SDH) are commonly done on frozen muscle tissue to visualize the distribution of

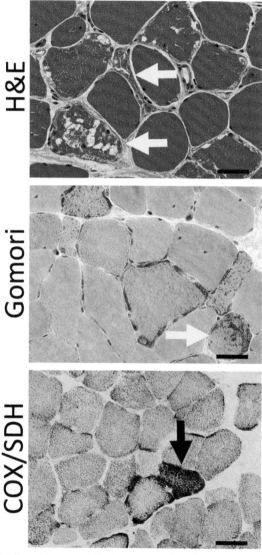

Fig. 3. Pathologic findings in severe MD. Severe mitochondrial disease can show alterations in fiber size, ragged red fibers (*yellow arrows*), and accumulations of mitochondria (here seen as *red-stained* subsarcolemmal areas on the Gomori trichrome stain). COX and SDH stains may show stains that are negative for COX, and some of these fibers may overexpress SDH (*black arrow*). Bar = 40 μm. COX, cytochrome oxidase; H&E, hematoxylin and eosin; SDH, succinate dehydrogenase.

mitochondria and other cellular elements. Although the nicotinamide adenine dinucleotide stain identifies the mitochondria and sarcotubular elements, staining patterns on COX and SDH stains identify mitochondria more specifically. Cases with ragged red fibers on Gomori trichrome stain should have visible mitochondrial aggregates on these stains, and other abnormalities of mitochondrial distribution may also be noted. The COX stain can specifically be useful because mitochondrial dysfunction can produce COX-negative fibers that fail to stain on this preparation. Although the number of COX-negative fibers increases even in normal muscle with increasing age, excessive numbers of COX-negative fibers may warrant further evaluation for MD. In cases where COX-negative fibers show overexpression of SDH, it may be useful to search for mtDNA mutations before testing the nuclear genome, because this staining pattern often corresponds to compensatory changes in SDH (which is predominantly nuclear-encoded) in response to significant alterations in COX (which is partially mitochondrial-encoded). In most cases of MD, however, it should be stressed that these helpful pathologic findings are likely absent, and that the key value of muscle biopsy lies in its potential to assess mitochondrial structure and function through multiple assays.

Electron microscopy
Electron microscopy is useful for the identification of structural abnormalities in mitochondria, because it can offer an excellent view of mitochondrial size, shape, and internal complexity, and allows the identification for abnormal inclusions that may be present within mitochondria (**Fig. 4**). Electron microscopy studies should be evaluated by a diagnostician accustomed to working with human muscle biopsy tissue, because

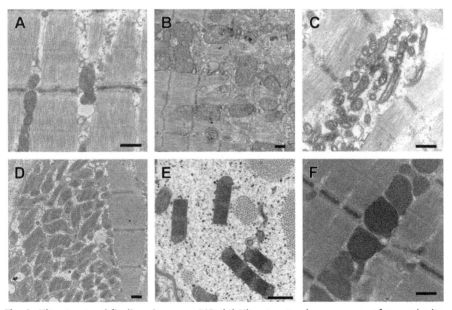

Fig. 4. Ultrastructural findings in severe MD. (*A*) Ultrastructural appearance of normal mitochondria in a patient without MD. (*B*) Low-power image illustrating mitochondrial enlargement and excessively complex internal architecture. (*C*) Other cases show abnormally small or hypocomplex mitochondria. (*D–F*) Some mitochondrial abnormalities create inclusions within mitochondria. These inclusions can appear paracrystalline (*D, E*), or may be less defined (*F*). Excessive numbers of mitochondria may also be seen in MD (*D*). Bar = 500 nm.

there is significant variation in normal mitochondrial morphology between species and even between different tissue types in humans. Many MD cases have only mild abnormalities of mitochondrial ultrastructure, and some appear entirely normal. Even mild ultrastructural abnormalities, however, are useful in determining the relevance of abnormal genetic or biochemical testing in these patients. Electron microscopy can also be useful for the distinction of mitochondrial aggregates from other types of pathologic aggregates that may be visible at the light microscopic level, including nemaline rods and myofibrillar inclusions.

Enzymatic testing
Because skeletal muscle biopsies harboring significant MD may not display structural abnormalities, the evaluation of mitochondrial RC enzymatic function can often be helpful in determining the likelihood of MD. These assays monitor the individual activity of the RC complexes by following the oxidation/reduction of specific substrates or substrate analogues. The most commonly used assay involves physically and chemically disrupting the muscle sample to liberate intact mitochondrial complexes. Artificial substrates are then added to this suspension and the rate of production of the product is measured using spectrophotometry. These results are typically normalized to a tricarboxylic acid cycle control, such as citrate synthase and/or mitochondrial complex II, to control for mitochondrial density. Although these assays are extremely helpful, there are numerous technical factors that make them complex to perform with significant inter-laboratory variation in "normal ranges".[7] They are typically performed as a send-out assay to one of several reference laboratories. The reports from these laboratories are helpful in assessing the activity of the RC, but there are a few key issues to consider when ordering and interpreting these assays:

- The biochemical activity of these enzymes is highly dependent on the interval between tissue removal and freezing, and may also be significantly affected by freeze/thaw cycles. Optimal results are obtained by using samples that were frozen within 30 minutes of removal from the patient. Specimens with excessive removal-to-freezing delays show poor function of the RC components and the internal control enzymes.
- The activity of RC complexes may be abnormal because of secondary effects of several disease states, so it is important to evaluate the biopsy for other disorders before sending out tissue for this assay.
- These assays evaluate the activity of mitochondrial RC complexes I to IV, but do not routinely evaluate the activity of complex V. We recommend contacting the reference laboratories performing this testing to determine the best way to evaluate complex V, if this is specifically suspected in a given patient.
- Some cases with significant MD may yield entirely normal mitochondrial electron transport chain activity results. This may be because the ratio of components is normal but there is a reduction in mitochondrial mass.

GENETIC TESTS

Definitive genetic diagnosis of MD may require evaluations of the mtDNA and the nDNA for mutations, either through targeted diagnostic DNA sequencing panels of the mtDNA or nDNA. Although the first described mutations in MD were found in the mtDNA, mtDNA-encoded defects only cause approximately 15% of all known MD and most mitochondrial proteins are actually coded in the nDNA. Thus, next-generation nDNA sequencing is a powerful tool for MD diagnosis.[8,9] Unfortunately, the interpretation of next-generation sequencing data for MD diagnosis is challenging, given the large number of target genes for sequencing and the potentially poor correlation between the genetic data and the clinical/biochemical phenotype.[10] Whole genome sequencing is on the horizon, but much more work is required to assign mutations to aspects of mitochondrial dysfunction and to identify which mutations are truly disease-causing.

EXPERIMENTAL/HIGHLY SPECIALIZED APPROACHES

Understanding global metabolism through analyses of the lipidome, metabolome, proteome, and transcriptome is progressing, and some disease-specific metabolites have been identified for some non-MD diseases.[11] The omics approach, however, is in need of substantial development before it approaches clinical utility. Improved bioinformatics tools are required to integrate the enormous amount of data yielded by omics methods.

Mechanistic information on MD has largely arisen from mitochondrial RC activity assays on complex components, isolated from their native matrix from fresh or frozen tissue, or from cultured cells. These assays are (like most clinical biochemical assays) performed under nonphysiologic basal conditions and with different substrate concentrations than are seen in vivo. Complex interactions between the substrates of these assays and other cellular components can lead to erroneous results.[12] Additionally, these assays cannot perform a functional assessment of processes that require intact mitochondrial structures (eg, those involved with mitochondrial membrane potential or coupling). Also, some components of the RC (eg, complex V) cannot be tested using this method. Thus, additional specialized methods of mitochondrial assessment may be used, some of which involve direct measurements of viable, functioning mitochondria. Although such assays offer the opportunity to measure phenotypes including oxygen consumption or ATP generation (reviewed in Ref.[13]), they also are limited to certain clinical sites because of their requirement for freshly isolated tissue. In all of the currently used assays, mitochondrial function is not assessed in its native-organ context and the need persists for a functional measurement of mitochondria in tissue. Our research group and others are working on new techniques for such assessments (including electron paramagnetic resonance spectroscopy[14]), which it is hoped will further improve the techniques available for understanding MD mechanisms and the relevance of abnormal genetic testing results in the near future.

SUMMARY

As a disease class with exceptional phenotypic and genetic variability, MD presents a diagnostic challenge in many patients. However, it is often possible to identify clinically relevant mitochondrial dysfunction using complementary diagnostic testing methods, even in mild cases. Although the development of improved diagnostic testing methods would be helpful, it may be possible to improve the diagnostic evaluation of MD in the short term through the employment of comprehensive, multidisciplinary diagnostic approaches, such as the three-strike approach that we have used over the past few years.

ACKNOWLEDGMENTS

The authors thank Ms Maggie Beatka and Dr Hui Meng for their artwork in the design of **Fig. 1**. Electron microscopy images were obtained at the Medical College of Wisconsin's Electron Microscopy Core Facility. This work was supported by grants from the Children's Hospital of Wisconsin Research Institute and the Clinical and Translational Science Institute of Southeastern Wisconsin (through funding provided by NCATS 8UL1 TR000055).

REFERENCES

1. Chinnery PF. Mitochondrial disorders overview. In: Pagon RA, Adam MP, Ardinger HH, et al, editors. GeneReviews. Seattle (WA): University of Washington, Seattle; 1993–2016.
2. Parikh S, Goldstein A, Koenig MK, et al. Practice patterns of mitochondrial disease physicians in North America. Part 1: diagnostic and clinical challenges. Mitochondrion 2014;14(1):26–33.
3. Gorman GS, Schaefer AM, Ng Y, et al. Prevalence of nuclear and mitochondrial DNA mutations related to adult mitochondrial disease. Ann Neurol 2015;77(5): 753–9.
4. Thorburn DR, Rahman S. Mitochondrial DNA-associated Leigh syndrome and NARP. In: Pagon RA, Adam MP, Ardinger HH, et al, editors. GeneReviews. Seattle (WA): University of Washington, Seattle; 1993–2016.
5. Wortmann SB, Kluijtmans LA, Rodenburg RJ, et al. 3-Methylglutaconic aciduria: lessons from 50 genes and 977 patients. J Inherit Metab Dis 2013;36(6):913–21.
6. Meyers DE, Basha HI, Koenig MK. Mitochondrial cardiomyopathy: pathophysiology, diagnosis, and management. Tex Heart Inst J 2013;40(4):385–94.
7. Gellerich FN, Mayr JA, Reuter S, et al. The problem of interlab variation in methods for mitochondrial disease diagnosis: enzymatic measurement of respiratory chain complexes. Mitochondrion 2004;4(5–6):427–39.
8. Goh V, Helbling D, Biank V, et al. Next-generation sequencing facilitates the diagnosis in a child with twinkle mutations causing cholestatic liver failure. J Pediatr Gastroenterol Nutr 2012;54(2):291–4.
9. Legati A, Reyes A, Nasca A, et al. New genes and pathomechanisms in mitochondrial disorders unraveled by NGS technologies. Biochim Biophys Acta 2016;1857(8):1326–35.
10. Kemp JP, Smith PM, Pyle A, et al. Nuclear factors involved in mitochondrial translation cause a subgroup of combined respiratory chain deficiency. Brain 2011; 134(Pt 1):183–95.
11. Gloerich J, Wevers RA, Smeitink JA, et al. Proteomics approaches to study genetic and metabolic disorders. J Proteome Res 2007;6(2):506–12.
12. Spinazzi M, Casarin A, Pertegato V, et al. Optimization of respiratory chain enzymatic assays in muscle for the diagnosis of mitochondrial disorders. Mitochondrion 2011;11(6):893–904.
13. Brand MD, Nicholls DG. Assessing mitochondrial dysfunction in cells. Biochem J 2011;435(2):297–312.
14. Bennett B, Helbling D, Meng H, et al. Potentially diagnostic electron paramagnetic resonance spectra elucidate the underlying mechanism of mitochondrial dysfunction in the deoxyguanosine kinase deficient rat model of a genetic mitochondrial DNA depletion syndrome. Free Radic Biol Med 2016;92:141–51.

Unusual Structural Autonomic Disorders Presenting in Pediatrics
Disorders Associated with Hypoventilation and Autonomic Neuropathies

Gisela Chelimsky, MD[a],*, Thomas Chelimsky, MD[b]

KEYWORDS

- Autonomic neuropathy • Fabry's disease • Familial dysautonomia • Hypoventilation
- Hereditary sensory and autonomic neuropathies

KEY POINTS

- Several disorders present with autonomic dysregulation and aberrant respiration. These include: familial dysautonomia, ROHHAD syndrome, congenital central hypoventilation, Rett syndrome and Prader Willie.
- Fabry disease is an x-linked disorder that can affect males as well as females. Pain is typically the first symptom. Fabry disease is often under diagnosed early in life and in females due to the nonspecific symptoms.
- There are 5 types of hereditary sensory and autonomic neuropathies (HSAN). HSAN II-V present in infancy or childhood and are autosomal recessive. HSAN I is autosomal dominant, with presentation mainly in adults and a few in adolescents.
- HSAN III (familial dysautonomia) affects mainly individuals of Ashkenazi or Eastern European Jewish descent. It is diagnosed by genetic testing. Early symptoms include poor feeding, oropharyngeal inoordination, decreased pain and temperature sensation, orthostatic hypotension, etc. Acquired autonomic ganglionopathies have antibodies to the ganglionic acetylcholine receptor, blocking the transmission in the sympathetic and parasympathetic branches, and present with moderate to severe orthostatic hypotension and absent axon reflexes.
- The autoimmune autonomic neuropathies affect the distal nerve endings, presenting with chronic pain starting usually in the feet. They can also develop gastrointestinal, urologic and cardiovascular symptoms.

Work partially supported by Advancing Healthier Wisconsin 5520298 grant.
Disclosures: T. Chelimsky is on the Advisory Board for Lundbeck and Ironwood (2014) Pharmaceutical.
[a] Division of Pediatric Gastroenterology, Department of Pediatrics, Medical College of Wisconsin, 8701 Watertown Plank Road, Milwaukee, WI 53226, USA; [b] Department of Neurology, Medical College of Wisconsin, 8701 Watertown Plank Road, Milwaukee, WI 53226, USA
* Corresponding author.
E-mail address: gchelimsky@mcw.edu

Structural autonomic disorders (producing structural damage to the autonomic nervous system or autonomic centers) are far less common than functional autonomic disorders (reflected in abnormal function of a fundamentally normal autonomic nervous system) in children and teenagers. This article focuses on this uncommon first group in the pediatric clinic. These disorders are grouped into 2 main categories: those characterized by hypoventilation and those that feature an autonomic neuropathy.

DISORDERS OF HYPOVENTILATION AND AUTONOMIC DYSREGULATION

Several disorders harbor both aberrant respiratory control and autonomic regulation, including familial dysautonomia (FD), rapid onset obesity with hypothalamic dysfunction, hypoventilation, and autonomic dysregulation (ROHHAD) syndrome, congenital central hypoventilation syndrome (CCHS), Rett syndrome, and Prader-Willi syndrome (PWS).[1] Two disorders present very early in life, CCHS and ROHHAD syndrome. The first is fairly well understood, most often due to a specific genetic mutation, whereas ROHHAD is currently diagnosed based on clinical presentation, with no clearly established pathophysiology. This article also briefly covers Rett syndrome and PWS to aid with the consideration of differential diagnosis (**Table 1**). Because an autonomic neuropathy dominates the pathophysiology of FD, it will be discussed in the second group.

Congenital Central Hypoventilation Syndrome

CCHS is a rare neurocristopathy that presents with impaired respiratory control, dysautonomia, sometimes neuroblastoma, and Hirschsprung disease.[2,3] The number of triplet repeats in the genetic mutation in large part dictates the severity of the presentation, which varies from the newborn period (severe cases) to later in life (even fifth and sixth decades). Impaired control of breathing owing to impaired responsiveness to CO_2, the biggest clinical threat in CCHS, may range from shallow breathing during sleep only to respiratory problems during both wakefulness and sleep.[3] The most common mutation affects the $PHOX_2B$ gene, which controls neuronal differentiation early in pregnancy and is strongly expressed in the retrotrapezoid nucleus, a key structure for respiratory control. $PHOX_2B$ is also expressed in other areas of the

Table 1
Summary of findings and onset of obesity, respiratory symptoms in different diagnoses with hypoventilation

	CCHS	ROHHAD	Rett Syndrome	PWS
Usual onset of disease	Usually birth, but can be later	~1.5–9 y	6–18 mo	At birth
Onset of breathing disorder	Birth	Variable	3–5 y of age	After 1 y of age
Obesity	No	Yes	No	Yes, starts between 12 mo and 6 y of age
Genetic mutation	$PHOX_2B$	Unknown	MECP2	Mutation in chromosome 15
Autonomic disorder	Fainting, ↓HF-HRV, OH	↑LF and LF/HF		↓LF meal response

neuraxis involved in breathing, such as the geniculate, petrosal, and nodose sensory ganglia and the nucleus of the solitary tract.[2]

The normal PHOX$_2$B gene contains 20 alanine repeats. About 90% of CCHS mutations are heterozygous for an expansion of alanine repeats.[3] The shortest alanine expansion of +5 has an incomplete penetrance for the respiratory issues, and no increased risk for neuroblastoma or Hirschsprung disease. These patients, when asymptomatic, may be at risk for respiratory decompensation when under stressful conditions, such as respiratory infections or anesthesia. Those with larger alanine expansions of +6 and more have abnormal control of breathing. These patients have moderate risk for Hirschsprung disease, and those with +7 are at high risk. Genotype also dictates the requirement for ventilator dependence.

Interestingly, neuroblastoma usually does not occur in these subjects. Tumors like ganglioneuromas and ganglioneuroblastomas, and less commonly neuroblastoma, develop in a small minority of subjects with CCHS and the longest polyalanine repeat expansion mutations. Neuroblastoma typically occurs in 8% of cases of CCHS due to nonalanine expansion mutations. These subjects are also at high risk for Hirschsprung disease[2] and have a generally worse clinical picture.[3]

Subjects with CCHS also manifest cardiac arrhythmias, with severity again directly correlating with the length of the polyalanine repeat expansion,[2] including sinus bradycardias, sinus pauses, and premature atrial and ventricular beats.[4] These subjects also have recurrent episodes of fainting, cor pulmonale/pulmonary hypertension, decreased heart rate variability (HRV), dizziness, and lack of nocturnal blood pressure dipping, and about 7% have orthostatic hypotension.[5]

Rapid Onset Obesity with Hypothalamic Dysfunction, Hypoventilation and Autonomic Dysregulation Syndrome

ROHHAD syndrome is characterized by rapid weight gain that starts between the ages of 1.5 and 9 years of age along with hypothalamic or hypophyseal dysfunction, with normal growth, development, and general health before to the onset of symptoms. Features may include hypernatremia with or without diabetes insipidus, growth hormone deficiency, hyperprolactinemia, hypothyroidism, adrenal dysfunction, and pubertal, behavioral, and developmental issues, which may be followed later by onset of alveolar hypoventilation[6–8] or obstructive sleep apnea. The breathing abnormalities can also develop before the onset of obesity.[9] Less than 100 cases have been reported.[8]

The cause of this disorder is still unclear. It usually presents later than CCHS, and obvious candidate genetic mutations, such as PHOX$_2$B, TRKB, and brain-derived neurotrophic factor (BDNF), are normal.[7] Furthermore, the evaluation for PWS[8] is also negative. So far, no genetic mutation accounts for the ROHHAD syndrome.[10]

Current theory postulates a paraneoplastic syndrome or an autoimmune disorder secondary to a neural crest tumor, perhaps in the context of a genetic predisposition. In one series, about 40% of the children with ROHHADs were found to have tumor of neural crest origin, but surgery to remove the tumor does not improve outcome.[11] Given the high frequency (HF) of the neural crest tumors, Bougneres and colleagues[12] proposed the acronym of ROHHADNET, which stands for *R*apid onset *O*besity, *H*ypoventilation, *H*ypothalamic and *A*utonomic *D*ysfunction, *NE*ural *T*umor.

Rett Syndrome

Rett syndrome is a disorder that affects mainly girls. In most cases, these children seem to be developing normally until the age of 6 to 18 months, before they start losing milestones in language, social skills, and cognitive areas with autistic-like behavior with stereotypic hand movement. Many children will also develop seizures, gastrointestinal issues, motor impairment, and a breathing disorder. The diagnosis of Rett syndrome is made mainly based on clinical features. A large deletion of the MECP2 gene typically causes Rett syndrome. The severity of the disease may relate to the associated BDNF polymorphisms, as the BDNF gene is regulated by MECP2.[13,14] Many MECP2 mutation types exist, probably accounting for the many phenotypes. The MECP2 gene occurs in all human tissues and more predominant in the brain, where it appears to regulate maturation and survival of neurons,[15] dendritic growth, and development of synapses.[16]

Subjects with Rett syndrome have prolonged QTc in about 30% to 55% of cases, with an increase in sympathetic tone.[16] Sympathetic tone, as measured by low-frequency (LF) heart rate variability (HRV) as well as the ratio of LF to parasympathetic HF HRV (LF/HF), correlated with leptin plasma levels, which are abnormally independent of body fat.[17,18] However, the cardiovascular response to active orthostatic challenge is not compromised in subjects with Rett syndrome.[19]

The breathing disorder starts with irregular respiration around ages 2 to 5 years. Breath-holding spells may be frequent, without following a specific pattern. Interestingly, the heart rate in subjects with Rett syndrome goes up during breath holding in contrast to healthy controls, in whom the heart rate changes little[20] during voluntary breath holding. Nocturnal changes are less prominent than those during the day and include tachypnea, erratic breathing, and heart rate dysregulation.[15] The uncoupling of respiratory and heart rate control has been taken as evidence of autonomic dyregulation.[21]

Subjects with Rett syndrome can manifest a large variety of movement disorders, epileptic and nonepileptic events, and aberrant breathing. Long-term video-polygraphic monitoring may improve the understanding of the diagnosis and underlying mechanism of the episodes.[22]

Prader-Willi Syndrome

PWS results from loss of expression of the paternally expressed genes from the 15q11-q13 region.[23] The phenotype of this disorder changes over time. Subjects present at birth with hypotonia, feeding difficulties that improve over time, characteristic facial features, hypogonadism, and dolichocephaly.[24] The short stature typically appears after 2 years and is due to growth hormone deficiency.[24] Hyperphagia with consequent weight gain develops between 1 and 6 years of age,[25] with daytime sleepiness, resembling idiopathic hypersomnolence,[26] perhaps related to obesity with obstructive apnea among several factors.[24] The orexin system, implicated in sleep, sustained wakefulness, and feeding behavior,[27] seems involved in subjects with PWS. Fourteen subjects with PWS had a moderate decrease in cerebral spinal fluid orexin levels, higher than in subjects with narcolepsy, but lower than in subject with idiopathic hypersomnia.[26] In the subjects with PWS, the level of orexin was negatively correlated with daytime sleepiness. Decreased orexin levels do not explain the obesity.[26]

Breathing abnormalities in PWS may begin at the age of 1 year,[28] related to respiratory muscle weakness, abnormal craniofacial features, and hypertrophy of the adenoids and tonsils. Some of these factors, along with obesity, contribute to obstructive apnea, but central apnea is also present in the younger subjects as well as other evidence of disordered central breathing control, such as an abnormal response to hypoxia and hypercapnia.[29] However, the increased sleep arousal threshold to hypercapnia may be due to abnormal peripheral chemoreceptor function and may contribute further to sleep-disordered breathing in PWS patients.[30] These changes probably constitute a subset of broader central autonomic dysregulation seen in decreased vagal tone independent of body mass.[31] When evaluating autonomic response to meals, subjects with PWS only showed a decreased LF-HRV response when compared with lean and obese controls, with no difference in the HF-HRV (vagal component) and the ratio of LF/HF.[32]

AUTONOMIC NEUROPATHIES
Hereditary Autonomic Neuropathies

Fabry disease

Fabry disease is an X-linked lysosomal storage inborn error of metabolism caused by a deficiency of the α-galactosidase A enzyme. Although classically thought to affect only men and boys, as for most X-linked disorders, women and girls may also be affected. Symptoms usually start in childhood, although the disease may start at birth or even in utero, and is often diagnosed later in life due to the variable phenotype.[33,34] Female manifestations range from asymptomatic to the severe disease seen in boys and men,[35] presumably due to lionization of the X chromosome.

The absence or decrease in amount of the α-galactosidase A enzyme results in an accumulation of globotriaosylceramide (GL-3) and other related glycosphingolipids in the lysosomes of endothelial cells, kidneys, heart, and nerve cells.[34]

Boys usually develop symptoms between the ages of 3 and 10 years, whereas girls may begin at any time of life into late adulthood or never. Pain is typically the earliest symptom. Two types of pain occur, a chronic burning and paresthesias sometimes associated with reduced ability to sense cold temperature[34,36] and an acute form labeled "Fabry crisis," with severe burning starting in the extremities and radiating proximally.[34] The accumulation of GL-3 may damage nerves by interfering with protein synthesis and perhaps affect ion channels. GL-3 accumulates in skin endothelium, smooth muscle, endoneural and perineural vessels and cells, axons, and blood vessels of the DRG. GL-3 also accumulates where the blood-brain barrier is more permeable, such as the preoptic, supraoptic, and preoptic hypothalamus nuclei and the dorsal nucleus of the vagus. Pain may improve over time because of permanent nerve damage, associated with reduced pain sensation and numbness.[36] Nerve damage affecting autonomic small fibers may lead to gastrointestinal, vasomotor, decreased pupillary constriction, decreased saliva, sweat, and tear production, and Raynaud phenomenon.[34,36] The neuropathy is length dependent; therefore, the symptoms usually start in the hands and feet.[36] Initially, the subjects have altered cold sensation, suggesting involvement of the A delta fibers.[37]

In children, the gastrointestinal symptoms, common in both female and male children,[38] usually include postprandial abdominal pain, early satiety, nausea and vomiting, and diarrhea. Hypohidrosis typically manifests as heat intolerance. Other classical complaints include fatigue, inability to gain weight, skin lesions (angiokeratomas), corneal changes, tinnitus, and hearing loss. In the teens, cardiac changes may appear with arrhythmias and a short PR interval. Kidney involvement begins in the teens as microalbuminuria and proteinuria.[34]

It is important to underscore that often Fabry disease is underdiagnosed early in life because of the nonspecific symptoms. On average, symptoms (by recall) start at age 9 in boys and age 13 in girls, with a median age of about 11 years before the diagnosis is made.[39] Therefore, pediatricians and gastroenterologists need to recognize that gastrointestinal symptoms, such as bloating, nausea, vomiting, episodic diarrhea, periumbilical abdominal pain, and constipation, may be the only symptom for many years. With normal endoscopies and colonoscopies, they may be considered a functional gastrointestinal disorder or otherwise misdiagnosed. The pathophysiology of the gastrointestinal symptoms is probably secondary to involvement of the autonomic nerves and subsequent development of a motility disorder. Small bowel bacterial overgrowth may occur because of dysmotility.

When attempting to obtain a diagnosis, it is important to use alpha-galactosidase enzyme levels as a screen only and to confirm the diagnosis with genetic testing. Some alleles may reduce the alpha-galactosidase content measured in blood, despite normal intracellular enzyme quantity and function. The authors recently reported such a case[40] based on one of these known nonpathogenic mutations.[41]

Hereditary sensory and autonomic neuropathies

Hereditary sensory and autonomic neuropathies (HSAN) include 5 types, HSAN I–V. HSAN II–V present in infancy or childhood and are autosomal recessive. HSAN I is autosomal dominant and has 6 responsible genes, but only 2 may present during adolescence with the remainder starting in adulthood.[42] This article focuses on HSAN II–V. HSAN III is also called FD and is discussed later. HSAN II–IV have complete penetrance but variable phenotypic expression. Although the disease starts in utero, the diagnosis may be delayed. Except for some cases of HSAN II, nearly all of these subjects have absent axon flare in response to intradermal histamine injection, which tests an axon reflex of C-fiber afferent fibers. Patients with HSAN V have preservation of this histamine flare response.[43]

HSAN II subjects present early in life. The disease is not progressive. Subjects have hypotonia, and sensory loss, which produces feeding difficulties, gastroesophageal reflux, and the development of injuries that go unrecognized because of the sensory deficit. Self-mutilation also occurs. Subjects usually have normal muscle mass.[43] So far, HSAN II has been associated with mutations in the HSN21WNK1, FAM134B, and KIF1A genes in adulthood.[42]

HSAN IV, also called congenital insensitivity to pain with anhidrosis, is due to a mutation in the NTRK1 gene.[42] Patients present with anhidrosis of the trunk and upper extremities, mental retardation, and decreased pain sensation. Autonomic nervous system involvement seems restricted to sweating; therefore, hypotension is not common. Other issues include thick palm skin, abnormal nails, and poor healing of ectodermal structures such as bone fractures.[43] Given the poor explanation of the injuries, occasionally these children may present with concerns of abuse.[44]

HSAN V has only loss of pain sensation, but the rest of the sensory responses are normal. Subjects have normal sweating and normal development.[42]

HSAN III or familial dysautonomia Also called Riley-Day syndrome and autonomic neuropathy type III, this autosomal recessive disorder affects primarily individuals of Ashkenazi or Eastern European Jewish descent. A chromosome 9q31 mutation distorts protein IKAP (elongator-1 protein) involved in myelination and neuronal development during embryogenesis. Although 3 mutations have been identified, a single mutation accounts for nearly all cases of FD. IKAP deficiency affects mainly sensory and autonomic functions,[45] and the affected individuals have significant autonomic cardiovascular, respiratory, pain, and temperature involvement as well as swallowing and gait problems.[46] Subjects with FD have abnormal brainstem reflexes with involvement of both peripheral and central neurons.[47] Although FD is present at birth with full penetrance, the phenotype is variable.[48]

Once made clinically, the diagnosis of FD now requires genetic testing. Patients may present in the neonatal period with poor feeding or increased caloric demand.

They may also have oropharyngeal incoordination with increased drooling and increased risk of aspiration pneumonias.[45] The feeding difficulties and aspiration are due to involvement of the brainstem reflexes needed to perform those functions.[48] FD children also have gastroesophageal reflux disease. Other features include absent emotional overflow tears, decreased pain and temperature perception, and decreased or absent tendon reflexes. Muscle tone is also decreased, and children have motor delays and learning disabilities.[45]

Autonomic nervous system involvement leads to orthostatic hypotension with unstable blood pressure and abnormal control of breathing with decreased CO_2 sensitivity and risk of apnea and death.[49] The respiratory sinus arrhythmia, a measurement of parasympathetic tone and cardiorespiratory coupling, is also decreased in FD subjects.[1] Afferent small sensory nerve involvement affects both the baroreflex and the chemoreflex feedback loops. Baroreflex impairment leads to common hypertensive episodes with everyday activity, starting in infancy, and is associated with increased sweating and blotching of the skin.[48] Cardiorespiratory dysregulation produces frequent episodes of labile heart rate, with higher rates paradoxically associated with higher blood pressures owing to the impaired baroreflex. These episodes may become "sympathetic storms" often triggered by stress, consisting of profound hypertension, diaphoresis, increased heart rate, piloerection, ileus, vomiting, and so forth. Constipation can also trigger these crises,[45] which can be managed in a similar way to autonomic dysreflexia in patients who have a spinal cord injury. The kidneys may also be involved in FD, with chronic renal failure, renal tubular acidosis, and hyperkalemia.[48]

Acquired Autonomic Ganglioneuropathies

Although less common in pediatrics, acquired neuropathies do occur and should be considered in the differential diagnosis. Here, acquired neuropathies seen more often in clinical pediatric practice are described. Clinical manifestations of autonomic diabetic neuropathy are uncommon in pediatrics, although the cardiovascular changes may develop early after diagnosis.[50,51]

Acquired ganglioneuropathies are divided into ganglionopathies affecting the proximal ganglion, either sensory or autonomic, and the more traditional neuropathies affecting the distal end of the axon, although some disorders, such as diabetes and Sjogren, may produce both simultaneously, are then termed a ganglioneuropathy.

Acquired sensory ganglionopathies

Also termed sensory neuronopathies, these disorders do not involve motor function, and therefore, do not truly belong under the classification of autonomic neuropathies, which are by definition, motor. They are discussed here for completeness and because they are part of the larger class of neuropathies involving small fibers. They are characterized by damage to the sensory (afferent) neurons of the dorsal root and the trigeminal ganglia. Dorsal root ganglia (DRG) are vulnerable to immune disorders because they are in close proximity to the border zone gap between oligodendroglia, which line nerves in the central nervous system, and Schwann cells, which take over in the peripheral nervous system. This gap provides greater than usual exposure of axons and nerve cell bodies to the immune system. The DRG contains myelinated and unmyelinated C fibers, which transmit pain and thermal sensation. These neuropathies typically present in a patchy (non-length-dependent) distribution because the abnormality occurs at the root level, not the distal nerve ending, the other major zone where axons are exposed to the immune system. Damage to the small fibers presents as patchy areas of severe pain, usually described as burning or aching and numbness, which can be located in the extremities, face, trunk, or scalp.[52,53] Many disorders can cause these acquired neuronopathies, including diabetes and glucose intolerance (more so in adults), infections, toxins, and immune processes, such as Sjogren disease.[54,55] In about half of the cases, the cause cannot be identified. Large myelinated fiber involvement will lead to additional symptoms and findings reflecting loss of proprioception and tactile sensation with gait and limb ataxia.

Acquired autonomic ganglionopathies

An antibody to the ganglionic acetylcholine receptor (AChR) may develop, blocking transmission across the autonomic ganglion in both the parasympathetic and the sympathetic branches. Patients typically present with moderate to severe orthostatic hypotension and have absent axon reflex responses on autonomic testing, because the axon reflex requires a functioning AChR receptor. When comparing patients with presumed auto-immune autonomic neuropathy associated with other causes (based on a postinfectious story) and patients with high AchR autoantibodies ($\geq$1.00 nmol/L), the latter have more cholinergic abnormalities, such as abnormal pupillary responses, sicca syndrome, and gastrointestinal symptoms.[56,57] Patients generally report an infection, usually viral, preceding the onset of the disease, with a subacute course. Chronic autoimmune autonomic neuropathy may also occur with lower AChR autoantibody levels, an insidious onset, and little cholinergic abnormality.[57]

Autoimmune autonomic neuropathies

In these disorders, the abnormality is located at the distal nerve ending and the symptoms reflect this pathologic process by being primarily distal, rather than patchy, as occurs in the ganglionopathies. Thus, these neuropathies present with chronic pain that usually begins in the feet and can have associated gastrointestinal, cardiovascular, and urologic symptoms, because these organs are also quite distal. The most common causes include diabetes (mainly in adults), Sjogren syndrome, celiac disease, and toxic or metabolic causes, with mitochondrial disorders producing a significant subset of this last group.[58] The idiopathic autonomic neuropathies typically do not have autoimmune or serologic markers.

In all of these disorders, diagnosis may require autonomic testing with evaluation of the sudomotor response, thermoregulatory sweat test, skin biopsies to evaluate epidermal nerve fiber density, and possibly surgical biopsies of sensory nerves (sural),[59,60] along with specific immunologic, metabolic, or genetic testing to establish a definitive cause.

REFERENCES

1. Carroll MS, Kenny AS, Patwari PP, et al. Respiratory and cardiovascular indicators of autonomic nervous system dysregulation in familial dysautonomia. Pediatr Pulmonol 2012;47(7):682–91.

2. Trang H, Brunet JF, Rohrer H, et al. Proceedings of the fourth international conference on central hypoventilation. Orphanet J Rare Dis 2014;9:194.

3. Rand CM, Carroll MS, Weese-Mayer DE. Congenital central hypoventilation syndrome: a neurocristopathy with disordered respiratory control and autonomic regulation. Clin Chest Med 2014;35(3):535–45.

4. Silvestri JM, Hanna BD, Volgman AS, et al. Cardiac rhythm disturbances among children with idiopathic congenital central hypoventilation syndrome. Pediatr Pulmonol 2000;29(5):351–8.

5. Movahed MR, Jalili M, Kiciman N. Cardiovascular abnormalities and arrhythmias in patients with Ondine's curse (congenital central hypoventilation) syndrome. Pacing Clin Electrophysiol 2005;28(11):1226–30.

6. Thaker VV, Esteves KM, Towne MC, et al. Whole exome sequencing identifies RAI1 mutation in a morbidly obese child diagnosed with ROHHAD syndrome. J Clin Endocrinol Metab 2015;100(5):1723–30.

7. Ize-Ludlow D, Gray JA, Sperling MA, et al. Rapid-onset obesity with hypothalamic dysfunction, hypoventilation, and autonomic dysregulation presenting in childhood. Pediatrics 2007;120(1):e179–88.

8. Cemeroglu AP, Coulas T, Kleis L. Spectrum of clinical presentations and endocrinological findings of patients with septo-optic dysplasia: a retrospective study. J Pediatr Endocrinol Metab 2015;28(9–10):1057–63.

9. Patwari PP, Wolfe LF. Rapid-onset obesity with hypothalamic dysfunction, hypoventilation, and autonomic dysregulation: review and update. Curr Opin Pediatr 2014;26(4):487–92.

10. Barclay SF, Rand CM, Borch LA, et al. Rapid-onset obesity with hypothalamic dysfunction, hypoventilation, and autonomic dysregulation (ROHHAD): exome sequencing of trios, monozygotic twins and tumours. Orphanet J Rare Dis 2015;10:103.

11. De Pontual L, Trochet D, Caillat-Zucman S, et al. Delineation of late onset hypoventilation associated with hypothalamic dysfunction syndrome. Pediatr Res 2008;64(6):689–94.

12. Bougneres P, Pantalone L, Linglart A, et al. Endocrine manifestations of the rapid-onset obesity with hypoventilation, hypothalamic, autonomic dysregulation, and neural tumor syndrome in childhood. J Clin Endocrinol Metab 2008;93(10): 3971–80.

13. Johnson CM, Cui N, Zhong W, et al. Breathing abnormalities in a female mouse model of Rett syndrome. J Physiol Sci 2015;65(5):451–9.

14. Glaze DG. Rett syndrome: of girls and mice–lessons for regression in autism. Ment Retard Dev Disabil Res Rev 2004;10(2):154–8.

15. Gallego J. Genetic diseases: congenital central hypoventilation, Rett, and Prader-Willi syndromes. Compr Physiol 2012;2(3):2255–79.

16. Lioy DT, Wu WW, Bissonnette JM. Autonomic dysfunction with mutations in the gene that encodes methyl-CpG-binding protein 2: insights into Rett syndrome. Auton Neurosci 2011;161(1–2):55–62.

17. Blardi P, de Lalla A, D'Ambrogio T, et al. Rett syndrome and plasma leptin levels. J Pediatr 2007;150(1):37–9.

18. Acampa M, Guideri F, Hayek J, et al. Sympathetic overactivity and plasma leptin levels in Rett syndrome. Neurosci Lett 2008;432(1):69–72.

19. Larsson G, Julu PO, Witt Engerstrom I, et al. Normal reactions to orthostatic stress in Rett syndrome. Res Dev Disabil 2013;34(6):1897–905.

20. Weese-Mayer DE, Lieske SP, Boothby CM, et al. Autonomic nervous system dysregulation: breathing and heart rate perturbation during wakefulness in young girls with Rett syndrome. Pediatr Res 2006;60(4):443–9.

21. Weese-Mayer DE, Lieske SP, Boothby CM, et al. Autonomic dysregulation in young girls with Rett syndrome during nighttime in-home recordings. Pediatr Pulmonol 2008;43(11):1045–60.

22. d'Orsi G, Trivisano M, Luisi C, et al. Epileptic seizures, movement disorders, and breathing disturbances in Rett syndrome: diagnostic relevance of video-polygraphy. Epilepsy Behav 2012;25(3):401–7.

23. Cassidy SB, Dykens E, Williams CA. Prader-Willi and Angelman syndromes: sister imprinted disorders. Am J Med Genet 2000;97(2):136–46.
24. Hurren BJ, Flack NA. Prader-Willi syndrome: a spectrum of anatomical and clinical features. Clin Anat 2016;29(5):590–605.
25. Holm VA, Cassidy SB, Butler MG, et al. Prader-Willi syndrome: consensus diagnostic criteria. Pediatrics 1993;91(2):398–402.
26. Omokawa M, Ayabe T, Nagai T, et al. Decline of CSF orexin (hypocretin) levels in Prader-Willi syndrome. Am J Med Genet A 2016;170(5):1181–6.
27. Tsujino N, Sakurai T. Orexin/hypocretin: a neuropeptide at the interface of sleep, energy homeostasis, and reward system. Pharmacol Rev 2009;61(2):162–76.
28. Williams K, Scheimann A, Sutton V, et al. Sleepiness and sleep disordered breathing in Prader-Willi syndrome: relationship to genotype, growth hormone therapy, and body composition. J Clin Sleep Med 2008;4(2):111–8.
29. Beauloye V, Dhondt K, Buysse W, et al. Evaluation of the hypothalamic-pituitary-adrenal axis and its relationship with central respiratory dysfunction in children with Prader-Willi syndrome. Orphanet J Rare Dis 2015;10:106.
30. Livingston FR, Arens R, Bailey SL, et al. Hypercapnic arousal responses in Prader-Willi syndrome. Chest 1995;108(6):1627–31.
31. DiMario FJ Jr, Bauer L, Volpe J, et al. Respiratory sinus arrhythmia in patients with Prader-Willi syndrome. J Child Neurol 1996;11(2):121–5.
32. Purtell L, Jenkins A, Viardot A, et al. Postprandial cardiac autonomic function in Prader-Willi syndrome. Clin Endocrinol (Oxf) 2013;79(1):128–33.
33. Ries M, Clarke JT, Whybra C, et al. Enzyme-replacement therapy with agalsidase alfa in children with Fabry disease. Pediatrics 2006;118(3):924–32.
34. Germain DP. Fabry disease. Orphanet J Rare Dis 2010;5:30.
35. Germain DP, Benistan K, Angelova L. X-linked inheritance and its implication in the diagnosis and management of female patients in Fabry disease. Rev Med Interne 2010;31(Suppl 2):S209–13.
36. Burlina AP, Sims KB, Politei JM, et al. Early diagnosis of peripheral nervous system involvement in Fabry disease and treatment of neuropathic pain: the report of an expert panel. BMC Neurol 2011;11:61.
37. Hilz MJ. Peripheral nervous system involvement in Fabry disease: role in morbidity and mortality. Clin Ther 2007;29(Suppl A):S11–2.
38. Politei J, Thurberg BL, Wallace E, et al. Gastrointestinal involvement in Fabry disease. So important, yet often neglected. Clin Genet 2016;89(1):5–9.
39. Wilcox WR, Oliveira JP, Hopkin RJ, et al. Females with Fabry disease frequently have major organ involvement: lessons from the Fabry Registry. Mol Genet Metab 2008;93(2):112–28.
40. Farooq SH, Hiner BC, Rhead C, et al. Characteristic pulvinar sign in pseudo-α-galactosidase deficiency syndrome. JAMA Neurol 2016;73(8):1020–1.
41. Yasuda M, Shabbeer J, Benson SD, et al. Fabry disease: characterization of alpha-galactosidase A double mutations and the D313Y plasma enzyme pseudo-deficiency allele. Hum Mutat 2003;22(6):486–92.
42. Auer-Grumbach M. Hereditary sensory and autonomic neuropathies. Handb Clin Neurol 2013;115:893–906.
43. Axelrod FB, Gold-von Simson G. Hereditary sensory and autonomic neuropathies: types II, III, and IV. Orphanet J Rare Dis 2007;2:39.
44. van den Bosch GE, Baartmans MG, Vos P, et al. Pain insensitivity syndrome misinterpreted as inflicted burns. Pediatrics 2014;133(5):e1381–7.
45. Gold-von Simson G, Axelrod FB. Familial dysautonomia: update and recent advances. Curr Probl Pediatr Adolesc Health Care 2006;36(6):218–37.

46. Norcliffe-Kaufmann L, Kaufmann H. Familial dysautonomia (Riley-Day syndrome): when baroreceptor feedback fails. Auton Neurosci 2012;172(1–2):26–30.
47. Gutierrez JV, Norcliffe-Kaufmann L, Kaufmann H. Brainstem reflexes in patients with familial dysautonomia. Clin Neurophysiol 2015;126(3):626–33.
48. Palma JA, Norcliffe-Kaufmann L, Fuente-Mora C, et al. Current treatments in familial dysautonomia. Expert Opin Pharmacother 2014;15(18):2653–71.
49. Maayan HC. Respiratory aspects of Riley-Day syndrome: familial dysautonomia. Paediatr Respir Rev 2006;7(Suppl 1):S258–9.
50. Karavanaki K, Baum JD. Coexistence of impaired indices of autonomic neuropathy and diabetic nephropathy in a cohort of children with type 1 diabetes mellitus. J Pediatr Endocrinol Metab 2003;16(1):79–90.
51. Verrotti A, Loiacono G, Mohn A, et al. New insights in diabetic autonomic neuropathy in children and adolescents. Eur J Endocrinol 2009;161(6):811–8.
52. Sheikh SI, Amato AA. The dorsal root ganglion under attack: the acquired sensory ganglionopathies. Pract Neurol 2010;10(6):326–34.
53. Dineen J, Freeman R. Autonomic neuropathy. Semin Neurol 2015;35(4):458–68.
54. Gorson KC, Herrmann DN, Thiagarajan R, et al. Non-length dependent small fibre neuropathy/ganglionopathy. J Neurol Neurosurg Psychiatry 2008;79(2):163–9.
55. Kuntzer T, Antoine JC, Steck AJ. Clinical features and pathophysiological basis of sensory neuronopathies (ganglionopathies). Muscle Nerve 2004;30(3):255–68.
56. Sandroni P, Vernino S, Klein CM, et al. Idiopathic autonomic neuropathy: comparison of cases seropositive and seronegative for ganglionic acetylcholine receptor antibody. Arch Neurol 2004;61(1):44–8.
57. Klein CM, Vernino S, Lennon VA, et al. The spectrum of autoimmune autonomic neuropathies. Ann Neurol 2003;53(6):752–8.
58. Luigetti M, Sauchelli D, Primiano G, et al. Peripheral neuropathy is a common manifestation of mitochondrial diseases: a single-centre experience. Eur J Neurol 2016;23(6):1020–7.
59. Vinik AI, Nevoret ML, Casellini C. The new age of sudomotor function testing: a sensitive and specific biomarker for diagnosis, estimation of severity, monitoring progression, and regression in response to intervention. Front Endocrinol (Lausanne) 2015;6:94.
60. Vernino S, Low PA, Fealey RD, et al. Autoantibodies to ganglionic acetylcholine receptors in autoimmune autonomic neuropathies. N Engl J Med 2000;343(12):847–55.

Usual and Unusual Manifestations of Systemic and Central Nervous System Vasculitis

James J. Nocton, MD

KEYWORDS

- Vasculitis • Pediatrics • Arteritis

KEY POINTS

- Diagnosis of vasculitis requires understanding and recognition of the clinical manifestations associated with each disease.
- The different vasculitides can be distinguished clinically, histologically, and with laboratory testing and imaging studies.
- Although there are common clinical patterns for each vasculitis, there are additional unusual clinical manifestations associated with these illnesses.
- Infectious, congenital, genetic, and metabolic diseases may mimic vasculitis.

INTRODUCTION

The idiopathic vasculitides are a complex group of immune-mediated illnesses that share blood vessel inflammation as the common primary feature.[1,2] These illnesses characteristically affect multiple organ systems, may present acutely or indolently, have overlapping clinical signs and symptoms, may mimic infectious illnesses and other systemic diseases, and respond variably to immunosuppressive and antiinflammatory treatment. Therefore, the vasculitides are frequently challenging to both diagnose and manage.[1] With the understanding that all of the forms of vasculitis in children are uncommon, this article discusses the primary pediatric vasculitides that pediatricians might encounter. Both characteristic and unusual manifestations are discussed.

DEFINITION AND CLASSIFICATION

There have been multiple attempts to define and classify the idiopathic vasculitides.[3–9] Vasculitis may be specified and organized based on the type of vessels affected, the

Disclosure: The author has nothing to disclose.
Department of Pediatrics, Medical College of Wisconsin, Children's Hospital of Wisconsin, 999 North 92nd Street, Suite C465, Milwaukee, WI 53226, USA
E-mail address: jnocton@mcw.edu

Pediatr Clin N Am 64 (2017) 185–204
http://dx.doi.org/10.1016/j.pcl.2016.08.013
0031-3955/17/© 2016 Elsevier Inc. All rights reserved.

pediatric.theclinics.com

size of vessels affected, the histopathology, or the presence of specific laboratory findings (eg, antineutrophil cytoplasmic antibodies [ANCA]). The American College of Rheumatology developed classification criteria for several types of vasculitis in adults in 1990.[4,5] Subsequently, consensus criteria for adult patients known as the Chapel Hill criteria were developed in 1994,[10] adopting a classification scheme primarily based on vessel size, which were revised most recently in 2012[3] (**Box 1**). In 2005, the Pediatric Rheumatology European Society (PRES) developed a classification scheme and classification criteria specifically for pediatric vasculitis.[6] This group also adopted a classification based on vessel size (**Box 2**). In 2008, the criteria for some of the most common pediatric vasculitides (Henoch-Schönlein purpura [HSP], granulomatosis with polyangiitis [GPA], polyarteritis nodosa [PAN], and Takayasu arteritis) were subsequently revised and validated with support from the Pediatric Rheumatology International Trials Organization (PRINTO)[7,8] (**Box 3**). Each of these attempts to organize, define, and classify these illnesses will remain imperfect and a work in progress until the specific causes, and perhaps the potential genetic associations, of the different vasculitides are fully understood.

DIAGNOSIS

The most common pediatric vasculitides, such as Kawasaki disease and HSP, present acutely with characteristic clinical manifestations and are not associated with specific diagnostic laboratory tests. The diagnosis therefore is most often based on clinical features alone. For the other idiopathic vasculitides, in addition to recognizing a pattern of clinical and consistent laboratory findings, the diagnosis also requires the identification of characteristic imaging findings, histopathology, or both. The ANCA-associated vasculitides are an exception, because these diagnoses may be made with reasonable certainty in the presence of characteristic clinical findings and a positive test for ANCA. The classification criteria developed for adults[3] and children[8] may be helpful when considering a diagnosis of vasculitis by allowing clinicians to match the features of an individual patient to the usual manifestations of the disease. However, it is important to recognize that classification criteria are generally based on typical and common manifestations of diseases, and strictly adhering to such criteria may, at times, result in diagnostic error or delay when some manifestations do not seem to fit the typical pattern.

A thorough history and physical examination are of paramount importance in helping to guide diagnostic testing. It is most helpful to carefully define the timing of onset of symptoms, the specific body or organ systems affected, and the severity of the systems. Many of the systemic vasculitides are associated with nonspecific constitutional symptoms, such as fever, fatigue, malaise, poor appetite, and weight loss, which may dominate the patient's and family's concerns, resulting in decreased awareness of the significance of additional symptoms and signs. A comprehensive review of systems should be performed with attention to even the most seemingly innocuous complaint. A review of medications, past history, family, and social history may provide clues to a specific diagnosis and also help to differentiate the vasculitides from infections, drug reactions, and other mimics of vasculitis (**Boxes 4–6**).[11] A careful and thorough physical examination is also essential, because there may be subtle findings that the patient and family either have not noticed or have overlooked. Particular attention to vital signs (eg, tachycardia, tachypnea, hypertension), skin findings (eg, palpable purpura, petechiae), peripheral pulses, the joint examination, and neurologic abnormalities are most helpful. Vital sign changes may be the only clue to the presence of significant heart, lung, or renal disease associated with a vasculitis.

Box 1
Classification of vasculitis in adult patients

Large vessel vasculitis

Takayasu arteritis

Giant cell arteritis

Medium vessel vasculitis

Polyarteritis nodosa (PAN)

Kawasaki disease

Small vessel vasculitis

ANCA-associated vasculitis
  Microscopic polyangiitis
  Granulomatosis with polyangiitis (GPA)
  Eosinophilic GPA

Immune complex
  Anti–glomerular basement membrane disease
  Cryoglobulinemic vasculitis
  Immunoglobulin A (IgA) vasculitis (Henoch-Schönlein purpura [HSP])
  Hypocomplementemic urticarial vasculitis

Variable vessel vasculitis

Behçet disease

Cogan syndrome

Single-organ vasculitis

Cutaneous leukocytoclastic angiitis

Cutaneous arteritis

Primary central nervous system vasculitis

Isolated aortitis

Vasculitis associated with systemic disease

Lupus vasculitis

Rheumatoid vasculitis

Sarcoid vasculitis

Vasculitis associated with probable cause

Hepatitis C virus–associated cryoglobulinemic vasculitis

Hepatitis B virus–associated vasculitis

Syphilis-associated aortitis

Drug-associated immune complex vasculitis

Drug-associated ANCA-associated vasculitis

Cancer-associated vasculitis

Adapted from Jennette JC, Falk RJ, Bacon PA, et al. 2012 revised International Chapel Hill Consensus Conference nomenclature of vasculitides. Arthritis Rheum 2013;65:5.

Box 2
Classification of pediatric vasculitis

Predominantly large vessel vasculitis

1. Takayasu arteritis

Predominantly medium-sized vessel vasculitis

1. Childhood PAN

2. Cutaneous polyarteritis

3. Kawasaki disease

Predominantly small vessels vasculitis

1. Granulomatous
   a. GPA
   b. Eosinophilic GPA

2. Nongranulomatous
   a. Microscopic polyangiitis
   b. HSP
   c. Isolated cutaneous leukocytoclastic vasculitis
   d. Hypocomplementemic urticarial vasculitis

Other vasculitides

1. Behçet disease

2. Vasculitis secondary to infection (including hepatitis B–associated PAN), malignancies, and drugs, including hypersensitivity vasculitis

3. Vasculitis associated with connective tissue diseases

4. Isolated vasculitis of the central nervous system

5. Cogan syndrome

6. Unclassified

Adapted from Ozen S, Ruperto N, Dillon MJ, et al. EULAR/PReS endorsed consensus criteria for the classification of childhood vasculitides. Ann Rheum Dis 2006;65:937.

Laboratory findings are often nonspecific and consistent with an acute or chronic inflammatory state. Leukocytosis, anemia, and thrombocytosis, and increased levels of acute phase reactants such as erythrocyte sedimentation rate (ESR) and C-reactive protein (CRP) are common. A urinalysis helps to determine the likelihood of glomerulonephritis. Likewise, blood urea nitrogen, creatinine, albumin, and transaminases may be indicators of specific organs affected. Antinuclear antibodies (ANA) and rheumatoid factor (RF) are not specific or sensitive for any of the vasculitides, but may be helpful to evaluate for potential systemic lupus erythematous (ANA) or immune complex disease (RF). Additional laboratory tests such as ANCA, imaging studies such as angiography, and biopsy for histopathology should be performed when considering specific diagnoses.

SPECIFIC VASCULITIDES
Henoch-Schönlein Purpura

Cardinal features
1. Purpura
2. Peripheral swelling

Box 3
Classification criteria for pediatric vasculitis

IgA vasculitis/HSP

- Purpura or petechia (mandatory) with lower limb predominance plus 1 of 4:
  - Abdominal pain
  - Histopathology (IgA deposit in a biopsy)
  - Arthritis or arthralgia
  - Renal involvement

Polyarteritis nodosa

- Histopathology or angiographic abnormalities (mandatory) plus 1 of 5:
  - Skin involvement
  - Myalgia/muscle tenderness
  - Hypertension
  - Peripheral neuropathy
  - Renal involvement

Granulomatosis with polyangiitis

- At least 3 of 6:
  - Histopathology (granulomatous inflammation)
  - Upper airway involvement
  - Laryngotracheobronchial stenosis
  - Pulmonary involvement
  - ANCA positivity
  - Renal involvement

Takayasu arteritis

- Angiographic abnormalities of the aorta or its major branches and pulmonary arteries showing aneurysm/dilatation (mandatory) plus 1 of 5:
  - Pulse deficit or claudication
  - Four limbs blood pressure discrepancy
  - Bruits
  - Hypertension
  - Increased acute phase reactant levels

Adapted from Eleftheriou D, Deniz Batu E, Ozen S, et al. Vasculitis in children. Nephrol Dial Transplant 2015;30:i95; with permission.

---

3. Abdominal symptoms
4. Renal disease

HSP is the most common vasculitis of childhood with an incidence of 10 cases per 100,000 children per year.[12] It is a small vessel vasculitis affecting arterioles, capillaries, and venules and histologically is a leukocytoclastic vasculitis, with evidence of leukocyte nuclear remnants within the vessel wall inflammation (**Fig. 1**). More specifically, there is predominant deposition of immunoglobulin A (IgA) within the inflammatory infiltrate. Many patients have a preceding viral illness or prior infection with group A *Streptococcus*.[13] HSP often begins with petechiae or palpable purpura of the buttocks and lower extremities (**Fig. 2**), although in some instances abdominal symptoms precede the other manifestations, and children may initially be thought to have a surgical abdomen.[14] Peripheral edema of the dorsa of the hands and feet and swelling around the large joints may occur. Approximately 40% to 50% of patients have evidence of glomerulonephritis and an equal number have abdominal pain or evidence of gastrointestinal bleeding during the course of the illness.[14] Intussusception

---

Box 4
Mimics of large vessel vasculitis

Infections

Syphilis

Tuberculosis

Human immunodeficiency virus

Leprosy

Mycotic aneurysms

Congenital and genetic vascular anomalies

Neurofibromatosis

Coarctation of the aorta

Middle aortic syndrome

Marfan syndrome

Ehlers-Danlos syndrome types IV and VI

Loeys-Dietz syndrome

Pseudoxanthoma elasticum

Fibromuscular dysplasia

Iatrogenic

After irradiation therapy

Adapted from Molloy ES, Langford CA. Vasculitis mimics. Curr Opinion Rheum 2008;20:30; with permission.

---

may occur, and less common but potentially severe complications of HSP include pulmonary hemorrhage[15] and central nervous system (CNS) vasculitis.[16] The diagnosis is most often based on the presence of characteristic clinical features, although histopathology showing leukocytoclastic vasculitis with predominant IgA deposition confirms a suspected diagnosis. The PRES/PRINTO diagnostic criteria (see **Box 3**) state that purpura or petechiae with lower limb predominance and at least 1 of either abdominal pain, histopathology, arthritis or arthralgia, or renal involvement, is 100% sensitive and 87% specific for a diagnosis of HSP.[8] Treatment is usually supportive, with most patients experiencing a resolution within 4 to 6 weeks. Less than 5% of patients develop chronic glomerulonephritis.[17] Treatment with glucocorticoids is controversial. There is evidence suggesting benefit for the gastrointestinal manifestations of HSP,[18,19] but glucocorticoids have not been proved to have a consistent effect on renal outcomes.[20]

Kawasaki Disease

Cardinal features
1. Fever
2. Conjunctivitis
3. Mucous membrane changes
4. Rash
5. Extremity changes (edema or erythema)
6. Single, enlarged cervical node

Kawasaki disease is the second most common vasculitis of childhood, although incidence varies widely among different ethnic groups.[21] Early descriptions of clinical

Box 5
Mimics of medium vessel vasculitis
Viral infection
Hepatitis B, C
Human immunodeficiency virus
Herpes viruses
Other infections
Endocarditis
Mycotic aneurysms
Malignancies
Leukemia
Lymphoma
Congenital and genetic vascular anomalies
Ehlers-Danlos syndrome type IV
Neurofibromatosis
Grange syndrome
Fibromuscular dysplasia
Hypercoagulable states
Antiphospholipid syndrome
Thrombotic thrombocytopenic purpura
Iatrogenic
Postprocedural
Adapted from Molloy ES, Langford CA. Vasculitis mimics. Curr Opinion Rheum 2008;20:30; with permission.

manifestations recognized the common cardinal features of the disease, but it is clear that the potential manifestations of Kawasaki disease are protean[22] and incomplete Kawasaki disease, in which only some of the cardinal features are present, is now well known.[22] Fever is daily, fairly high, and only transiently remits with antipyretics. Without treatment, the fever persists for an average of 11 days. The conjunctivitis is bilateral, bulbar predominantly, with an absence of exudate, is painless, and often spares the limbus. Mucous membrane changes include pharyngeal erythema, fissuring, erythema, or peeling of the lips, and prominent papillae of the tongue (so-called strawberry tongue). There is no characteristic rash, and most often it is diffuse; erythematous; and macular, papular, or patchy; but may also be urticarial, scarlatini-form, or erythema multiforme. Early in the disease there may be prominent erythema and desquamation within the perineum. The extremity changes are characteristically either diffuse erythema of the palms and soles or edema of the dorsa of the hands and feet. The least common cardinal feature of Kawasaki disease is unilateral anterior cervical adenopathy, with at least 1 node being 1.5 cm in diameter. Laboratory testing often reveals mild leukocytosis, mild anemia, and after the first week of illness a marked thrombocytosis. Inflammatory markers such as the ESR and CRP are usually at increased levels, and there may be increased transaminase levels, low albumin

Box 6
Mimics of central nervous system vasculitis

Sarcoidosis

Susac syndrome

Infections (bacterial, mycobacterial, fungal, viral, protozoal)

Malignancies (lymphoma)

Vasospasm

Fibromuscular dysplasia

Antiphospholipid antibody syndrome

Thrombotic thrombocytopenic purpura

Cerebral autosomal dominant arteriopathy with subcortical infarcts and leukoencephalopathy (CADASIL)

Mitochondrial disease

Fabry disease

Sneddon syndrome

Sickle cell disease

Leukoencephalopathies

Adenosine deaminase-2 deficiency

Cerebral hemorrhage

Moyamoya disease

Thrombus

Endocarditis

Myxoma

Adapted from Molloy ES, Langford CA. Vasculitis mimics. Curr Opinion Rheum 2008;20:32; with permission.

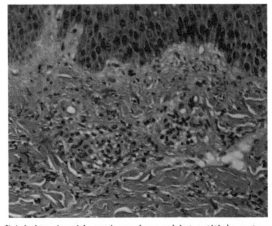

Fig. 1. HSP: superficial dermis with perivascular and interstitial neutrophils, nuclear dust, and extravasated erythrocytes (hematoxylin-eosin, original magnification ×10). (*Courtesy of* Annette Segura, MD, Medical College of Wisconsin.)

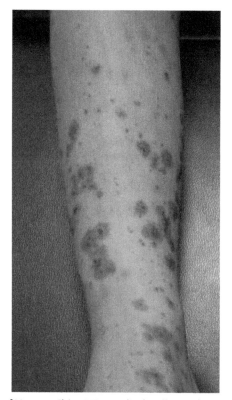

Fig. 2. HSP. (*Courtesy of* Yvonne Chiu, MD, Medical College of Wisconsin.)

level, and pyuria. Cerebrospinal fluid (CSF) testing may show a lymphocytic pleocytosis. However, none of these laboratory tests are diagnostic or present in all cases. The diagnosis is therefore clinical, with no single clinical feature or laboratory result that is sufficiently sensitive or specific. The presence of fever plus the characteristic findings for 4 of the other 5 cardinal features of the disease has been proposed as diagnostic.[22,23] These criteria were adopted in the recent PRES/PRINTO consensus classification of pediatric vasculitis, with the inclusion of perineal desquamation with extremity changes as a modified criterion.[6] The diagnosis is challenging when only a few of the cardinal features are present. A consensus guideline has been published, which proposes an algorithm to follow for patients who have incomplete features of Kawasaki disease.[22] If several criteria consistent with Kawasaki are present in the absence of a reasonable alternative explanation, treatment of Kawasaki disease is recommended to decrease the likelihood of the development of coronary artery aneurysms. These aneurysms, the most concerning potential complication of Kawasaki disease, develop in 15% to 25% of untreated patients and place patients at risk for potential thrombosis, or less often rupture, and subsequent myocardial ischemia or infarction.[22] Treatment with intravenous immunoglobulin and aspirin has been shown to decrease this risk to less than 5%,[24] and treatment should be administered in all patients suspected of having either complete or incomplete Kawasaki disease. Treatment should ideally be administered within the first 10 days of illness, because coronary artery aneurysms are most likely to develop after that time.[25]

Takayasu Arteritis

Cardinal features (highly variable)
1. Absent pulses
2. Hypertension
3. Claudication
4. Syncope/dizziness
5. Headaches
6. Abdominal pain

Takayasu arteritis is a vasculitis of the aorta and its major branches, such as the carotid, subclavian, celiac, mesenteric, renal, and iliac arteries.[26] The disease is most common in young female patients,[27] with an increased incidence in Asians,[28] but may occur in children as young as 2 years[29] and in all ethnic groups.[28] Inflammation may occur throughout the aorta and in multiple large arteries, or it may be restricted to a segment of the aorta and a few large arteries. Accordingly, the clinical symptoms and signs are variable, depending on which portions of the aorta and which branches are affected. Inflammation within the arterial walls leads to stenosis, poststenotic dilatation, and a reduction in blood flow, and subsequently the symptoms that patients manifest are ischemic. For example, if the proximal aorta and carotids are affected, symptoms of headache, dizziness, vertigo, or syncope may be predominant. If the distal aorta and iliac arteries are affected, patients may have claudication. When inflammation is isolated to the renal arteries, patients may be asymptomatic but have hypertension. Associated nonspecific constitutional symptoms, such as fatigue, malaise, fever, decreased appetite, and weight loss, are present in some, but not all, cases. In 2 reviews of a total of 40 children with Takayasu arteritis, headache, abdominal pain, and claudication were common presenting symptoms and hypertension, absent pulses, and bruits were common physical findings.[26,29] The typical signs that usually alert clinicians to the possibility of systemic vasculitis, such as palpable purpura, arthritis, evidence of inflammation within the airway or gastrointestinal tract, or abnormal urinary sediment, are often absent with Takayasu arteritis.[26] Laboratory testing is also nonspecific, and although most patients have increased inflammatory markers, the presence of active vasculitis secondary to Takayasu with a normal ESR and CRP has been described.[29] The variability of symptoms, the nonspecific symptoms associated with the disease, the lack of cutaneous or organ inflammation, the lack of specific or sensitive diagnostic tests, and the unfamiliarity that many pediatricians have with ischemic disease, such as claudication, all result in Takayasu arteritis being a challenge to diagnose. The diagnosis, according to PRES/PRINTO classification criteria, is made with angiographic abnormalities and 1 of the following: decreased pulses or claudication, blood pressure discrepancy in the limbs, bruits, hypertension, or increased acute phase reactant levels[8] (see **Box 3**). Contrast enhancement of the wall of the aorta or arteries on angiography is consistent with inflammation. Stenosis of vessels alone may be associated with active inflammation but may also be residual from previous inflammation (**Fig. 3**). Examination of arterial or aortic tissue may also confirm the diagnosis, but this is rarely feasible.

In patients with unexplained fevers, constitutional symptoms, hypertension, or symptoms suggestive of ischemia, the possibility of Takayasu arteritis should be considered. If there is an unexplained increase in the levels of inflammatory markers, imaging should be performed. Magnetic resonance angiography (MRA), computed tomography (CT) angiography, and conventional angiography have each been shown to be sufficiently sensitive. MRA and CT angiography should be performed with contrast. MRA has the advantage of limiting radiation exposure, but CT angiography may be

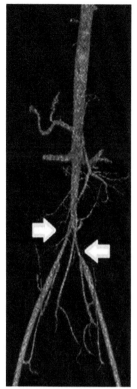

Fig. 3. Computed tomography (CT) angiogram reconstruction of images from a patient with Takayasu arteritis; note narrowing of the distal aorta and common iliac arteries (*arrows*).

performed in less time and therefore may be more practical. Treatment of Takayasu arteritis includes glucocorticoids, often in combination with another immunosuppressive agent such as methotrexate or cyclophosphamide.

Antineutrophil Cytoplasmic Antibody–Associated Vasculitis

The ANCA-associated vasculitides are a group of diseases that share several common features, including inflammation of the airways, rapidly progressive and pauci-immune glomerulonephritis, and increased ANCA levels. They are often described as pulmonary-renal syndromes because of the organs affected.

Granulomatosis with polyangiitis

Cardinal features
1. Upper airway inflammation
2. Lower airway inflammation
3. Renal disease (glomerulonephritis)
4. ANCA:predominant anti–proteinase 3 antibodies

GPA is a vasculitis affecting vessels within the upper and lower airways and the glomeruli. Chronic upper airway inflammation is often the first manifestation and patients may initially be treated with multiple courses of antibiotics for presumed infection before the diagnosis of GPA is considered.[30] Inflammation of the nasal passages results in refractory rhinorrhea or bloody nasal discharge,[31] with the inflammation sometimes eroding the nasal septum and leading to perforation and a so-called saddle nose. Inflammation within the trachea may cause subglottic stenosis,[32] and lung inflammation typically causes bilateral cavitating pulmonary nodules, pulmonary hemorrhage, or both.[30] The lung disease may be silent, with nodules apparent only on imaging studies. Rapidly progressive glomerulonephritis with hematuria, proteinuria, hypertension, and renal insufficiency are frequent.[30,31,33] Biopsy reveals glomerulonephritis, often with crescent formation and a characteristic paucity of immunoglobulin or complement deposition (**Fig. 4**). Fever, malaise, fatigue, anorexia, and weight loss are common,[30,31,34] and additional clinical manifestations may include peripheral neuropathies, palpable purpura, arthritis, and scleritis or episcleritis.[34] Gastrointestinal and CNS vasculitis are uncommon.[30,31] The diagnosis may be made in the presence of characteristic clinical findings along with increased ANCA level. The PRES/PRINTO criteria state that at least 3 of the following 6 criteria must be present: characteristic histopathology, upper airway inflammation, laryngotracheobronchial inflammation, pulmonary involvement, renal involvement, and an increased ANCA level[8] (see **Box 3**). There are 2 different antigens recognized by the ANCAs associated with vasculitis: proteinase 3 and myeloperoxidase (MPO).[35] GPA is more often associated with anti–proteinase 3 antibodies and microscopic polyangiitis (MPA) is more often associated with anti-MPO antibodies. Eosinophilic GPA (EGPA) may be associated with either antibody. Histology may confirm the diagnosis, with the kidney revealing pauci-immune glomerulonephritis and other tissues showing granulomatosis inflammation. Treatment of GPA often requires immunosuppression with cyclophosphamide and corticosteroids, although limited forms of the disease may be effectively treated with methotrexate.[36–38] Recent studies in adult patients have shown that rituximab is as effective as cyclophosphamide in inducing and maintaining remission.[39,40]

Microscopic polyangiitis

Cardinal features
1. Pulmonary hemorrhage
2. Renal disease (glomerulonephritis)
3. ANCA:predominant anti-MPO antibodies

MPA is a vasculitis that affects the capillaries of the lungs and the glomeruli, leading to pulmonary hemorrhage and rapidly progressive pauci-immune glomerulonephritis.

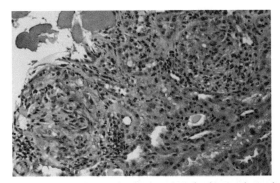

Fig. 4. Antineutrophil cytoplasmic antibody–associated glomerulonephritis: 2 glomeruli with focal fibrinoid necrosis and karyorrhectic debris compressed by epithelial crescents (hematoxylin-eosin, original magnification ×10). (*Courtesy of* Annette Segura, MD, Medical College of Wisconsin.)

Unlike GPA and EGPA, upper airway involvement is unusual, with no patients from recently described French cohorts experiencing upper airway manifestations.[30,31] Patients may present acutely with pulmonary hemorrhage (**Fig. 5**), at which time renal insufficiency is often discovered. Prodromal symptoms of fever, weight loss, arthralgias, and myalgias, are commonly reported[30,31,41] and palpable purpura may be present.[31] CNS disease has been described in some series,[31] but often represents effects secondary to hypertension or the posterior reversible encephalopathy syndrome rather than vasculitis. Ocular[31,41] and gastrointestinal involvement[30,31] have also been described, but these manifestations are less common. Laboratory testing reveals the presence of anti-MPO antibodies in most cases.[31] Renal biopsy typically reveals a necrotizing, pauci-immune glomerulonephritis identical to that seen in GPA. If lung tissue is biopsied, capillaritis with alveolar hemorrhage is characteristic. Unlike GPA and EGPA, the inflammation of MPA is not granulomatous. Treatment is similar to that of GPA with corticosteroids, cyclophosphamide, or rituximab.

Eosinophilic granulomatosis with polyangiitis

Cardinal features
1. Chronic, refractory reactive airway disease
2. Upper airway inflammation
3. Eosinophilia
4. ANCA; neither type predominant

EGPA is a granulomatous vasculitis that typically has a long prodromal course consisting of chronic upper airway inflammation (allergic rhinitis, sinusitis, nasal polyposis) and chronic refractory symptoms and signs of reactive airway disease.[42] After several years, patients develop peripheral eosinophilia and eosinophilic pulmonary infiltrates, followed eventually by pulmonary vasculitis. Not all patients follow this sequence and vasculitis may occur before symptoms of asthma.[43] Cutaneous, cardiac, gastrointestinal, and peripheral neurologic system involvement may occur.[42,43] Mononeuritis

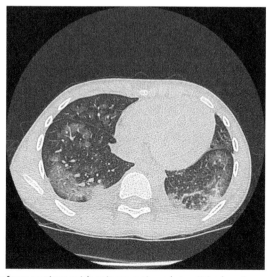

Fig. 5. CT of chest from patient with microscopic polyangiitis showing opacities consistent with diffuse pulmonary hemorrhage.

multiplex is the most common peripheral neuropathy.[42] Unlike GPA and MPA, glomerulonephritis is an uncommon feature of EGPA. Renal disease was not present in any patients in the largest cohort of pediatric patients described to date,[42] and, when present, it is usually milder than the renal disease of GPA and MPA.[43] Because of the long prodrome, and because histology at an earlier stage does not necessarily reveal vasculitis, the diagnosis of EGPA may be difficult, particularly distinguishing EGPA from allergic bronchopulmonary aspergillosis and other hypereosinophilic syndromes. ANCAs are also discovered less commonly with EGPA than with GPA or MPA, particularly in childhood,[42] making diagnosis challenging. Histology reveals necrotizing granulomas and vasculitis, if performed at a late enough stage of the disease, often with striking eosinophilic inflammation. Treatment is usually with corticosteroids and immunosuppressive agents,[43] similar to the treatment of the other ANCA-associated vasculitides.

Polyarteritis Nodosa

PAN is a vasculitis of small and medium-sized arteries. It may occur as a systemic disease or as disease isolated to the skin and subcutaneous tissue. Cutaneous PAN is more common in childhood than systemic PAN. It remains unclear whether these are separate conditions or different forms of the same vasculitis.

Systemic PAN

Cardinal features
1. Abdominal pain and gastrointestinal symptoms
2. Hypertension

Systemic PAN is commonly associated with fever, malaise, anorexia, weight loss, palpable purpura, abdominal pain, and hypertension.[30,44] In male patients, testicular pain may occur,[45] and cardiac disease, joint symptoms, and central and peripheral nervous system involvement have been described.[30,44] The PRES/PRINTO criteria state that childhood PAN is defined by histopathology or angiographic abnormalities plus 1 of the following: skin involvement, myalgia or muscle tenderness, hypertension, peripheral neuropathy, or renal involvement[8] (see **Box 3**). Because of the abdominal pain and palpable purpura, the disease may be confused with HSP. There are no diagnostic laboratory findings, but thrombocytosis, and increased levels of inflammatory markers are typical.[44] Imaging with angiography (MRA, CT angiography, or conventional angiography) reveals aneurysms and stenosis along medium-sized and small arteries, occasionally with collateral vessel formation in long-standing disease. Biopsy of affected tissues is not always practical, but reveals a necrotizing arteritis. Treatment is similar to that of other systemic vasculitides, with a combination of corticosteroids and cytotoxic agents being effective in most cases.[30]

Cutaneous PAN

Cardinal feature
1. Painful subcutaneous nodules

Cutaneous PAN is nearly always limited to cutaneous tissue. Some patients have fever, myalgia, and arthralgia,[46] but, unlike the systemic form of PAN, there is no internal organ vessel involvement. Some patients have been described with neuropathies and rarely inflammatory bowel disease.[47] There have been some reports of cutaneous PAN as a poststreptococcal condition.[48,49] Patients present with painful subcutaneous nodules that may have overlying purpura[47] (**Fig. 6**). Livedo reticularis is also

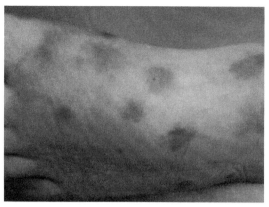

Fig. 6. Cutaneous PAN. (*Courtesy of* Yvonne Chiu, MD, Medical College of Wisconsin.)

commonly associated.[46,47] The diagnosis is usually made by skin biopsy revealing necrotizing small vessel vasculitis (**Fig. 7**). Treatment with corticosteroids is often effective, with some patients requiring additional immunomodulating or immunosuppressive agents.[46]

Central Nervous System Vasculitis

CNS vasculitis may be idiopathic, for which the term childhood primary angiitis of the CNS (cPACNS) has been applied,[50] or it may occur secondary to infections, malignancies, medications, or other inflammatory diseases. The idiopathic forms of CNS vasculitis, cPACNS, may affect either large arteries[51] or small vessels. These two forms of vasculitis have different clinical presentations, different imaging findings, and often require different treatments.[52]

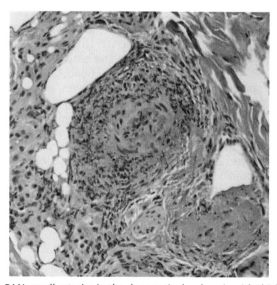

Fig. 7. Cutaneous PAN: small arteries in the deep reticular dermis with thickened walls, fibrinoid necrosis, and perivascular inflammatory cells (hematoxylin-eosin, original magnification ×10). (*Courtesy of* Annette Segura, MD, Medical College of Wisconsin.)

Large vessel cPACNS (angiography positive)

Cardinal features
1. Stroke
2. Other focal findings

Large vessel cPACNS usually presents with focal deficits and headaches.[51] Movement disorders, cranial neuropathies, and ischemic syndromes corresponding with the vascular distribution of the vessels affected are common. Laboratory features include increased ESR and CRP level in most, but not all patients, and abnormalities of the CSF only occasionally.[51] Angiography reveals stenosis of affected vessels. Large vessel disease may be progressive, with additional lesions appearing over time, or may occur in an isolated large vessel and remain stable. When interpreting angiography, it is critical to be aware that some visualized narrowing of cerebral vessels may be reversible, and the result of vasospasm rather than a fixed inflammatory lesion. This condition has been reported to occur in children and adults,[53] with the diagnosis confirmed by repeat imaging revealing resolution of the narrowed segment. Other conditions that might appear similar to vasculitis on angiography include moyamoya disease, fibromuscular dysplasias, and congenital vascular diseases.[52] Clinical syndromes that may present similar to vasculitis include metabolic diseases such as mitochondrial encephalopathy, lactic acidosis and stroke, hypercoagulable states, infections, and CNS lymphomas. These conditions may need to be excluded with additional testing while the diagnosis of cPACNS is considered. Treatment of progressive large vessel disease generally requires cyclophosphamide and corticosteroids. Treatment of nonprogressive disease is controversial, with limited data suggesting benefit with corticosteroids and anticoagulation.[52]

Small vessel cPACNS (angiography negative)

Cardinal features
1. Encephalopathy
2. Seizures

Small vessel cPACNS usually presents with seizures, encephalopathy with global neurologic deficits, and/or behavior changes.[50,54] Cognitive dysfunction and mood disorders may occur. Focal neurologic symptoms are less common. Children with small vessel cPACNS usually have increased ESR and CRP levels and most have abnormal CSF with pleocytosis, increased protein levels, or both.[55] Angiography is normal, and the diagnosis requires brain biopsy. Most patients should be evaluated for other inflammatory brain diseases, such as those with encephalitis associated with infection, lymphoma, N-methyl-D-aspartate receptor antibodies, or neuromyelitis optica associated with aquaporin-4 antibodies.[52] Biopsy should be performed of leptomeninges, gray matter, and subcortical white matter. Patients with small vessel cPACNS have a predominantly lymphocytic inflammatory infiltrate within the walls of arterioles, capillaries, and venules and most patients have involvement of multiple vessels in different layers of the brain and meninges.[54,56,57] Treatment requires cyclophosphamide and corticosteroids, followed by maintenance treatment with an immunosuppressive.[52,55]

RARE ASSOCIATIONS WITH VASCULITIS
Adenosine Deaminase 2 Deficiency

Adenosine deaminase (ADA) 2 deficiency is a recently described syndrome that may mimic PAN and CNS vasculitis.[58,59] Patients develop a combination of recurrent fevers, livedoid rashes, hepatosplenomegaly, ischemic and/or hemorrhagic strokes, and vasculitis similar to PAN. Genetic testing reveals loss-of-function mutations in *CECR1*, the gene encoding the ADA 2 protein. Treatment with tumor necrosis factor inhibitors or interleukin-1 inhibitors, as well as hematopoietic stem cell transplant, may have some promise.[60]

Cerebral Autosomal Dominant Arteriopathy with Subcortical Infarcts and Leukoencephalopathy

Cerebral autosomal dominant arteriopathy with subcortical infarcts and leukoencephalopathy (CADASIL) is a syndrome that may mimic isolated CNS vasculitis and has been described in children as young as 3 years of age.[61,62] The clinical presentation is variable, but migraine headaches, strokes, mood disturbances, and cognitive impairment have been commonly reported. Seizures have been reported in 5% to 10% of patients.[62] MRI may reveal lacunar infarcts and signal abnormalities and biopsy of brain tissue characteristically reveals an arteriopathy of small arteries with thickened arterial wall and the presence of granular osmiophilic material within the vessel wall. Similar osmiophilic granules may be seen in skin and other organs, even though the clinical manifestations are isolated to the CNS.[62] Genetic testing reveals mutations in the NOTCH3 gene, encoding a transmembrane receptor.

Posterior Reversible Encephalopathy Syndrome

Posterior reversible encephalopathy syndrome may develop in patients with underlying glomerulonephritis or who have been treated with immunosuppression, features that are common in those with an underlying systemic vasculitis.[63] Recognition of this syndrome is critical, because it should not be mistaken for the development of CNS vasculitis. Patients typically develop acute-onset seizures with or without cortical visual disturbances, and are often acutely hypertensive.[63] Neuroimaging studies are characteristic and reveal subcortical edema without evidence of infarction. The condition is reversible and best managed by controlling the blood pressure.

REFERENCES

1. Weiss PF. Pediatric vasculitis. Pediatr Clin North Am 2012;59(2):407–23.
2. Eleftheriou D, Deniz Batu E, Ozen S, et al. Vasculitis in children. Nephrol Dial Transplant 2015;30:i94–103.
3. Jennette JC, Falk RJ, Bacon PA, et al. 2012 Revised international Chapel Hill consensus conference nomenclature of vasculitides. Arthritis Rheum 2013;65:1–11.
4. Hunder GG, Arend WP, Bloch DA, et al. The American College of Rheumatology 1990 criteria for the classification of vasculitis. Introduction. Arthritis Rheum 1990;33:1065–7.
5. Bloch DA, Michel BA, Hunder GG, et al. The American College of Rheumatology 1990 criteria for the classification of vasculitis. Patients and methods. Arthritis Rheum 1990;33:1068–73.
6. Ozen S, Ruperto N, Dillon MJ, et al. EULAR/PReS endorsed consensus criteria for the classification of childhood vasculitides. Ann Rheum Dis 2006;65:936–41.
7. Ruperto N, Ozen S, Pistorio A, et al. EULAR/PRINTO/PRES criteria for Henoch-Schonlein purpura, childhood polyarteritis nodosa, childhood Wegener granulomatosis and childhood Takayasu arteritis: Ankara 2008. Part I: Overall methodology and clinical characterisation. Ann Rheum Dis 2010;69:790–7.
8. Ozen S, Pistorio A, Iusan SM, et al. EULAR/PRINTO/PRES criteria for Henoch-Schönlein purpura, childhood polyarteritis nodosa, childhood Wegener

granulomatosis and childhood Takayasu arteritis: Ankara 2008. Part II: final classification criteria. Ann Rheum Dis 2010;69:798–806.

9. Waller R, Ahmed A, Patel I, et al. Update on the classification of vasculitis. Best Pract Res Clin Rheumatol 2013;27:3–17.

10. Jennette JC, Falk RJ, Andrassy K, et al. Nomenclature of systemic vasculitides: the proposal of an international consensus conference. Arthritis Rheum 1994; 37:187–92.

11. Molloy ES, Langford CA. Vasculitis mimics. Curr Opin Rheumatol 2008;20:29–34.

12. Saulsbury FT. Clinical update: Henoch-Schonlein purpura. Lancet 2007;369: 976–8.

13. Weiss PF, Klink AJ, Luan X, et al. Temporal association of *Streptococcus*, *Staphylococcus*, and parainfluenza pediatric hospitalizations and hospitalized cases of Henoch-Schonlein purpura. J Rheumatol 2010;37:2587–94.

14. Saulsbury FT. Henoch-Schonlein purpura in children. Report of 100 patients and review of the literature. Medicine (Baltimore) 1999;78:395–409.

15. Rajagopala S, Shobha V, Devaraj U, et al. Pulmonary hemorrhage in Henoch-Schönlein purpura: case report and systematic review of the English literature. Semin Arthritis Rheum 2013;42(4):391–400.

16. Bérubé MD, Blais N, Lanthier S. Neurologic manifestations of Henoch-Schönlein purpura. Handb Clin Neurol 2014;120:1101–11.

17. Stewart M, Savage JM, Bell B, et al. Long term renal prognosis of Henoch-Schonlein purpura in an unselected childhood population. Eur J Pediatr 1988; 147:113–5.

18. Weiss PF, Feinstein JA, Luan X, et al. Effects of corticosteroid on Henoch-Schonlein purpura: a systematic review. Pediatrics 2007;120:1079–87.

19. Weiss PF, Klink AJ, Localio R, et al. Corticosteroids may improve clinical outcomes during hospitalization for Henoch-Schonlein purpura. Pediatrics 2010; 126:674–81.

20. Dudley J, Smith G, Llewellyn-Edwards A, et al. Randomised, double-blind, placebo-controlled trial to determine whether steroids reduce the incidence and severity of nephropathy in Henoch-Schonlein Purpura (HSP). Arch Dis Child 2013;98:756–63.

21. Singh S, Vignesh P, Burgner D. The epidemiology of Kawasaki disease: a global update. Arch Dis Child 2015;100(11):1084–8.

22. Newburger JW, Takahashi M, Gerber MA, et al. Diagnosis, treatment, and long-term management of Kawasaki disease: a statement for health professionals from the Committee on Rheumatic Fever, Endocarditis, and Kawasaki Disease, Council on Cardiovascular Disease in the Young, American Heart Association. Pediatrics 2004;114:1708–33.

23. Dajani AS, Taubert KA, Gerber MA, et al. Diagnosis and therapy of Kawasaki disease in children. Circulation 1993;87:1776–80.

24. Newburger JW, Takahashi M, Beiser AS, et al. A single intravenous infusion of gamma globulin as compared with four infusions in the treatment of acute Kawasaki syndrome. N Engl J Med 1991;324:1633–9.

25. Newburger JW, Takahashi M, Gerber MA, et al. Diagnosis, treatment, and long-term management of Kawasaki disease: a statement for health professionals from the Committee on Rheumatic Fever, Endocarditis and Kawasaki Disease, Council on Cardiovascular Disease in the Young, American Heart Association. Circulation 2004;110:2747–71.

26. Cakar N, Yalcinkaya F, Duzova A, et al. Takayasu arteritis in children. J Rheumatol 2008;35(5):913–9.

27. Vanoli M, Daina E, Salvarani C, et al. Takayasu's arteritis: a study of 104 Italian patients. Arthritis Rheum 2005;53:100–7.
28. Numano F, Okawara M, Inomoto H, et al. Takayasu's arteritis. Lancet 2000;356: 1023–5.
29. Hahn D, Thomson PD, Kala U, et al. A review of Takayasu's arteritis in children in Gauteng, South Africa. Pediatr Nephrol 1998;12(8):668–75.
30. Iudici M, Puechal X, Pagnoux C, et al. Childhood-onset systemic necrotizing vasculitides: long-term data from the French vasculitis study group registry. Arthritis Rheum 2015;67(7):1959–65.
31. Sacri A, Chambaraud T, Ranchin B, et al. Clinical characteristics and outcomes of childhood-onset ANCA-associated vasculitis: a French nationwide study. Nephrol Dial Transplant 2015;30:i104–12.
32. Guardiani E, Moghaddas H, Lesser J, et al. Multilevel airway stenosis in patients with granulomatosis with polyangiitis (Wegener's). Am J Otolaryngol 2015;36(3): 361–3.
33. Kosalka J, Bazan-Socha S, Ignacak M, et al. Clinical manifestation of pediatric granulomatosis with polyangiitis - the experience of two regions in Poland. Folia Med Cracov 2014;54(1):5–12.
34. Cabral DA, Uribe AG, Benseler S, et al. Classification, presentation, and initial treatment of Wegener's granulomatosis in childhood. Arthritis Rheum 2009; 60(11):3413–24.
35. Rasmussen N, Wiik A, Jayne D. A historical essay on detection of anti-neutrophil cytoplasmic antibodies. Nephrol Dial Transplant 2015;30:i8–13.
36. Villa-Forte A, Clark TM, Gomes M, et al. Substitution of methotrexate for cyclophosphamide in Wegener granulomatosis: a 12-year single-practice experience. Medicine (Baltimore) 2007;86(5):269–77.
37. De Groot K, Rasmussen N, Bacon PA, et al. Randomized trial of cyclophosphamide versus methotrexate for induction of remission in early systemic antineutrophil cytoplasmic antibody-associated vasculitis. Arthritis Rheum 2005;52:2461–9.
38. Hoffman GS, Leavitt RY, Kerr GS, et al. The treatment of Wegener's granulomatosis with glucocorticoids and methotrexate. Arthritis Rheum 1992;35:1322–9.
39. Stone J, Merkel P, Spiera R, et al. Rituximab versus cyclophosphamide for ANCA-associated vasculitis. N Engl J Med 2010;363:221–32.
40. Guillevin L, Pagnoux C, Karras A, et al. Rituximab versus azathioprine for maintenance in ANCA-associated vasculitis. N Engl J Med 2014;371:1771–80.
41. Siomou E, Tramma D, Bowen C, et al. ANCA-associated glomerulonephritis/systemic vasculitis in childhood: clinical features–outcome. Pediatr Nephrol 2012; 27(10):1911–20.
42. Gendelman S, Zeft A, Spalding SJ. Childhood-onset eosinophilic granulomatosis with polyangiitis (formerly Churg-Strauss syndrome): a contemporary single-center cohort. J Rheumatol 2013;40(6):929–35.
43. Comarmond C, Pagnoux C, Khellaf M, et al. Eosinophilic granulomatosis with polyangiitis (Churg-Strauss): clinical characteristics and long-term followup of the 383 patients enrolled in the French Vasculitis Study Group cohort. Arthritis Rheum 2013;65(1):270–81.
44. Eleftheriou D, Dillon MJ, Tullus K, et al. Systemic polyarteritis nodosa in the young: a single-center experience over thirty-two years. Arthritis Rheum 2013; 65(9):2476–85.
45. Hernández-Rodríguez J, Tan CD, Koening CL, et al. Testicular vasculitis: findings differentiating isolated disease from systemic disease in 72 patients. Medicine (Baltimore) 2012;91(2):75–85.

46. Fathalla BM, Miller L, Brady S, et al. Cutaneous polyarteritis nodosa in children. J Am Acad Dermatol 2005;53(4):724–8.
47. Daoud MS, Hutton KP, Gibson LE. Cutaneous periarteritis nodosa: a clinicopathological study of 79 cases. Br J Dermatol 1997;136(5):706–13.
48. Fink C. The role of the streptococcus in post-streptococcal reactive arthritis and childhood polyarteritis nodosa. J Rheumatol 1991;18(Suppl 29):14–20.
49. Till S, Amos R. Long term follow-up of juvenile onset cutaneous polyarteritis nodosa associated with streptococcal infection. Br J Rheumatol 1997;36:909–11.
50. Benseler SM, deVeber G, Hawkins C, et al. Angiography-negative primary central nervous system vasculitis in children: a newly recognized inflammatory central nervous system disease. Arthritis Rheum 2005;52:2159–67.
51. Benseler SM, Silverman E, Aviv RI, et al. Primary central nervous system vasculitis in children. Arthritis Rheum 2006;54:1291–7.
52. Twilt M, Benseler SM. CNS vasculitis in children. Mult Scler Relat Disord 2013; 2(3):162–71.
53. Probert R, Saunders DE, Ganesan V. Reversible cerebral vasoconstriction syndrome: rare or underrecognized in children? Dev Med Child Neurol 2013;55(4): 385–9.
54. Cellucci T, Tyrrell PN, Sheikh S, et al. Childhood primary angiitis of the central nervous system; identifying disease trajectories and early risk factors for persistently higher disease activity. Arthritis Rheum 2012;64:1665–72.
55. Hutchinson C, Elbers J, Halliday W, et al. Treatment of small vessel primary CNS vasculitis in children: an open-label cohort study. Lancet Neurol 2010;9:1078–84.
56. Yaari R, Anselm IA, Szer IS, et al. Childhood primary angiitis of the central nervous system: two biopsy-proven cases. J Pediatr 2004;145:693–7.
57. Lanthier S, Lortie A, Michaud J, et al. Isolated angiitis of the CNS in children. Neurology 2001;56:837–42.
58. Zhou Q, Yang D, Ombrello AK, et al. Early-onset stroke and vasculopathy associated with mutations in ADA2. N Engl J Med 2014;370(10):911–20.
59. Navon Elkan P, Pierce SB, Segel R, et al. Mutant adenosine deaminase 2 in a polyarteritis nodosa vasculopathy. N Engl J Med 2014;370:921–31.
60. Van Eyck L Jr, Hershfield MS, Pombal D, et al. Hematopoietic stem cell transplantation rescues the immunologic phenotype and prevents vasculopathy in patients with adenosine deaminase 2 deficiency. J Allergy Clin Immunol 2015;135(1): 283–7.
61. Benabu Y, Beland M, Ferguson N, et al. Genetically proven cerebral autosomal-dominant arteriopathy with subcortical infarcts and leukoencephalopathy (CADASIL) in a 3-year-old. Pediatr Radiol 2013;43(9):1227–30.
62. Chabriat H, Joutel A, Dichgans M, et al. Cadasil. Lancet Neurol 2009;8(7): 643–53.
63. Hinchey J, Chaves C, Appignani B, et al. A reversible posterior leukoencephalopathy syndrome. N Engl J Med 1996;334(8):494–500.

Fever of Unknown Origin in Childhood

Michael J. Chusid, MD

KEYWORDS

- Fever of unknown origin • Diagnostic evaluation • Cancer • Infection • Inflammation

KEY POINTS

- Evaluation of fever of unknown origin (FUO) in children requires documentation of fever in the medical setting and repetitive reassessment of history and physical evaluation.
- Most childhood FUOs have an infectious cause, but in some cases, underlying neoplastic, rheumatologic, or inflammatory conditions are diagnosed.
- Diagnostic evaluation of childhood FUO should be performed in a staged manner, leaving expensive imaging and invasive procedures for last.
- Molecular genetic techniques are playing an increasingly important role in the diagnosis of childhood FUO.

INTRODUCTION

Elevation of body temperature beyond the normal range is characteristic of a wide variety of abnormal conditions in adults and children. Body temperature is maintained within a normal range through a complex interactive array of physiologic processes. Derangement of these processes, frequently induced by a wide variety of infectious agents, leads to elevation in body temperature beyond the normal physiologic range, called "fever." In addition to infectious agents, a variety of autoimmune, metabolic, oncologic, neurologic, developmental, and inflammatory conditions also produces fever. Diagnostic assessment of a persistently febrile child may become daunting when the child's clinical and laboratory findings do not match one of the common causes of febrile disease. Evaluation of such children, especially when the child manifests persistent or progressive illness, calls upon the physician to construct a comprehensive, sometimes unfamiliar, differential diagnosis. A persistently febrile child, lacking an obvious source of fever, can be one of the most perplexing and worrisome puzzles encountered in clinical pediatrics and can be highly stressful for the child, his parents, and his physician.

Disclosure Statement: M.J. Chusid, sole author of this article, has no relevant financial or nonfinancial relationships to disclose.
Infectious Diseases, Department of Pediatrics, Medical College of Wisconsin, Suite C450, 999 North 92nd Street, Wauwatosa, WI 53226, USA
E-mail address: mchusid@mcw.edu

Pediatr Clin N Am 64 (2017) 205–230
http://dx.doi.org/10.1016/j.pcl.2016.08.014
0031-3955/17/© 2016 Elsevier Inc. All rights reserved.
pediatric.theclinics.com

TEMPERATURE CONTROL AND HUMAN DISEASE

Elevation of body temperature beyond the normal range is an ancient weapon in the armamentarium of complex multicellular organisms against microbial invasion and other disease processes. Despite a high metabolic cost, fever, as a response to an invasive microbial attack, has been retained as a basic host defense mechanism through hundreds of millions of years of natural selection. Its preservation speaks to its fundamental importance in host defense.[1,2]

Endothermal ("warm blooded") vertebrates establish their own internally maintained temperature-controlled environments via a variety of physiologic and behavioral mechanisms.[1,2] Endogenous pyrogenic cellular cytokines released in response to an inflammatory process have the capacity of advancing upward the central thermoregulatory "set point." Constant monitoring of blood temperature by thermosensitive cells within in the anterior hypothalamus serves as a biologic thermostat. Body temperature is regulated through a centrally controlled efferent system of physiologic responses to a negative disparity (blood temperature below set point) between blood temperature and central set point that includes increased heat production due to motor activity (shivering) and brown fat catabolism, augmented by increased heat retention secondary to peripheral vasoconstriction.[1–3] In the presence of a positive disparity between blood temperature and set point, body temperature is reduced through vasodilation and perspiration.[1–3] Behavioral activities, such as adjusting room temperature, clothing selection, body positioning, and ingestion of warm or cool liquids, play a secondary role in temperature control.

Currently, the mammalian thermoregulatory system remains a black box from a molecular point viewpoint. However, it is clear that tumor necrosis factor-α (TNF-α) and interleukin-6 (IL-6), in conjunction with interleukin-1Aβ (IL-1Aβ) are major contributors in the upregulation of the central nervous system's thermoregulatory set point.[4,5] No single cytokine seems to efficiently increase the central set point. Both IL-1 and IL-6 seem to be required for greatest effectiveness, perhaps in conjunction with other agents.[4,5] The major effect of IL-1 and IL-6 in thermoregulation is on the elaboration of prostaglandin E in the cyclooxygenase-2 and STAT3 metabolic pathways.[6] Inhibition of prostaglandin E synthesis is the mechanism of action through which most antipyretics, including acetaminophen and nonsteroidal anti-inflammatories (NSAIDs), reduce the central set point.[7]

Fever is an important sign in alerting parents and physicians that the child is experiencing an infection or other significant cause of upregulation of the hypothalamic set point. Parents, and to a lesser degree, professional caregivers, are often concerned about the potential harm that fever may have upon the health of the febrile child. Such concern can reach a crescendo, dubbed "fever phobia," describing the exaggerated fear about the height to which fever can spiral in an otherwise physiologically intact child.[8]

Ironically, the most available evidence leads to the conclusion that elevated body temperature is a major host defense mechanism, evolved and conserved through the eons by natural selection. Fever appears to play a nonspecific, but significant role in protection of the host against microbial invasion. Studies have repeatedly demonstrated that critically ill patients in intensive care units, whose body temperatures are aggressively maintained at normothermic levels by suppressing fever through pharmacologic or external environmental means, are significantly more likely to expire than matched patients whose body temperatures are allowed to increase freely.[9,10] At least one study had to be terminated for ethical concerns because death rates in the fever-controlled group so significantly exceeded that of the unsuppressed fever group.[10]

The reason for the beneficial effect of increased body temperature in ameliorating infection and other inflammatory processes is likely multifactorial. Growth of certain human pathogens such as *Treponema pallidum* and *Mycobacterium leprae* are directly inhibited by an increase in body temperature. Interestingly, these infectious agents tend not to induce fevers in infected individuals, presumably as a defensive measure.

Increased body temperature is associated with nonspecific enhancement of a wide array of host defense responses. In most infections, it is likely the mammalian host response's increased efficiency at higher body temperature is most responsible for the salubrious effect of increased body temperature. Most mammalian immune functions are significantly more effective at temperatures above the normal range. Polymorphonuclear neutrophils (PMNs) move more quickly toward an infectious target at higher temperatures, phagocytose more efficiently, and kill pathogenic agents in vitro more quickly at higher temperatures.[11] Adherence of T-helper lymphocytes, immunoglobulin production, and TNF-α cytotoxicity is significantly more efficient at elevated temperatures than at normal host temperature.[12,13] Increased body temperature also leads to improved immune response to immunizing agents and may even play a role in more efficient immune-mediated tumor defense.[14]

THE FEBRILE CHILD

Parents become greatly concerned about the presence of a fever in their child because this sign often suggests to them that their child has a significant illness. Setting aside the issue of infants younger than 3 months of age, where any elevation of core temperature greater than 37°C must be considered potentially significant, there is less agreement about what represents a fever in older children. Assessment protocols used in emergency departments and urgent care centers have led to various definitions of fever in children. In many cases, fever is defined as a temperature of 38.5°C, although in other settings, readings higher than 38°C are considered significant.[15]

The normal child has a body temperature that demonstrates a daily circadian rhythm, with temperature as low as 36°C in the early morning hours and as high as 37.5°C in the late afternoon. Most parents are unaware of this cycle and may report their child as having "low-grade fever" in the afternoon. Others, taking their child's temperature in the early morning, may report the child as always having a "low" baseline temperature.[15] There are, of course, rare individuals whose hypothalamic set point may be consistently higher or lower than the average child.

The means by which a child's temperature is obtained affects the level recorded. Oral temperatures are generally 0.5°C lower than core temperatures measured rectally. Newer modalities in temperature assessment include infrared devices for measuring skin temperature, liquid crystal skin strips, and aural electronic devices. The cutaneous devices can be accurate but depend on dry skin. Aural thermometry can be inaccurate and is difficult to use properly.[16] If the device's infrared beam falls upon cerumen in the ear canal, the temperature may be recorded inaccurately low. If the tympanic membrane is inflamed, measured temperatures may exceed true core temperature, sometimes to an alarming level.

Because fever is such a common sign in a vast array of illnesses, it is critical to distinguish between children with a febrile illness likely to be significant and those likely to be minor. High-risk illnesses require closer follow-up, more intensive assessment, and more detailed laboratory workup. One of the most difficult tasks for even the most experienced practitioner is to distinguish between fever related to a transient intercurrent infection and that produced by serious illness. History, physical examination, and basic screening laboratory results are often helpful in making this distinction.

At one time the term, "fever of unknown origin" (FUO) referred primarily to adult patients who had demonstrated fever without a definable source for at least 3 weeks, including 1 week in the hospital, with negative evaluation by routine testing.[17] Cleary, given current financial constraints and the development of modern imaging and rapid molecular diagnostic techniques, such an approach is no longer feasible in either adults or children. Workup of such patients is much more intensive and rapid than formerly.

FUO is a confusing term in pediatric medicine, and the requirement for 3 weeks of fever never gained much traction. Instead, children are sometimes described as having FUO after the fever has been present for just a few days and simple screening tests are negative, although some pediatricians require as long as 2 weeks of fever before using the term "FUO."[15,18–22] In part, because of the disparity in definition of FUO in adults and children, but also because of a difference in the prevalence of different types of febrile conditions, there is a significant difference in the diagnosed causes of FUOs in adults and children.[18,20,23] Although infection accounts for the greatest proportion of underlying diagnoses in adults (35%), infection accounts for more than 50% of FUOs in children. Conversely, malignancy accounts for a higher percentage (11%) of FUOs in adults than it does in children (6%).[20,23] Rheumatologic conditions (16%) are also a more important cause of fever in adults than in children (9%).[20,23] About one-quarter of children with FUO have fevers that resolve without diagnosis.[18,20] This presumably relates to undiagnosed viral processes.[24]

The diagnostic evaluation of a child with a prolonged fever of uncertain cause can be taxing and perplexing. Most serious infections rapidly declare themselves through clinical course and routine laboratory studies and cultures, particularly in young infants in whom detailed protocols have been developed to prospectively distinguish those febrile infants likely to have serious invasive bacterial infections from those with less serious conditions. Such protocols take into account the age of the patient, vital signs, and basic laboratory tests, including assessment of inflammatory markers. Assessment of older infants and children is less standardized and requires more individualization of evaluation. There are certain initial historical, physical, and laboratory findings that help discriminate between children with benign and those with more serious underlying processes (**Box 1**).

One of the most useful bits of information available in the evaluation of febrile children is serologic inflammatory markers. In febrile children, significant elevation of these markers indicates a potentially serious inflammatory process. Several familiar measures of inflammation may be important in this assessment, including white blood cell count, absolute neutrophil count, differential, platelet count, erythrocyte sedimentation rate (ESR), C-reactive protein (CRP), and procalcitonin.[23,25–28] Serum immunoglobulin levels, ferritin, and fibrinogen concentrations may also be beneficial, although none of these assays are perfect in assessing inflammatory status because of the varied lengths of time it takes for each of the assays to become elevated and/or return to baseline levels. Newer assays like procalcitonin level are highly useful in assessing the presence of an inflammatory condition in its earliest stages, but even procalcitonin and CRP levels may be subject to false negativity early in the course of illness. Conversely, assays like the ESR and platelet count suffer from being quite delayed in their elevations, sometimes as long as a week after the disease onset, and then may be quite slow to return to normal during recovery, which hampers their diagnostic utility during the early stage of an inflammatory illness and limits usefulness in assessing response to therapy. Frequently it is beneficial to use more than one of these markers in helping

Box 1
Childhood fever of unknown origin: discriminants between likely innocuous and potentially serious febrile conditions

History:

Prolonged appetite change

Weight loss

Sleep perturbation

Focal complaints

High fever longer than 5 days

Physical examination:

Organomegaly

Lymphadenopathy

Rash

Clubbing

Focal findings

Screening laboratory tests:

Anemia

Hypoalbuminemia

Lactate dehydrogenase or uric acid elevation

Immunoglobulin elevation

Elevated inflammatory markers:

Marked leukocytosis

Bandemia

Pronounced thrombocytosis or thrombocytopenia

Markedly elevated:

Erythrocyte sedimentation rate

C-reactive protein

Ferritin

Fibrinogen

determine the severity and significance of a prolonged fever. Determination of the patient's level of systemic inflammation and duration of fever allows dividing patients among those with minimal signs of inflammation and those with very elevated levels, who are at higher risk of having a more serious underlying illness.[8,9] Following these assays serially can help assess the patient's response to therapy and resolution or progression of inflammation.

DOCUMENTATION OF FEVER

Many patients seen in the ambulatory setting who are reported to have fever actually are afebrile. Before embarking on a detailed diagnostic workup, it is critical to demonstrate the presence of fever in a controlled setting. Review of prior medical records may help document that the child has been febrile. If the child does not have a documented fever during the initial visit, he or she should return when a fever is present. It is often useful to have the parents initiate a "fever diary."[15] Temperature should be recorded at least twice a day, at least 8 hours apart at the same times, by the same method, each day, for later assessment.[29–32] Review of a fever diary by the primary care provider with parents is often useful in demonstrating the lack of significant fever in their child and often leads to a discussion of circadian rhythms and definition of fever. In many cases, the use of a fever diary establishes that the child is not actually febrile or has resolved an earlier illness.

If fever is confirmed, a fever diary can provide clues regarding the potential underlying cause of the fever. Persistently high fevers are frequently the sign of a serious ongoing systemic process requiring further investigation. The presence of a single daily fever spike, particularly in the late afternoon, may be an indication of the presence of a localized inflammatory process like an abscess (**Box 2**). Intermittent periods of fever occurring every 2 to 3 days may be seen in infections like malaria. Fevers associated with a transient increase in systemic inflammation for several days, then completely remitting, with recurrences after at least 3 to 4 weeks, are concerning for a noninfectious autoinflammatory periodic fever syndrome (see John M. Routes and James W. Verbsky's article, "Immunodeficiency Presenting as an Undiagnosed Disease," in this issue).[29–31] Patients with cyclic neutropenia can display a similar pattern.[33] Rheumatologic conditions such as juvenile idiopathic arthritis (JIA) and systemic lupus erythematosus (SLE) can sometimes show such a periodic fever pattern, but patient symptoms often do not totally remit during afebrile periods nor inflammatory markers totally normalize.

In some situations, fever continues to be reported at home, but is never observed in a controlled medical environment. In this situation, an alternative measuring device should be used for taking the temperatures at home. If fever persists at home but is never seen in a medical setting, the reliability of the individual reporting the fever should be critically assessed. Such individuals may be exaggerating the character

---

Box 2
Childhood fever of unknown origin: cyclic symptoms and periodicity

Short (days):

Malaria

Borreliosis

Medium (weeks):

FMF, Hibernian fever

Hyper IgD, TRAPS, PFAPA

Cyclic neutropenia

Long (months):

Lupus erythematosus

Juvenile idiopathic arthritis

Acute rheumatic fever

Chronic recurrent multifocal osteomyelitis

Abbreviations: FMF, familial mediterranean fever; PFAPA, periodic fever, aphthous stomatitis, pharyngitis and adenitis syndrome; TRAPS, tumor necrosis factor associated syndrome.

of the illness because of obsessive concern about the health of the child. In unusual instances, caregivers may induce fevers or falsify reports of fever in the child for ulterior motives, as in the Munchausen-by-proxy syndrome (see Hillary W. Petska and colleagues' article, "The Intersection of Medical Child Abuse and Medical Complexity," in this issue).

INDIVIDUALIZED MEDICAL HISTORY

Once determined that a child actually has FUO, evaluation of the child requires a rigorous reassessment of the child's history and physical examination. Frequently, repeated intensive history reviews and physical examinations by an experienced clinician can result in rapid diagnosis of a previously perplexing case (**Box 3**).

A child who appears to have had an extended febrile illness may simply be experiencing a "pseudo-FUO," a consecutive series of self-limited minor infections.[15] This is especially likely if the child is an only child in the home attending *school* for the first time, or who has older siblings who bring home infectious agents. *Daycare* attendance is a common cause of frequent viral infections as well as bacterial infections caused by pneumococci or Kingella.[34] *Adopted* children may have been infected before adoption in their country of origin with a variety of infectious agents including tuberculosis, human immunodeficiency virus (HIV), hepatitis B or C, or even malaria or typhoid in their country of origin.[35]

Some children consume unsafe food products that may be conduits of infectious agents. *Unpasteurized milk* can transmit intestinal tuberculosis, brucellosis, listeriosis, Campylobacter, enteropathogenic *Escherichia coli*. or Salmonella infections.[36] *Goat's milk* and *soft cheeses* are fed to children and are associated with brucellosis, listeriosis, and salmonellosis.[37] Recent immunization with *live vaccines* can produce a delayed fever in children without other symptoms. Although the widespread use of pneumococcal and *Haemophilus influenzae* B (HIB) vaccines has markedly reduced rates of invasive infection with those pathogens, many children now are

---

Box 3
Childhood fever of unknown origin: frequently overlooked historical clues

Adoption, domestic or international

Sole child, newly attending daycare or school

Informal home daycare

Older siblings attending school or daycare

Ethnicity

Unrecognized underlying medical conditions

Diet: Goat's milk, unpasteurized products, raw meat

Immunizations: Modified schedule or recent

Animal exposure: Pets, farm, wildlife

Blood product exposure

Tuberculosis exposure: Reservation, elderly coughers, former prisoners, HIV, recent immigrants

Drug use: prescription, over the counter, illicit

Piercings and tattoos

Sexual activity or abuse

undervaccinated because of parental fear, and invasive infections with these agents may be overlooked.

Animal exposure should be explored in detail (**Table 1**). Zoonoses are on the increase.[38] Exposure to common household pets like *cats* is associated with Bartonellosis, a relatively frequent but unrecognized cause of unexplained fever. *Dog* contact can be associated with Salmonella infection. Pet *lizards*, *snakes*, and *turtles* are notorious for infecting children with Salmonella, even without direct contact with infants and toddlers because of contamination of the child's environment with fecal material. *Fish and turtle food* is often contaminated with Salmonella.

Although *blood products* are now tested for most known infectious agents, new transmissible agents are emerging, such as Chikungunya and Zika virus.[39] Herpesviruses like Epstein-Barr virus (EBV), cytomegalovirus (CMV), and human herpesvirus 6 (HHV6) can also be transmitted to blood product recipients. Tuberculosis may not be recognized as a potential cause of fever in a child. Situations of risk for tuberculosis transmission include exposure of the child to Native American *reservations*, *recent immigrant or visitors* from developing countries, or *debilitated elderly* individuals.

Careful review of a febrile child's drug use needs to be performed. *Illicit drug* use by the parenteral route can be associated with sepsis and intravascular or cardiac infection. *Drug fever* due to hypersensitization can occur with any pharmaceutical taken chronically, including over-the-counter agents. Many antibiotics, but particularly sulfa drugs, can be associated with drug fever, and although such individuals may also develop other more typical manifestations of a hypersensitivity reaction, fever can be the sole symptom. Accidental organophosphate poisoning or exposure to acetylcholinesterase inhibitors can induce fever.[40] A history of *piercings* and *tattoos* should alert the examiner to possible blood-borne infections like HIV or hepatitis as well as infectious endocarditis (IE). A history of *sexual activity* similarly increases the possibility of sexually transmitted infections or pelvic disease related to tubo-ovarian infection or missed abortion.

In children with FUO, a detailed history of potentially overlooked environmental clues should be sought. Residence in areas of known *endemic infections* needs to be considered. Prominent areas in the United States for infection spread through the pulmonary route include California's San Joaquin Valley and Sonoran Desert areas of the Southwest (coccidiodomycosis), the Ohio and Mississippi River Valleys (histoplasmosis), and the northern tier of the Upper Midwest and New York (blastomycosis). Recent *foreign travel* increases the risk of acquisition of infections endemic to areas visited including malaria, hepatitis E, dengue, leptospirosis, Chikungunya and Zika virus infection, visceral leishmaniasis, acute schistosomiasis, tuberculosis, and yellow and

Table 1	
Childhood fever of unknown origin: common zoonoses	
Infection	**Reservoir**
Leptospirosis	Canines
Tuberculosis (enteric)	Cattle
Brucellosis	Goats, cattle
Q-fever (Coxiella)	Sheep
Salmonella	Reptiles, birds, amphibians
Ornithosis (Chlamydophila)	Birds
Rat bite fever (Streptobacillus)	Rats
Lymphocytic choriomeningitis	Mice
Cat scratch disease (Bartonella)	Cats

typhoid fevers.[41] Contact with *arthropod vectors*, including mosquitoes and ticks, needs to be carefully sought when encountering a febrile child. Arthropods transmit a wide variety of infections, including Lyme disease, ehrlichiosis, anaplasmosis, babesiosis, and other rickettsial infections.[42] Exposure to a *farm* environment raises the possibility of acquisition by the child of animal-borne infections including salmonellosis, brucellosis, Q-fever, ornithosis, and tularemia.[37,38,43] Rural children are more likely to ingest unpasteurized cow and goat milk products. When assessing febrile children, one needs to consider the family's *drinking water* source. Private *wells* can become contaminated with fecal agents like Salmonella or Giardia and are capable of producing long-standing febrile illnesses in children, especially because reinfection can occur.

FOCUSED PHYSICAL EXAMINATION

Assessment by physical examination of the child with undiagnosed fever requires a detailed and directed assessment (**Box 4**). *Documentation* of fever is critical. The relationship between height of fever and heart rate should be assessed. Patients with typhoid fever or other enteric fevers may have a *relative bradycardia* for their recorded temperature. *Height and weight* need to be obtained and compared with previously plotted measurements. Decreases in growth velocity or weight loss may help identify an unrecognized chronic underlying process. The more chronic the process, the more likely it becomes a noninfectious cause of FUO.

Although *generalized lymphadenopathy* can be associated with a wide spectrum of causes of fever, including infections, neoplasms, and rheumatologic causes, regional or *localized adenopathy* is usually related to a contiguous infectious process. *Facial pain*, particularly over the mastoid, malar, or frontal areas, may be indicative of sinusitis or mastoiditis, common causes of unexplained fever in children. *Dental* pain on tooth percussion can be indicative of a dental abscess, whereas *pharyngeal asymmetry* and pain can be a sign of a peritonsillar or parapharyngeal infection.

Examination of the neck of the febrile child needs to include careful assessment for *meningismus*. Children presenting with subtle meningismus may have subacute or

---

Box 4
Childhood fever of unknown origin: focused physical examination

Vital signs: Heart rate and temperature association

General: Decreased growth velocity

Nodes: Generalized or regional adenopathy

Face: Localized pain, erythema, or swelling

Mouth: Dental or pharyngeal pain, asymmetry

Neck: Cervical pits, associated inflammation

Eyes: Visual disturbances, abnormal movements, opsoclonus

Heart: Arrhythmias, rubs, distant sounds, new murmurs

Abdomen: Pain, organomegaly, masses

Extremities: Clubbing, splinters

Neuromuscular: Muscle or bone pain

Joints: Effusions, decreased range of motion

Skin: Transient or persistent rash, petechiae, tattoos, piercings

chronic meningitis caused by fungal or tuberculous agents. A parameningeal focus of infection like mastoiditis, sinusitis, or vertebral osteomyelitis can present with fever and mild meningeal irritation. Neck masses associated with cutaneous pits can indicate an infected bronchial cleft or thyroglossal duct cyst. Painful lateral neck masses may indicate Lemierre disease or inflammatory entities such histiocytic necrotizing lymphadenitis (Kikuchi-Fujimoto disease).[44,45] Rarely, Kawasaki disease (KD) presents with fever and an isolated cervical mass that can be confused with a pyogenic cervical abscess failing to respond to standard antibiotic and surgical therapy.[46] An enlarged mass in the anterior neck can be indicative of an enlarged thyroid with thyroid storm or suppurative thyroiditis.

Examination of the *eyes* may demonstrate scleral hemorrhages or retinal Roth spots indicative of endovascular infection or rheumatologic conditions. The darting movements of *opsiclonus* can be a clue to the presence of neuroblastoma, a tumor sometimes associated with fever in young children. Examination of the heart can reveal *arrhythmias* seen with febrile conditions, including rheumatic fever, Lyme disease, and myocardial abscess. New *murmurs* may be a sign of IE. *Pericardial rubs*, adventitial sounds, or distant heart sounds are suggestive of pericardial infection or an effusion related to postinfectious immune reaction or to a rheumatologic process like SLE. Careful examination of the abdomen is required to exclude the presence of *organomegaly*, *masses*, or localized *pain*. The percussive *flank pain* of renal infection needs to be sought. In appropriate populations, a careful *rectal examination* may help alert the examiner to the presence of a periappendiceal abscess or pelvic infection.

Tattoos and *piercings* may indicate the presence of blood-borne infections. Children with clubbing of nails may have chronic underlying conditions capable of causing fever, including IE, hepatitis, and cystic fibrosis. Careful examination may reveal generalized *muscular pain* as seen in influenza-related myositis or pain localized to one muscle as noted in pyogenic myositis.[47] Bone *pain*, indicative of osteomyelitis or tumor should be assessed. *Joint effusions* should be sought. If present in multiple joints, these may indicate the presence of an immune or autoimmune process. *Transient rashes* may be suggestive of JIA or other vasculitides.

SYNDROMIC CHARACTERIZATION OF CHILDHOOD FEVER OF UNKNOWN ORIGIN

Many children with FUO do not present with fever as their sole symptom. After taking a comprehensive history and performing a careful physical examination, other signs and symptoms may be noted allowing placement of the patient into one of several broad syndromic categories and the clinician to focus attention on the most likely diagnostic entities. Such categorizations should be tentative and nonexclusive. Both noninfectious and infectious febrile childhood conditions present in a syndromic manner in children with FUO.

SYNDROMIC FEVER: NONINFECTIOUS CAUSES

One of the more common syndromes associated with a noninfectious cause is isolated fever, sometimes in association with systemic inflammatory response syndrome (SIRS).[48] Fever can be the sole presenting symptom of common childhood malignancies, particularly acute leukemia and lymphoma (**Box 5**) that may be the result of the release of cytokines by a malignant tumor clone or secondary to host response to the tumor. A related process may be operative in hemophagocytic lymphocytic histiocytosis (HLH) and macrophage activation syndromes (MAS).[49,50] Neuroblastoma also can present primarily with fever, possibly related to vasoactive neuroendocrine tumor products.

Box 5
Childhood fever of unknown origin: noninfectious causes

Sepsis/shock/SIRS: HLH, MAS, acute leukemia, lymphoma, neuroblastoma, drug fever, lupus

Cervical lymphadenopathy (predominant): Kikuchi, HLH, KD, ALPS

Pharyngitis/tonsillitis: IBD

Meningitis: Ruptured craniopharyngioma, IVIG, or NSAID use

Cardiovascular: KD, PAN

Pericarditis: Postinfectious (*N meningitidis*, Mycoplasma), SLE

Pneumonitis: Sarcoid, Wegener syndrome, aspiration

Hepatitis/hepatomegaly: IBD, autoimmune hepatitis, drug hypersensitivity

Gastroenteritis/abdominal pain: IBD, pancreatitis

Musculoskeletal: Histiocytosis, ankylosing spondylitis, relapsing multifocal osteomyelitis, malignancy, JIA, postinfectious (GABS, *N meningitidis*, HIB)

Dermatologic: Lupus, JIA, KD, IBD

Abbreviations: ALPS, autoimmune lymphoproliferative syndrome; GABS, group Aβ hemolytic streptococcus; IBD, Inflammatory bowel disease; IVIG, intravenous immune globulin; MAS, macrophage activation syndrome; PAN, polyarteritis nodosa.

A wide variety of apparently noninfectious febrile conditions in children is associated with prominent cervical lymphadenopathy, sometimes accompanied by generalized lymphadenopathy. KD variant disease can manifest as isolated cervical lymphadenitis with fever.[46] Other noninfectious febrile syndromes presenting with cervical adenopathy, such as Kikuchi-Fujimoto disease and autoimmune lymphoproliferative syndrome (ALPS) appear to have an immune or autoimmune pathogenesis and demonstrate distinctive histopathologic changes and cell marker analysis of affected nodes.[44,51]

As the oropharynx is part of the gastrointestinal (GI) track, noninfectious, febrile inflammatory conditions involving the GI track may demonstrate pharyngeal involvement with pain, pharyngitis, and mucosal ulceration. On occasion, oropharyngeal lesions antedate more distal GI symptoms, confusing diagnosis. Inflammatory bowel disease (IBD) should be considered in any child presenting with unexplained fever and oral or pharyngeal lesions. In older children, fever, weight loss, and abdominal pain are a common presentation for IBD, frequently without diarrhea. Idiopathic, obstructive, or drug-induced pancreatitis is also a relativity common cause of childhood FUO associated with patients with fever and poorly localized, severe abdominal pain.

Generalized or focal osseous lesions associated with fever are not always of infectious cause. Common primary hematologic malignancies like leukemia or the secondary metastatic lesions of tumors such as neuroblastoma or rhabdomyosarcoma can present with such prominent bone and joint symptoms that malignancy can be confused with infection. Febrile children with aleukemic leukemia may be treated empirically for presumed septic joints or osteomyelitis until the correct diagnosis is made. Drug-induced hypersensitivity fever may be associated with significant neck pain.[52] Other febrile, noninfectious processes like histiocytosis X, chronic recurrent multifocal osteomyelitis, and rheumatologic conditions such as ankylosing spondylitis can be confused with an infection.[53]

Fevers associated with noninfectious cardiovascular disease include both immune-mediated conditions like poststreptococcal acute rheumatic fever, or myopericarditis related to SLE or polyarteritis nodosa (PAN). KD-associated myocarditis may one day be recognized to be immune mediated. Fever characterizes a variety of autoimmune syndromes involving the renal system and lung, including granulomatosis with polyangiitis (Wegener granulomatosis) and PAN.[54,55] Fever with skin manifestations as a primary symptom may be seen with the evanescent rash of JIA, the photosensitivity eruption of SLE, or necrotic skin lesions associated with granulomatosis with polyangiitis, PAN, or IBD.

SYNDROMIC FEVER: INFECTIOUS CAUSES

Primary infections or secondary immunologic reactions to infection account for 60% to 70% of FUOs in those children in whom a diagnosis is made.[18,20] Many cases of FUO relate to unusual presentations of common infections. Results of laboratory testing may be altered by empiric use of antibiotic or anti-inflammatory agents, complicating diagnosis. A proportion of children with FUO do suffer from infections with unusual agents, requiring expansion of differential diagnoses and use of unfamiliar diagnostic tests and procedures. Because many children with FUO present with signs and symptoms other than simply fever, it is useful to construct a differential diagnosis based on affected organ systems. This allows the clinician to focus on those laboratory assays and imaging procedures most likely to provide a prompt diagnosis.

Fever can be associated with infections affecting virtually every organ system (**Box 6**). Fever, sometimes associated with SIRS can be the dominant finding before significant organ involvement is recognized. Widespread use of routine Haemophilus, Pneumococcal and *Neisseria meningitidis* vaccines has markedly reduced febrile occult bacteremias with these agents, but such bacteremias still do occur. The infecting organism may be a serotype not included in the vaccines or in infants in whom immunization is incomplete. Any of the these organisms, as well as *Staphylococcus aureus* (SA) Group A (GABS), and Group B (GBBS) β hemolytic strep can produce a confusing clinical picture of shock associated with fever and SIRS, with marked leukopenia or leukocytosis, DIC, thrombocytopenia, and purpuric skin lesions. If antibiotic therapy is initiated before obtaining blood cultures, the clinical picture may be quite confusing in the presence of negative cultures. A similar picture can occur with enteric organisms and Pseudomonas. Septicemic infection with Pseudomonas and *N meningitidis* is sometimes associated with host immune defects. Rickettsial agents, especially Rocky Mountain Spotted Fever (RMSF) and ehrlichiosis, can present with fever and a shocklike state with negative blood cultures. The infection will be unresponsive to standard broad-spectrum empiric antibiotic therapy.[42] Recognition of the possibility of rickettsial infection is critical in such cases, because there is a 10% mortality in untreated patients with many rickettsial agents. Malaria has become more common with increased international travel of children due to inconsistent use of prophylaxis and travel to areas with drug resistant strains. New, unfamiliar infectious agents like Chikungunya virus, Hantavirus, and Zikavirus are constantly emerging and may present only with prolonged fever.[56,57]

FUO with prominent cervical lymphadenopathy, with or without pharyngitis, is a rather common scenario in which most physicians will test for EBV infection. If the Monospot test is used for diagnosis, there is a high false negativity rate, especially in children less than 5 years of age. Young children also frequently fail to display the atypical monocytosis so commonly observed in the peripheral blood of older children and young adults. CMV, HIV, and toxoplasmosis produce a clinical and laboratory picture identical to EBV infection. Adenovirus infection is recognized as capable of producing isolated high fever of 2 or 3 weeks in duration.[58] Although GABS infection is the

Box 6
Childhood fever of unknown origin: infectious causes

Sepsis/shock/SIRS:

Gram-positive organisms: *S pyogens, Staphylococcus aureus,* Pneumococcus

Gram-negative organisms: *N meningitidis,* enteric Gram negatives, pseudomonas

Rickettsial agents (RMSF, Ehrlichiosis)

Hanta virus

Dengue

Malaria

Cervical lymphadenopathy (predominant):

Viral: EBV, CMV, HIV, adenovirus

Parasitic: Toxoplasmosis

Pharyngitis/tonsillitis:

Non-group A streptococcus: Groups C and G

Arcanobacterium

Lemierre syndrome (Fusobacterium, other anaerobes)

Peritonsillar or parapharyngeal abscess

Ludwig angina

Meningitis:

Parameningeal infection: Mastoiditis, subdural/epidural abscess, vertebral osteomyelitis, discitis

Fungal agents: Cryptococcosis, coccidiodomycosis, histoplasmosis, blastomycosis

Bacterial agents: Leptospirosis, *Mycobacteria tuberculosis*

Parasitic: Naegleria, Baylisascaris

Viral: Lymphocytic choriomeningitis

Cardiovascular:

Endocarditis: HACEK bacteria, Bartonella, Coxiella, Legionella, Streptobacillus, culture negative

Peripheral venous infection: CONS, enterococci, enteric gram-negative bacteria, SA

Pericarditis: Pyogenic organisms, mycobacteria, fungal, viral

Pneumonitis:

Foreign body, sequestered lobe

Obstructive: Tumor, ring, sling

Endemic agent: Legionella, Histoplasma, Blastomyces, Cryptococcus, Coccidiodomyces

Unrecognized Immune deficiency: Aspergillus, Mucor, Cryptococcus, Nocardia

Reflux, Aspiration

Unrecognized agents: *Chlamydophila pneumoniae* or *C psittaci; Pneumocystis jiroveci,* Legionella

Hepatitis/hepatomegaly:

Virus: Hepatitis B, C, E, EBV, CMV, HSV

Fungus: Histoplasmosis, Candida

Bacterial: Solitary hepatic abscess, Bartonella, Leptospira, GB disease, cholangitis

Parasitic: Toxoplasmosis

Gastroenteritis/abdominal pain/renal:

Parasitic: Giardia, Cryptosporidium, Entamoeba

Bacterial: Yersinia, *C difficile*, *E coli*, Brucella, Aeromonas

Mycobacterial: *M bovis* and tuberculosis

Periappendiceal or pelvic abscesses

UTI: *S hominis*, anaerobes, Mycobacteria, Adenovirus

Pyelonephritis, renal abscess

Musculoskeletal:

Osteomyelitis: long bones, vertebral, discitis

Subacute osteomyelitis: Group β streptococcus, kingella, salmonella

Pyomyositis: *S aureus*, gram-negative enteric agents

Myositis: Influenza A and B

Dermatologic:

Pustular: Streptobacillus, *S aureus*

Necrotic: Pseudomonas, *N meningitidis*

Bullae: SA

Sandpaper: Group Aβ streptococcus

Abbreviations: CONS, coagulase negative staphylococci; HACEK, haemophilus, aggregatibacter, cardiobacterium, eikenella, kingella; HSV, herpes simplex virus; UTI, Urinary tract infections.

most commonly diagnosed bacterial infection of the pharynx associated with fever and pharyngitis, serogroup groups C and G streptococcal infections are able to produce a febrile infection undetectable by routine rapid testing. Standard testing of pharyngeal swabs will also overlook the presence of *Arcanobacterium haemolyticum*, a bacterial agent capable of producing a febrile illness with pharyngitis and rash. It is clinically indistinguishable from GABS pharyngitis, but nonresponsive to β-lactam therapy.[59]

At times, a common bacterial or viral pharyngeal infection precedes a more invasive secondary infection of anatomic structures and spaces within the neck. Peritonsillar and parapharyngeal infection may initially go unrecognized, especially if the child is receiving antibiotics for a primary pharyngitis. Invasion of large veins in the neck after a viral or bacterial pharyngitis by the anaerobe, *Fusobacterium necrophorum*, results in painful cervical masses in Lemierre syndrome.[45] These patients develop bacterial thrombophlebitis of cervical veins. This infection is usually associated with anaerobic bacteremia with septic pulmonary embolization and pneumonia.[45]

Bacterial and viral meningitis are common causes of febrile illness with meningismus and are usually easily diagnosed. However, diagnosis of FUO associated with cerebrospinal fluid (CSF) pleocytosis in which bacterial cultures of the CSF are negative can be troublesome. Bacterial parameningeal infections induce CSF pleocytosis and elevated CSF protein with normal glucose concentrations. The most common locations for the primary infection are sinuses and mastoids. Such infections may be chronic, producing epidural and subdural empyemas and a sterile, inflammatory CSF response.[60] A similar picture in the CSF is noted with parenchymal brain abscesses. Fungal meningitis, due to cryptococcosis, blastomycosis, histoplasmosis, and coccidioidomycosis, results in the clinical and laboratory picture of subacute or chronic meningitis. The CSF formula is often suggestive of a bacterial infection, but bacterial cultures are persistently negative. Tuberculous meningitis produces a similar subacute or chronic meningitis, although often with prominent cranial nerve abnormalities.[61] In both tuberculous and fungal meningitis, inapparent pneumonitis is often found.

Severe aseptic meningitis can be seen in toddlers after ingestion of raccoon feces due to the raccoon roundworm *Baylisascaris*. This parasite induces a profound eosinophilic meningitis.[62] Leptospirosis is associated with aseptic meningitis, often preceded by fever and hepatitis.[63] The mouse-associated agent, lymphocytic choriomeningitis virus, produces a chronic lymphocytic meningitis.[64] If a child with FUO and undiagnosed meningitis has been swimming in ponds or ditches in warmer climates, amebic meningitis must be considered.[65]

The presence of IE must be considered in any child with FUO. Most, although not all cases of IE, occur in children with existing anatomic cardiac abnormalities or develop soon after surgical correction of cardiac lesions.[66] Murmurs may be absent, and the infected area may not be evident on routine transthoracic echocardiographic studies. Unless multiple high-volume blood cultures are obtained before the initiation of antibiotic therapy, IE caused by bacteria like α streptococci and enterococci can be missed. Some cases of IE may be difficult to confirm microbiologically despite the presence of obvious vegetations, resulting in "culture-negative infective endocarditis." Routine cultures may remain negative because of infection with particularly fastidious "nutritionally deficient" bacterial strains or those in the "HACEK" spectrum (Haemophilus, Aggregatibacter, Cardiobacterium, Eikenella, and Kingella). Other agents difficult to cultivate in standard commercial blood culture media include Bartonella, Streptobacillus, Brucella, Legionella, Chlamydophila, Coxiella, and Mycoplasma.[66] Molds like Aspergillus produce large vegetations, but blood cultures are frequently negative. Many patients with IE demonstrate characteristic embolic left-sided pulmonary lesions and/or ischemic systemic lesions due to arterial emboli, depending on location of the infection and anatomy of the infected heart.

Infections of the peripheral vascular system are common. Any organism can invade a sterile thrombus, resulting in persistent intravascular infection. Such infection often occurs as a consequence of current or prior use of an indwelling venous catheter.[67] The usual clinical picture of such infection is persistent hectic fever with persistently positive blood cultures, often with embolization of end arteries in the pulmonary or peripheral vascular systems. A similar picture of septic thrombophlebitis without prior catheter use is a complication of SA infections of bone and soft tissues.[68] The pericardium can be secondarily infected by the pyogenic organisms causative of both community- and hospital-associated pneumonias, but can also be an unrecognized site of infection due to bacteremia with organisms like *S aureus*, *N meningitides*, and *Streptococcus pneumoniae*.

FUO associated with recurrent or chronic pulmonary infiltrates in a distinct anatomic area suggests an obstructive bronchial lesion. Lesions may be congenital due to bronchomalacia or stenosis or due to vascular slings and rings or sequestered lobes. Other obstructive lesions are acquired, such as aspirated foreign bodies or tumors. Obstruction can result in chronic or recurrent bacterial infection and development of bronchiectasis with destruction of pulmonary parenchyma. Recurrent diffuse alveolar infiltrates may be seen with chronic aspiration secondary to neurologic or developmental abnormalities, esophageal dysfunction, or reflux. In the appropriate geographic setting, pulmonary infection with epidemic or endemic agents like

Legionella, Histoplasma, Blastomyces, and Coccidioides may be present. Pulmonary infection with unusual agents like Aspergillus, Nocardia, or Cryptococcus may be the first indicator of unrecognized immunodeficiency. Diffuse pneumonias unresponsive to empiric antibiotic therapy are sometimes caused by Chlamydophila and Mycoplasma.

Patients with FUO and hepatomegaly and/or hepatitis need to be carefully evaluated for not only the common causes of viral hepatitis (hepatitis A, B, C) but also infection with other common viruses, which may produce significant hepatocellular damage like herpesviruses EBV, CMV, herpes simplex virus (HSV), and adenovirus. Disseminated fungal infection with Histoplasma or Candida can produce numerous small hepatosplenic inflammatory lesions.[69] Similar granulomatous lesions can be seen in cat scratch disease, due to *Bartonella henslae*.[70] Hepatitis and renal failure occur in leptospirosis. Acute toxoplasmosis or toxacariasis can present with fever and marked hepatosplenomegaly. Solitary liver abscess, most frequently associated with *S aureus* infection or gram-negative enteric agents, can be a particularly difficult febrile condition to diagnose when the abscess is small. Liver function abnormalities are uncommon, even with multiple or large abscesses. Solitary bacterial hepatic abscess is a common presentation for phagocytic cell abnormalities such chronic granulomatous disease.[71] Unsuspected anatomic abnormalities of the biliary system or gallbladder disease can also present with an ascending cholangitis and secondary liver abscesses. Splenic abscesses may be solitary or multiple and are often associated with infection elsewhere.[72]

Children with FUO accompanied by diarrhea and abdominal pain may be infected with an unanticipated agent or a microorganism the microbiology laboratory may be unable to detect by routine means. Some laboratories do not routinely assess stool for the presence of Vibrio or Yersinia unless specifically requested. *Clostridium difficile* toxin disease can produce a confusing and unrecognized secondary febrile illness in children treated with antibiotics for an antecedent febrile illness, especially if the child's diarrhea is misidentified as a side effect of antibiotic use. Aeromonas infection also can produce a confusing picture of febrile colitis because the organism is frequently not recognized as pathogenic. Although most intestinal parasitic infections are not associated with fever, patients infected with Giardia, Cryptosporidium, and *Entamoeba histolytica* can be febrile. Intestinal infection due to *Mycobacteria tuberculosis* or *Mycobacterium bovis* can produce a chronic febrile illness with notable abdominal pain. When evaluating young children with fever and poorly localized abdominal pain because of their age, periappendiceal or pelvic abscesses may be overlooked, particularly in the absence of a rectal examination.

Infections of the renal system are a frequent cause of FUO in children. Urinary tract infections (UTI) may be caused by bacterial agents not recognized as pathogens, including coagulase-negative staphylococci species, α streptococci, and Lactobacilli. Some infectious agents are not detectable by techniques used to assess patients for UTI, such as anaerobes, mycobacteria, and viruses like Adenovirus and BK virus. The sensitivity of the urine culture is also not absolute in diagnosing upper track urinary infections. Patients with fever can have pyelonephritis despite negative urine cultures or those whose positivity does not reach diagnostic criteria for UTI. This can occur because of intrarenal obstruction of urine flow from the infected renal papillae. Children with FUO may have renal abscesses with low urinary bacterial concentrations, particularly following antibiotic treatment for a presumed uncomplicated UTI.

Unsuspected infections of the musculoskeletal system can be a cause of FUO in childhood, especially young children unable to localize discomfort. In infants, osteomyelitis due to GBBS, Salmonella, and *S aureus* can be a result of silent bacteremias, presenting as a new febrile illness, days or even weeks later. Only the most careful physical examination may detect localized discomfort upon palpation of infected bones or movement of infected joints. Focused observation may be required to observe subtle decreased movement of affected limbs in infants. In the toddler, joint and bone infections due to Kingella have become recognized as occurring in epidemics among young children attending daycare centers or preschools.[34] Identification of Kingella requires a high index of suspicion and the use of molecular diagnostic techniques. Children with sickle syndromes can develop bone and joint infections difficult to distinguish from thrombo-occlusive crises. Vertebral osteomyelitis or discitis can present a confusing picture in the febrile child, particularly in the presence of nerve root or spinal cord compression by abscesses or inflammatory masses. Pyomyositis can be difficult to diagnose in the febrile child because of poor pain localization. These infections sometimes occur following traumatic or overuse injury to a muscle, allowing leakage of hematogenous pathogens into the muscle to establish infection.[47] When the infected muscle lies in the pelvic floor or supportive muscles of the hip, physical examination can be misleading, and radiologic studies misinterpreted if pyomyositis is not considered. Diffuse myositis with fever is a relatively common complication of influenza A or B infection, and on occasion, can dominate symptoms in patients infected with these viral agents.

Children with FUO may have rashes, but many are nonspecific in appearance. Cutaneous petechiae and hemorrhagic "splinters" are seen under the nails in intravascular infections, especially IE.[66] There may also be palatal and scleral hemorrhages in such patients. Sepsis with *S aureus* and other pyogenic agents can demonstrate similar lesions without a definable intravascular focus. Large irregular necrotic purpuric lesions, the results of obstruction of cutaneous end arterioles, are associated with infections capable of inducing intravascular thrombosis. This eruption is most often seen in meningococcemia, an organism sometimes impossible to isolate from blood, if even a single antibiotic dose has been administered before culture acquisition. Similar eruptions are seen occasionally in severe *S pneumoniae* and *H influenzae* sepsis and can occur with almost any agent capable of producing sepsis. Fever and erythema with prominent blistering and bullae formation are observed with infection with exotoxin A-producing strains of *S aureus*, in staphylococcal scalded skin syndrome. At times this diagnosis is not considered, because the eruption is in response to a toxin and often not to an invasive infection. Therefore, blood and cultures of the skin and fluid with vesicles are often negative. The causative organism may be colonizing an umbilical stump in infants or the nose or other mucous membranes in older children. A rough erythematous rash similar to the texture of sandpaper is typical of group A beta streptococcal infection and often exfoliates. In patients with rodent exposure and FUO with a pustular eruption, infection with *Streptobacillus moniliformis*, the agent of rat bite fever, must be considered.[73] Ecthyma gangrenosum (EG), large round or ovoid painful necrotic purpuric cutaneous lesions with a thin erythematous collar, is most commonly associated with bacteremic infections with gram-negative agents, particularly Pseudomonas. These lesions are most frequently seen in febrile children with an underlying immune deficiency or neoplasm, although EG has been noted in infants with Pseudomonas sepsis without definable immune deficiency.

LABORATORY AND RADIOLOGIC EVALUATION

Laboratory evaluation of a child with FUO should be performed in a staged manner, with more invasive tests reserved for children with evidence suggestive of serious disease (**Box 7**). The most helpful initial screening tests in patients with FUO are usually

---

Box 7
Childhood fever of unknown origin: staged workup

Initial:

CBC, manual differential

ESR, CRP

Urinalysis

Blood, urine, stool and throat cultures

Chest radiograph

Chemistry panel

Secondary (as appropriate):

IgM, IgG, IgA

Albumin

PCRs: Adenovirus, mycoplasma

Serologies: EBV, CMV, HIV, ANA, others as appropriate

Sinus CT

Abdominal ultrasound

Whole-body NMRI

Cardiac echocardiography in selected patients

Tertiary (as indicated):

Bone marrow with cultures

Radionuclide leukocyte or gallium scan

Biopsy of abnormal tissues with comprehensive cultures

rRNA analysis of culture negative tissue

Abbreviations: ANA, antinuclear antibody; CBC, complete blood count; CT, Computer-assisted tomography; rRNA, ribosomal RNA.

---

urinalysis and urine culture, inflammatory markers, blood culture, and chest radiograph. If inflammatory markers are in the normal to near normal range and fever has been clearly documented, one needs to consider the patient might have a noninflammatory cause of fever (**Box 8**). Noninflammatory fevers can be secondary to processes that disrupt thermoregulatory function related to damage to critical anatomic areas in the

---

Box 8
Childhood fever of unknown origin: noninflammatory causes

Dysautonomia syndromes: Genetic or acquired

Abnormal eccrine gland function: Burns, ichthyosis, hypernatremia, cystic fibrosis

Neurologic damage: Vascular, traumatic, postinfectious, autoimmune

Drugs: Anticholinergics

Poisoning: Aspirin, anticholinesterases, organophosphates, heavy metals

Endocrine: Hyperthyroidism, hyperadenocorticalism

hypothalamus. "Central fever" is a term often used for such elevations, and such a mechanism should be suspected when multiple inflammatory markers fail to increase with fever. Another clue to a fever of noninflammatory cause is disassociation of autonomic functions with height of the child's fever, that is, heart rate and respiratory rate fail to increase with fever spikes or the presence episodes of hypothermia interspersed with those of hyperthermia. Other causes of noninflammatory fevers include conditions that affect the ability of the child to perspire normally, reducing effectiveness of heat loss through evaporation due to abnormal or traumatized skin. Reduction in perspiration rate due to the effect of drugs or poisons and metabolic or endocrine conditions that reduce efficiency of perspiration (cystic fibrosis) or produce a sustained increase in basal metabolic activity (thyrotoxicosis) can also produce fever.

If inflammatory markers are suggestive of an active inflammatory process, further assessment requires serologic evaluation for causes of FUO. Viral infections associated with prolonged fever include EBV, CMV, and adenovirus. Specific EBV serologies including anti-EBV immunoglobulin G (IgG) and IgM should always be obtained rather than the Monospot test, especially in young children. Early HIV infection can present with fever and a mononucleosis-like picture, and an HIV screen should be sought in children where there is sexual activity or possible abuse. Mycoplasma and Adenovirus nasopharyngeal polymerase chain reaction (PCR) helps rule out these agents as causes of FUO.

A wide variety of zoonoses affect children. If exposure to certain animals is found, specific serologic or cultures should be obtained as appropriate for those agents (see **Table 1**). The increased prevalence of nontraditional household pets requires the physician to assess the possibility that animals may have been the source of the child's FUO. Reptiles and birds are a particular risk to young infants and toddlers. Excrement from these animals is frequently found on floors or rugs where infants are placed, allowing transmission of infectious agents without direct contact. The increased frequency of rats as pets has led to an increasing number of Streptobacillus infections, an organism not easily isolated in standard culture media. Pet birds or trips to an aviary can result in ornithosis due to *Chlamydophila psittaci*, even without direct contact with birds. Petting zoos are notorious for outbreaks of salmonellosis, enteropathogenic *E coli*, and Campylobacter infection among child visitors. Asymptomatic cats carry Bartonella in their mouths and on their claws. Even the most minor of scratches or contamination of minor abrasions with feline saliva can be associated with bartonellosis. Most clinicians are familiar with the usual manifestations of "cat scratch fever," a peripheral nodular lesion at the initial site with associated regional lymphadenitis and fever. Few recognize the hepatosplenic form of the infection without lymphadenopathy. Exposure to farm animals should lead to consideration of assessment for salmonellosis, Q fever, Campylobacter infection, and intestinal tuberculosis if unpasteurized milk has been ingested.

If a child with FUO resides in an area endemic for environmental or tick-borne infections, testing should be considered for those pathogens. Patients with persistent pulmonary infiltrates should be tested for fungal antigenuria for Coccidioidomycosis, Histoplasmosis, and Blastomycosis if they have spent significant time in areas endemic for those infections. If the child has had contact with an individual with a chronic unexplained cough, or exposure to a high-risk environment for pulmonary tuberculosis, a tuberculin skin test should be placed or an interferon-gamma release assay performed. Ticks are known to be carriers of a variety of infections, many with prolonged fever as a major symptom, including RMSF, Lyme disease, Anaplasmosis, Ehrlichiosis, and Babesiosis. Many infections with these agents present primarily with fever, and rashes may be absent or forgotten. In a large proportion of cases of tick-borne infections, a prior tick bite is not reported. Testing for infection with these agents is often through a "Tick Panel" incorporating a variety of testing methods for the diverse causes of infections associated with arthropod bites. Many tick-borne infections are associated with simultaneous coinfection with a second or even third tick-borne agent, complicating the clinical picture and therapy. It is important to be aware of health alerts issued by state and national bodies regarding epidemic febrile infections occurring in the United States or in popular travel destinations. Recent examples of unfamiliar febrile illnesses occurring in the United States among travelers to areas of outbreak include infections with Hantavirus, Rubeola, and Zika virus.

The chronicity of the inflammatory process can be assessed by obtaining quantitative immunoglobulin levels, which tend to elevate when inflammatory conditions are present for more than a couple of weeks. Similarly, serum albumin and hemoglobin levels tend to drop in chronically ill children over the same period. These results help the clinician deduce whether an inflammatory process is chronic or acute. The antinuclear antibody (ANA) test is a reasonable screen for autoimmune conditions, but is not adequate for diagnosis of many rheumatologic diseases. Antistreptolysin O and anti-DNase B titers may help exclude rheumatic fever as a cause of FUO, especially if antibiotics have been recently used in patient therapy.

The development of sensitive noninvasive imaging techniques has revolutionized the evaluation of children with FUO by allowing detection of occult infection, inflammation, anatomic abnormalities, or tumors. Computer-assisted tomography (CT) of the chest and abdomen, with and without contrast, is helpful in assessing those areas for inflammatory lesions, lymphadenopathy, and tumors, but is rapidly being replaced by whole-body nuclear MRI (NMRI). NMRI has the advantages of not exposing the child to radiation and allowing assessment of areas either not usually CT scanned (central nervous system) or not easily evaluable by CT (soft tissues). CT of the sinuses still should be considered before a whole-body NMRI if there are any suggestions of sinus disease, because occult sinusitis is a relatively common cause of FUO in children. Rarely, Gallium-67 scan or radiolabeled PMNs may be able to detect localized inflammatory lesions or demonstrate diffuse uptake in the marrow or nodes consistent with neoplasm. These methods have fallen out of favor because of the amount of radiation to which they expose the child and difficulties in interpretation.

In the current medicolegal climate, most children with significant fever of more than several days' duration require an echocardiogram to assess coronary artery status to help determine the need for intravenous immune globulin infusions (IVIG) for empiric treatment of incomplete or atypically presenting KD. Dramatic response of fever and inflammation to empiric IVIG infusion is considered by some to be evidence for KD. However, IVIG contains antibodies to many infectious agents, and IVIG is an immunomodulator, which may nonspecifically inhibit inflammation in febrile patients, regardless of the cause of underlying inflammatory process.

If areas of inflammation, granulomatous reaction, fluid collection, suppuration, or suspected malignancy are found on imaging, it is often possible to obtain tissue for culture and histology via minimally invasive radiologic techniques. Some lesions, particularly cardiac and hepatic, may be approachable via a transvascular approach. Osseous or lymphatic tissue near to body surface can be sampled by thin-needle aspiration. Routine histology with special tissue stains for mycobacteria, bacteria, and fungi, in association with bacterial cultures for such pathogens, is usually sufficient for analysis of tissue. At times, electron microscopy of the tissue may be helpful. In selected cases, viral cultures or PCRs or probes of tissue may be of benefit.

Marrow aspiration is useful in ruling out malignancy, and bone marrow culture may be helpful in making the diagnosis of intracellular infections, like brucellosis, tuberculosis, and salmonellosis. If cultures yield unidentifiable microorganisms, modern microbiologic techniques, such as matrix-assisted laser desorption/ionization time-of-flight mass spectrometry, allows rapid identification of unusual organisms.[74] Emerging microbiologic techniques such as 16s ribosomal RNA genetic bacterial or 28s fungal sequencing allows detection of nonculturable microorganisms from infected tissue.[75] New, more sensitive, and broader genetic techniques, which assess the entire microbial genome, are on the near horizon and will have a huge impact on the diagnosis of infections in children with FUO. They potentially allow diagnosis of infection anywhere in the body through detection of microbial genetic material in infected tissues, but potentially also in peripheral blood or other fluids like urine and CSF.[76]

Therapeutic "trials" with antibiotics are ineffective in the evaluation of the patient with FUO. The "shotgun" use of antibiotics in patients with fevers of unknown cause may delay the ultimate diagnosis. In cases where diagnosis of the cause of the fever is not apparent, if the child is not critically ill, it is appropriate to simply follow the patient closely. Sometimes fever resolves permanently.[22] At other times fever recurs with new symptoms, or if fever persists, new symptoms or laboratory abnormalities appear, allowing the underlying diagnosis to be made. Frequent re-examination often results in successful diagnosis. With some processes in which diagnosis by exclusion is the rule or for which no definitive diagnostic test exists, like JIA and recurrent multifocal osteomyelitis, diagnosis can be made only after repeated febrile episodes.

THE FUTURE

In the near future, advancements in diagnostic procedures will shorten the interval required to diagnose FUOs in children and increase accuracy of diagnosis. Some of these assays and procedures are currently being critically evaluated for general use. Direct direction and quantitation of fever-inducing cytokines in blood and tissues will facilitate identification of inflammatory stimuli, helping determine whether the illness is infectious, immune, neoplastic, or of an alternative cause. Omics (metabolomics, proteomics, and genomics), the qualitative and quantitative assessment of host genome, associated proteins and metabolic products, and subsequent alteration by fever-inducing processes, will allow detailed determination of the nature of the host response to specific infectious agents and noninfectious processes.[77]

Advances in imaging techniques and wider utilization methods already available, such as PET, will result in better assessment of abnormalities of metabolic function in organs of children with FUO. Safer invasive tissue sampling, particularly via the transvascular route, will allow direct sampling of tissue for diagnostic purposes from previously inaccessible locations. Diagnostic microbiologic techniques will continue migration from classic methodologies toward metabolic and genetic ones. Such techniques will require only the presence of microbial genetic material within tissues and fluids for pathogen identification, allowing definitive, rapid etiologic diagnosis of infections impossible to diagnose by older methodologies. Novel pathogens will be identified in this manner as the causative agents of illnesses now not even recognized to be infections. These advances will revolutionize the workup, diagnosis, and therapy of illnesses associated with childhood FUO, making the process safer, faster, more accurate, and more economical.

SUMMARY

Evaluation of FUO in children requires confirmation of fever in a medical setting. Careful repeated reassessment of the child's medical history and physical examination may provide important clues regarding the underlying cause of fever. Although most childhood FUOs have an infectious cause, a significant minority are related to neoplasms, collagen vascular disease, or a variety of underlying inflammatory conditions. In some cases, the fever simply resolves, never to appear again.

Initial assessment of FUO, using nonspecific measures of systemic inflammation like the complete blood count, ESR, and CRP, helps identify those children likely to have a serious condition related to their prolonged fever. Workup of childhood FUO should be staged, with expensive imaging and invasive surgical or biopsy procedures done last. Assessment of the child with FUO for laboratory and physical findings demonstrating involvement of a particular organ system can help focus diagnostic testing. Molecular genetic techniques are playing an increasingly important role in the diagnosis of infectious and noninfectious conditions associated with childhood FUO.

REFERENCES

1. Earn DJ, Andrews PW, Bolker BM. Population-level effects of suppressing fever. Proc Biol Sci 2014;281:20132570.
2. Evans SS, Repasky EA, Fisher DT. Fever and the thermal regulation of immunity: the immune system feels the heat. Nat Rev Immunol 2015;15:335–49.
3. Romanovsky AA. Thermoregulation: some concepts have changed. Functional architecture of the thermoregulatory system. Am J Physiol Regul Integr Comp Physiol 2007;292:R37–46.
4. Sundgren-Andersson AK, Ostlund P, Bartfai T. IL-6 is essential in TNF-α-induced fever. Am J Physiol 1998;275:R2028–34.
5. Kozak W, Kluger MJ, Soszynski D, et al. IL-6 and IL-1β in fever: studies using cytokine-deficient (knockout) mice. Ann N Y Acad Sci 1998;856:33–47.
6. Rummel C, Sachot C, Poole S, et al. Circulating interleukin-6 induces fever through a STAT3-linked activation of Cox-2 in the brain. Am J Physiol Regul Integr Comp Physiol 2006;291:R1316–26.
7. Ivanov AI, Romanovsky AA. Prostaglandin E_2 as a mediator of fever: synthesis and catabolism. Front Biosci 2004;9:1977–93.
8. Schmitt BD. Fever phobia: misconceptions of parents about fevers. Am J Dis Child 1980;134(2):176–81.
9. Launey Y, Nesseler N, Malledant Y, et al. Clinical review: fever in septic ICU patients-friend or foe? Crit Care 2011;15:222–9.
10. Schulman CI, Namias N, Doherty J, et al. The effect of antipyretic therapy upon outcomes in critically ill patients: a randomized, prospective study. Surg Infect (Larchmt) 2005;6:369–75.
11. Van Oss CJ, Absolom DR, Moore LL, et al. Effect of temperature on the chemotaxis, phagocytic engulfment, digestion and O2 consumption of human polymorphonuclear leukocytes. J Reticuloendothel Soc 1980;27(6):561–5.
12. Knippertz I, Stein MF, Dorrie J, et al. Mild hyperthermia enhances human monocyte-derived dendritic cell functions and offers potential for applications in vaccination strategies. Int J Hyperthermia 2011;27:591–603.
13. Roberts NF, Steigbigel RT. Hyperthermia and human leukocyte functions: effects on response of lymphocytes to mitogen and antigen and bactericidal capacity of monocytes and neutrophils. Infect Immun 1977;18(3):673–9.
14. Ostberg JR, Ertel BR, Lanphere JA. An important role for granulocytes in the thermal regulation of colon tumor growth. Immunol Invest 2005;34:259–72.

15. Marshall GS. Prolonged and recurrent fevers in children. J Infect 2014;68(Suppl 1):S83–93.

16. Dodd SR, Lancaster GA, Craig JV, et al. In a systematic review, infrared ear thermometry for fever diagnosis in children finds poor sensitivity. J Clin Epidemiol 2006;59:354–7.

17. Petersdorf RG, Beeson PB. Fever of unknown origin: report on 100 cases. Medicine (Baltimore) 1961;40(1):1–30.

18. Chusid MJ. Fever. In: Wedgewood RJ, Davis SD, Ray CG, et al, editors. Infections in Children. Philadelphia: Harper and Row; 1982. p. 228–38.

19. Arora R, Mahajan P. Evaluation of child with fever without source. Review of literature and update. Pediatr Clin North Am 2013;60:1049–62.

20. Chow A, Robinson JL. Fever of unknown origin in children: a systemic review. World J Pediatr 2011;7:5–10.

21. McCarthy P. Fever without apparent source on clinical examination. Curr Opin Pediatr 2005;17:93–110.

22. Tolan RW Jr. Fever of unknown origin: a diagnostic approach to this vexing problem. Clin Pediatr (Phila) 2010;49(3):207–13.

23. Gaeta GB, Fusco FM, Nardiello S. Fever of unknown origin: a systemic review of the literature for 1995-2004. Nucl Med Commun 2006;27:205–11.

24. Colvin JM, Muenzer JT, Jaffe DM, et al. Detection of viruses in young children with fever without an apparent source. Pediatrics 2012;130(6):e1455–62.

25. Andreola B, Bressan S, Callegaro S, et al. Procalcitonin and C-reactive protein as diagnostic markers of severe bacterial infections in febrile infants and children in the Emergency Department. Pediatr Infect Dis J 2007;26(8):672–7.

26. Maheshwari N. How useful is C-reactive protein in detecting occult bacterial infection in young children with fever without apparent focus? Arch Dis Child 2006;91:533–5.

27. Sanders S, Barnett A, Correa-Velez C, et al. Systemic review of the diagnostic accuracy of C-reactive protein to detect bacterial infection in nonhospitalized infants and children with fever. J Pediatr 2008;153:570–4.

28. Schimmelpfennig RW Jr, Chusid MJ. Illnesses associated with extreme elevation of the erythrocyte sedimentation rate in children. Clin Pediatr (Phila) 1980;19:175–8.

29. Caorsi R, Pelagatti MA, Federici S, et al. Periodic fever, apthous stomatitis, pharyngitis and adenitis syndrome. Curr Opin Rheumatol 2010;22:579–84.

30. Federici S, Sormani MP, Ozen S, et al, Paediatric Rheumatology International Trials Organisation (PRINTO) and Eurofever Project. Evidence-based provisional clinical classification criteria for autoinflammatory periodic fevers. Ann Rheum Dis 2015;74:799–805.

31. Long SS. Distinguishing among prolonged, recurrent, and periodic fever syndromes: approach of a pediatric infectious diseases subspecialist. Pediatr Clin North Am 2005;52(3):811–35.

32. Eishout G, Monteny M, van der Wouden JC, et al. Duration of fever and serious bacterial infections in children: a systemic review. BMC Fam Pract 2011;12:33.

33. Dale DC. Cyclic and chronic neutropenia: an update on diagnosis and treatment. Clin Adv Hematol Oncol 2011;9(11):868–9.

34. Yagupsky P, Porsch E, St Geme JW 3rd. Kingella kingae: an emerging pathogen in young children. Pediatrics 2011;127(3):557–65.

35. Ampofo K. Infectious disease issues in adoption of young children. Curr Opin Pediatr 2013;25(1):78–87.

36. Committee on Infectious Diseases, Committee on Nutrition, American Academy of Pediatrics. Consumption of raw or unpasteurized milk and milk products by pregnant women and children. Pediatrics 2014;133(1):175–9.

37. Chusid MJ, Perzigian RW, Dunne WM, et al. An unusual cause of FUO in a child: brucellosis. Wis Med J 1989;88:11–3.

38. Lieberman JM. North American zoonoses. Pediatr Ann 2009;38(4):193–8.

39. Walsh GM, Shih AW, Solh Z, et al. Blood-borne pathogens: a Canadian Blood Services Centre for innovation symposium. Transfus Med Rev 2016;30(2):53–68.

40. Gordon CJ, Rowsey PJ. Poisons and fever. Clin Exp Pharmacol Physiol 1998; 25(2):145–9.

41. Tolle MA. Evaluating a sick child after travel to developing countries. J Am Board Fam Med 2010;23(6):704–13.

42. Chapman AS, Bakken JS, Folk SM, et al, Tickborne Rickettsial Diseases Working Group, CDC. Diagnosis and management of tick-borne rickettsial diseases: Rocky Mountain spotted fever, ehrlichiosis, and anaplasmosis—United States. A practical guide for physicians and other health-care and public health professionals. MMWR Recomm Rep 2006;55:1–29.

43. Anderson A, Bijlmer H, Fournier PE, et al. Diagnosis and management of Q fever—United States, 2013. Recommendations from CDC and the Q fever Working Group. MMWR Recomm Rep 2013;62:1–30.

44. Kang HM, Kim JY, Choi EH, et al. Clinical characteristics of severe histiocytic necrotizing lymphadenitis (Kikuchi-Fujimoto Disease) in children. J Pediatr 2016;171:208–12.

45. Ramirez S, Hild TG, Rudolph CN, et al. Increased diagnosis of Lemierre syndrome and other Fusobacterium necrophorum infections at a Children's Hospital. Pediatrics 2003;112:e380–5.

46. Kanegaye JT, Van Cott E, Tremoulet AH, et al. Lymph-node-first presentation of Kawasaki disease compared with bacterial cervical adenitis and typical Kawasaki disease. J Pediatr 2013;162(6):1259–63.

47. Chusid MJ, Hill WC, Bevan JA, et al. Proteus pyomyositis of the piriformis muscle in a swimmer. Clin Infect Dis 1998;26:194–5.

48. Scott HF, Deakyne SJ, Woods JM, et al. The prevalence and diagnostic utility of systemic inflammatory response syndrome vital signs in a pediatric emergency department. Acad Emerg Med 2015;22(4):381–9.

49. Zhang L, Zhou J, Sokol L. Hereditary and acquired hemophagocytic lymphohistiocytosis. Cancer Control 2014;21(4):301–12.

50. Ravelli A, Davì S, Minoia F, et al. Macrophage activation syndrome. Hematol Oncol Clin North Am 2015;29(5):927–41.

51. Li P, Huang P, Yang Y, et al. Updated understanding of autoimmune lymphoproliferative syndrome (ALPS). Clin Rev Allergy Immunol 2016;50(1):55–63.

52. Morís G, Garcia-Monco J. The challenge of drug-induced aseptic meningitis revisited. JAMA Intern Med 2014;174(9):1511–2.

53. Van Howe RS, Starshak RJ, Chusid MJ. Chronic recurrent multifocal osteomyelitis: case report and review of the literature. Clin Pediatr 1989;28:54–9.

54. Bohm M, Gonzalez Fernandez MI, Ozen S, et al. Clinical features of childhood granulomatosis with polyangiitis (Wegener's granulomatosis). Pediatr Rheumatol Online J 2014;12:18.

55. Eleftheriou D, Dillon MJ, Tullus K, et al. Systemic polyarteritis nodosa in the young: a single-center experience over thirty-two years. Arthritis Rheum 2013; 65(9):2476–85.

56. Harter KR, Bhatt S, Kim HT, et al. Chikungunya fever in Los Angeles. West J Emerg Med 2014;15(7):841–4.
57. Summers DJ, Acosta RW, Acosta AM. Zika virus in an American recreational traveler. J Travel Med 2015;22(5):338–40.
58. Tabain I, Ljubin-Sternak S, Cepin-Bogović J, et al. Adenovirus respiratory infections in hospitalized children: clinical findings in relation to species and serotypes. Pediatr Infect Dis J 2012;31(7):680–4.
59. Carlson P, Seppänen M, Tarvainen K, et al. Pharyngitis and exanthema caused by Arcanobacterium haemolyticum. Acta Derm Venereol 2001;81(2):143–4.
60. Quraishi H, Zevallos JP. Subdural empyema as a complication of sinusitis in the pediatric population. Int J Pediatr Otorhinolaryngol 2006;70(9):1581–6.
61. Miftode EG, Dorneanu OS, Leca DA, et al. Tuberculous meningitis in children and adults: a 10-year retrospective comparative analysis. PLoS One 2015;10(7): e0133477.
62. Gavin PJ, Kazacos KR, Shulman ST. Baylisascariasis. Clin Microbiol Rev 2005; 18(4):703–18.
63. Rajajee S, Shankar J, Dhattatri L. Pediatric presentations of leptospirosis. Indian J Pediatr 2002;69(10):851–3.
64. Bonthius DJ. Lymphocytic choriomeningitis virus: an under-recognized cause of neurologic disease in the fetus, child, and adult. Semin Pediatr Neurol 2012; 19(3):89–95.
65. Lopez C, Budge P, Chen J, et al. Primary amebic meningoencephalitis: a case report and literature review. Pediatr Emerg Care 2012;28(3):272–6.
66. Baltimore RS, Gewitz M, Baddour LM, et al, American Heart Association Rheumatic Fever, Endocarditis, and Kawasaki Disease Committee of the Council on Cardiovascular Disease in the Young and the Council on Cardiovascular and Stroke Nursing. Infective endocarditis in childhood: 2015 update: a scientific statement from the American Heart Association. Circulation 2015;132(15):1487–515.
67. Brennan C, Wang VJ. Management of fever and suspected infection in pediatric patients with central venous catheters. Pediatr Emerg Med Pract 2015;12(12):1–17.
68. David MZ, Daum RS. Community-associated methicillin-resistant Staphylococcus aureus: epidemiology and clinical consequences of an emerging epidemic. Clin Microbiol Rev 2010;23(3):616–87.
69. Rammaert B, Desjardins A, Lortholary O. New insights into hepatosplenic candidosis, a manifestation of chronic disseminated candidosis. Mycoses 2012;55(3): e74–84.
70. Malatack JJ, Jaffe R. Granulomatous hepatitis in three children due to cat-scratch disease without peripheral adenopathy. An unrecognized cause of fever of unknown origin. Am J Dis Child 1993;147(9):949–53.
71. Chusid MJ. Pyogenic hepatic abscess in infancy and childhood. Pediatrics 1978; 62:554–9.
72. Keidl CM, Chusid MJ. Splenic abscesses in childhood. Pediatr Infect Dis J 1989; 8:368–73.
73. Elliott SP. Rat bite fever and Streptobacillus moniliformis. Clin Microbiol Rev 2007; 20(1):13–22.
74. Dierig A, Frei R, Egli A. The fast route to microbe identification: matrix assisted laser desorption/ionization-time of flight mass spectrometry (MALDI-TOF MS). Pediatr Infect Dis J 2015;34(1):97–9.
75. Jenkins C, Ling CL, Ciesielczuk HL, et al. Detection and identification of bacteria in clinical samples by 16S rRNA gene sequencing: comparison of two different approaches in clinical practice. J Med Microbiol 2012;61(Pt 4):483–8.

76. Gyarmati P, Kjellander C, Aust C, et al. Metagenomic analysis of bloodstream in-fections in patients with acute leukemia and therapy-induced neutropenia. Sci Rep 2016;6:23532.
77. Liu X, Ren H, Peng D. Sepsis biomarkers: an omics perspective. Front Med 2014; 8(1):58–67.

Differentiating Familial Neuropathies from Guillain-Barré Syndrome

Brett J. Bordini, MD[a],*, Priya Monrad, MD[b]

KEYWORDS

- Guillain-Barré syndrome • Acute inflammatory demyelinating polyradiculoneuropathy
- Congenital neuropathy • Charcot-Marie-Tooth hereditary neuropathy

KEY POINTS

- Guillain-Barré syndrome is the most common cause of acute flaccid paralysis in childhood. Acute inflammatory demyelinating polyneuropathy is the most common variant of Guillain-Barré syndrome and is diagnosed based on clinical presentation, as well as the presence of albuminocytologic dissociation in the cerebrospinal fluid and demyelinating changes on electromyography.
- Numerous variants of Guillain-Barré exist and may mimic other causes of acquired peripheral neuropathy or inherited neuropathy.
- Key to diagnosing a seemingly acquired peripheral neuropathy as an inherited neuropathy is recognizing subtle systemic manifestations, signs of long-standing neuromuscular disease, or a positive family history.

INTRODUCTION

The acute onset of flaccid limb weakness or sensory dysfunction in children and young adults prompts consideration of acquired peripheral neuropathies, the differential diagnosis of which includes Guillain-Barré syndrome (GBS), which is best conceptualized as a collection of clinically-related disorders characterized by peripheral nerve fiber dysfunction secondary to an acute inflammatory and presumed autoimmune mechanism. The most common form of GBS is acute inflammatory demyelinating polyradiculoneuropathy (AIDP), in which immune-mediated peripheral nerve fiber demyelination leads to weakness, areflexia, and paresthesia beginning in the distal extremities and progressing proximally. In addition to these distinctive findings, patients with AIDP variably experience autonomic dysfunction, neuropathic pain, voiding

[a] Department of Pediatrics, Section of Hospital Medicine, Nelson Service for Undiagnosed and Rare Diseases, Children's Hospital of Wisconsin, Medical College of Wisconsin, Milwaukee, WI, USA; [b] Department of Child and Adolescent Neurology, Medical College of Wisconsin, Milwaukee, WI, USA
* Corresponding author. Children's Hospital of Wisconsin Children's Corporate Center, Suite 560, Milwaukee, WI 53226.
E-mail address: bbordini@mcw.edu

pediatric.theclinics.com

dysfunction, and progression of weakness to involve respiratory insufficiency and even failure. Diagnosis is contingent on recognizing the peripheral nerve as the source of the patient's neuromuscular symptoms and subsequently undertaking an appropriate evaluation that shows the characteristic findings of albuminocytologic dissociation in the cerebrospinal fluid, peripheral nerve fiber demyelination on electromyography (EMG), and nerve root enhancement on MRI of the spine. The disorder typically develops within weeks of a benign gastrointestinal or respiratory illness, is monophasic, reaches a nadir within several weeks of symptom onset, and responds to immunomodulatory therapy, with many patients experiencing full recovery within several months of onset. However, up to 20% of patients with GBS are left with some degree of residual disability.[1]

Although AIDP is the most common presentation of GBS in pediatrics, numerous variant forms have been described that differ with respect to immunologic target and symptom constellation. Variants such as Miller Fisher syndrome are characterized by prominent ophthalmoplegia, ataxia, and areflexia with absent weakness, whereas patients with the polyneuritis cranialis variant experience multiple cranial nerve palsies and severe peripheral sensory loss. Patients with axonal, rather than demyelinating, variants may lack sensory and autonomic symptoms but are at higher risk of respiratory failure. Diagnosis under these circumstances is more challenging, because these variant presentations may mimic other causes of acquired peripheral neuropathy. Furthermore, localization of the disorder to the peripheral nerve may be challenging when motor or sensory symptoms are subtle, multifocal, or seemingly not restricted to a readily identifiable peripheral nerve distribution. Despite these variations, the disorder still typically follows a monophasic course and responds to immunomodulation, with symptoms reaching a nadir within weeks and resolving within months.

The natural and treated history of GBS may at times confound certainty in the diagnosis. Up to 7% of patients with GBS experience recurrent attacks in the years following the initial event, despite receiving immunomodulatory therapy[2]; more acutely, up to 16% of patients with GBS experience treatment-related fluctuations, in which an initial improvement after treatment is followed by subsequent worsening of symptoms within the first 2 months of symptom onset.[3] Furthermore, up to 5% of patients with presumed GBS ultimately meet diagnostic criteria for acute-onset chronic inflammatory demyelinating polyneuropathy (CIDP), with persistent or recurrent symptoms lasting longer than 2 months.[3] In addition to recurrent episodes, treatment-related fluctuations, and acute-onset CIDP, the persistence of symptoms following immunomodulatory therapy should prompt consideration of an alternative cause of acute-onset acquired peripheral neuropathy, with a broad differential diagnosis that includes infectious, rheumatic, endocrinologic, toxic, nutritional, and other causes. Furthermore, in addition to chronic acquired conditions, the presence of atypical, persistent, or systemic symptoms should prompt consideration of inherited peripheral neuropathies. Many of these disorders develop insidiously and show systemic involvement that more overtly suggests an underlying genetic cause; however, some patients present with acute or subacute symptoms of peripheral neuropathy and subtle systemic symptoms. These presentations may mimic GBS, at least in initial presentation.

Patients with the acute onset of peripheral nervous system dysfunction are most likely to have an acquired cause of their disorder. Patients whose symptoms, physical findings, and diagnostic evaluation are consistent with GBS are often appropriately managed empirically with immunomodulatory therapy. Patients presenting atypically, either in terms of the timing of symptom development or with respect to symptom constellation, may have a variant of GBS, may have an alternative cause for their acquired peripheral neuropathy, or may have a rare and likely genetic cause for their symptoms. On occasion, patients with inherited peripheral neuropathies present acutely, although historical features and physical examination findings can reveal subtle signs of chronic, progressive nerve fiber dysfunction or systemic illness that indicate an underlying genetic cause for their symptoms.

ACUTE INFLAMMATORY DEMYELINATING POLYRADICULONEUROPATHY AND THE DIFFERENTIAL DIAGNOSIS OF ACQUIRED PERIPHERAL NEUROPATHY

The annual incidence of GBS in pediatrics is as high as 1.34 cases per 100,000 in individuals less than 15 years of age, with a slight male predominance.[4] Up to two-thirds of cases are preceded by a mild respiratory or gastrointestinal illness in the weeks before the onset of symptoms, with typical infections including *Campylobacter jejuni* enteritis and cytomegalovirus.[1] Acute inflammatory demyelinating polyradiculoneuropathy accounts for approximately 90% of cases of GBS in North America.[1] The typical presentation of AIDP is of a person who complains of numbness or tingling in the legs and feet before developing progressive clumsiness and weakness that seems to ascend symmetrically up the legs over a matter of several days. In children, this may be mistaken for fatigue, growing pains, joint problems, or clumsiness caused by illness. Symptoms generally peak within 2 to 4 weeks of onset, and as the disease progresses, the patient develops an ascending flaccid paralysis with areflexia that may affect the hands, cranial nerves, and ultimately the diaphragm, which may lead to respiratory failure. Most patients develop gait unsteadiness or an inability to ambulate and most complain of neuropathic pain, whereas approximately half have bulbar symptoms and half show autonomic dysfunction.[5] The most common manifestation of autonomic dysfunction is sinus tachycardia, although additional manifestations may include bradycardia, blood pressure lability, and less commonly urinary retention or gastrointestinal symptoms.[6]

Timely and appropriate diagnosis requires recognizing the peripheral nerve as the source of the patient's symptoms and differentiating peripheral neuropathy from myelopathy, myopathy, or lesions in the brain. Key historical features and physical examination findings suggestive of peripheral nerve fiber dysfunction include a distal-to-proximal progression of symptoms and findings, because both demyelinating and axonal disorders affect the peripheral nerves in a length-dependent fashion. Sensory symptoms tend to predominate early in the course of illness, although they may be vague at first, consisting of numbness and tingling in a stocking-glove distribution. As paresthesia and pain progress proximally, flaccid weakness and diminished or absent tendon reflexes develop. Severe sensory involvement may lead to sensory ataxia, wherein a loss of proprioceptive input and joint position sensation leads to clumsiness and poor coordination when the patient closes the eyes and eliminates visual feedback from the regulation of movement. Differentiating sensory ataxia from weakness requires performing movements in a plane of motion that does not require resistance against gravity. The symptoms of peripheral neuropathy in AIDP tend to be symmetric and progress in an ascending fashion, and although some variations in this presentation are possible, major deviations from this pattern, such as unilateral findings or proximal-to-distal progression, should prompt consideration of alternative causes. Hyperreflexia, spasticity, and cerebellar ataxia indicate central, rather than peripheral, involvement, and specifically indicate intracranial or upper motor neuron disorders. Proximal weakness tends to predominate rather than distal weakness in myopathies, and myelopathies tend to present with sensory levels or dermatomally-distributed symptoms.

With the peripheral nerve fiber identified as the source of the patient's symptoms, the typical evaluation for suspected GBS includes lumbar puncture and an electromyogram. MRI of the brain or spine may be indicated if there are concerns about intracranial disorders or if the speed of symptom progression or distribution of symptoms suggests disorder in the spinal cord, as opposed to the peripheral nerve. Albuminocytologic dissociation, in which the cerebrospinal fluid protein level is increased but the total nucleated cell count remains within normal limits, is somewhat specific for GBS but is fairly insensitive, being present in up to half of affected patients in the first week of illness and up to 75% of affected patients by the third week of illness.[1] Patients who have a history of infection with human immunodeficiency virus may show cerebrospinal fluid pleocytosis in the context of GBS; otherwise, the presence of pleocytosis suggests an alternative diagnosis.[1] Contrast-enhanced MRI of the spine may show enhancement of the nerve roots and cauda equina, a finding which has a sensitivity greater than 90% for GBS but which is fairly nonspecific.[7]

EMG may distinguish whether a neuropathic process is demyelinating, axonal, or a combination of both, and nerve conduction velocity studies should be performed on at least 2 nerves to confirm findings. The critical measures are the amplitude of the compound motor action potential (CMAP) at a proximal and distal site, the conduction velocity along the tested nerve, and the qualities of the F-wave. Demyelinating processes show the following 4 characteristic changes on EMG: (1) reduced maximum motor conduction velocity and (2) partial conduction block or abnormal temporal dispersion leading to (3) prolonged motor distal latency and (4) prolonged or absent F-wave latencies. A reduction of conduction velocity by 30%, an increase in temporal dispersion by 30%, and a distal CMAP and F-wave latency of 150% of normal limits has a sensitivity of 72% for detecting AIDP.[8] However, in demyelinating diseases such as AIDP, some patients have normal responses early in the disease course and an EMG should be repeated in those patients after 1 to 2 weeks for maximum diagnostic yield if there is ongoing uncertainty in the diagnosis. The reported order in which abnormalities appear is absence or decrease in the tibial H-wave, dispersion of the F-wave, abnormal CMAP dispersion, prolonged CMAP and F-wave latencies, and then decrease in CMAP conduction velocity.[8] In axonal disorders, the EMG reveals normal conduction velocities but decreased distal CMAP amplitudes; sensory nerve action potential amplitudes may be normal or decreased depending on the presence of sensory symptoms.

Patients whose presentation and evaluation are consistent with AIDP receive supportive care and undergo treatment targeted at curbing the aberrant immunologic response presumed to be driving the peripheral nerve fiber dysfunction. Intravenous immunoglobulin is the treatment modality of choice in pediatrics, although plasmapheresis may be used. In general, AIDP is a monophasic illness with a good prognosis. However, up to 20% of patients with GBS require assisted ventilation for respiratory insufficiency or failure, and mortality approaches 4%, either from respiratory or autonomic causes.[9]

Patients whose history, physical examination findings, or results of diagnostic evaluation are inconsistent with AIDP may have a variant of GBS or may have an alternative cause of acquired peripheral neuropathy. The differential diagnosis of acquired peripheral neuropathy in pediatrics is presented in **Box 1**.[10–18]

VARIANT PRESENTATIONS OF GUILLAIN-BARRÉ SYNDROME

Variant presentations of GBS, their clinical distinctions from AIDP, and pertinent diagnostic findings are presented in **Table 1**.[19,20] Atypical presentations, particularly

Box 1
Causes of pediatric-onset acquired peripheral neuropathy

Infectious
Chronic Chagas disease
Diphtheria
Human immunodeficiency virus
Leprosy
Lyme disease
Rabies
West Nile virus[a]

Noninfectious inflammatory
Celiac disease
CIDP
GBS
Eosinophilic granulomatosis with polyangiitis
Henoch-Schönlein purpura[a]
Inflammatory bowel disease[a]
Juvenile idiopathic arthritis[a]
Polyarteritis nodosa
Sarcoidosis
Sjögren syndrome
Systemic lupus erythematosus
Granulomatosis with polyangiitis

Endocrine
Diabetes mellitus
Hypothyroidism

Medications
Bortezomib
Chloramphenicol
Cisplatin
Cytarabine
Isoniazid
Lamivudine
Metronidazole
Paclitaxel
Penicillin
Phenytoin
Stavudine
Sulfonamides
Thalidomide

Vincristine

Zidovudine

Nutritional

Vitamin B_1 (thiamine) deficiency

Vitamin B_2 (riboflavin) deficiency

Vitamin B_6 (pyridoxine) deficiency or toxicity

Vitamin B_{12} (cobalamin) deficiency

Vitamin E (tocopherol) deficiency

Other

Critical illness polyneuropathy/myopathy

Bone marrow transplant–related graft-versus-host disease

Lymphoma[a]

Neurofibromatosis

Porphyria

Traumatic neuropathy

Uremia

Toxic

Arsenic

Gold

Lead

Mercury

N-hexane (glue huffing)

Organophosphates

Thallium

[a] Rare manifestation.

in those variants involving the cranial nerves or lacking prominent sensory findings, may make localization to the peripheral nerve challenging. However, most variants can be categorized based on the primary symptom constellation: those variants that present with ophthalmoplegia, ataxia, and areflexia without limb weakness; or those that present with plegia or paresis with variable sensory and autonomic symptoms.

Miller Fisher syndrome is the prototypical variant of the ophthalmoplegia-ataxia-areflexia constellation and accounts for up to 10% of GBS cases in Western countries, although in certain eastern Asian populations it accounts for up to 25% of cases of GBS.[21] Up to 10% of patients with Miller Fisher syndrome have additional findings of encephalopathy and hyperreflexia consistent with Bickerstaff brainstem encephalitis.[22] Some patients in this spectrum may lack ataxia or ophthalmoplegia, and some have symptoms that overlap with the plegia-paresis constellation and include features of both constellations.[20]

Symptomatically, patients in the plegia-paresis constellation often seem to have findings similar to AIDP, although with incomplete anatomic distributions or variability

Table 1
Variant forms of Guillain-Barré syndrome in pediatrics. Clinical features that distinguish from acute inflammatory demyelinating polyradiculoneuropathy and key diagnostic features, including antiganglioside antibody profiles

Variant	Clinical Distinctions from AIDP	Diagnostic Features
Ophthalmoplegia-Ataxia-Areflexia Constellation		
Miller Fisher syndrome	Ophthalmoplegia, ataxia out of proportion to sensory loss, absent weakness	EMG/NCV studies showing axonopathy, although some patients may have demyelinating features, also with reduced or absent sensory nerve action potentials; antibodies isolated include anti-GT_{1a}, GQ_{1b}, GD_{1b}
Bickerstaff brainstem encephalitis	Considered a subtype of Miller Fisher syndrome; includes ophthalmoplegia, ataxia, encephalopathy, and hyperreflexia	EMG/NCV studies similar to Miller Fisher; MRI findings variable but may include hyperintense foci in the brainstem on T2-weighted imaging, thalamic or cerebellar lesions possible; antibodies isolated include anti-GT_{1a}, GQ_{1b}, GD_{1b}
Plegia/Paresis With or Without Sensory and Autonomic Symptoms Constellation		
Paraparetic GBS	Weakness and paresthesia restricted to the lower extremities	EMG/NCV studies similar to AIDP
Facial diplegia and distal limb paresthesia	Similar to AIDP but with bifacial weakness; rare in children but may present in adolescents	EMG/NCV studies similar to AIDP; antibodies isolated include anti-GM_2; association with cytomegalovirus infection
Polyneuritis cranialis	Multiple bilateral cranial nerve palsies (often sparing the optic nerve); severe peripheral sensory loss	MRI showing enhancement of cranial nerves; antibodies isolated include anti-GQ_1, GT_1
Pharyngeal-cervical-brachial weakness	Swallowing dysfunction; weakness of oropharyngeal, neck, and shoulder muscles	EMG/NCV studies showing axonopathy; antibodies isolated include anti-GT_{1a}, GQ_{1b}, GD_{1a}
Acute motor axonal neuropathy	Absence of sensory or autonomic symptoms; rapid progression of ascending symmetric weakness; higher likelihood of respiratory failure	EMG/NCV studies showing motor axonopathy without demyelinating features; antibodies isolated include anti-GM_1, GM_{1b}, GD_{1a}, GalNac-GD_{1a}; strong association with *C jejuni* infection

(continued on next page)

Table 1 (continued)		
Variant	Clinical Distinctions from AIDP	Diagnostic Features
Acute motor-sensory axonal neuropathy	Absence of autonomic symptoms; prolonged course with possible muscle wasting; rare in children	EMG/NCV studies showing motor and sensory axonopathy without demyelinating features; antibodies isolated include anti-GM_1, GM_{1b}, GD_{1a}; strong association with C jejuni infection
Pure sensory GBS	Significant sensory ataxia with absent reflexes and minor motor involvement	EMG/NCV studies with demyelinating features; antibodies isolated include anti-GD_{1b}

Abbreviation: NCV, nerve conduction velocity.

in the degree or completeness of sensory, motor, and autonomic findings. For example, patients with paraparetic GBS have findings restricted to the lower extremities, whereas patients with pharyngeal-cervical-brachial GBS have weakness in a capelike distribution that also includes the pharyngeal musculature, leading to swallowing dysfunction. Patients with acute motor axonal neuropathy lack sensory and autonomic symptoms, whereas patients with sensory GBS have minimal, if any, weakness.

Neurophysiologically, there is variability both within and between the ophthalmoplegia-ataxia-areflexia constellation and the plegia-paresis constellation with respect to underlying disorder, with some variants showing a demyelinating pattern and others showing an axonal pattern. Although the specific immunologic target in AIDP is not known, specific antiganglioside antibodies have been identified for many GBS variants.[19] The formation of antiganglioside antibodies is thought to underlie the immune-mediated axonopathy seen in axonal variants, and the distribution of particular gangliosides throughout the peripheral nervous system is thought to underlie the variability in the distribution of symptoms.[1] Although these immunohistologic distinctions provide valuable information regarding the pathophysiology of GBS, distinguishing variants of GBS by symptom constellation may ultimately prove more valuable in the immediate clinical evaluation period.[20] It is further worth noting that diagnosis of these variants is based on clinical grounds and the results of neuroimaging and neurophysiologic investigations and does not require demonstration of antiganglioside antibodies, which may not be widely available for testing in clinical settings or which may require significant time to complete and lead to delays in therapy.

Patients who lack an infectious prodrome and whose symptoms persist beyond 2 months may have acute-onset CIDP, as opposed to GBS. Treatment of CIDP is still designed to curb aberrant immunologic activity via immunomodulation, although many patients experience chronic, stable symptoms, or have a prolonged relapsing-remitting course. Alternatively, patients with more chronic or persistent symptoms, or whose history and physical examination reveal systemic involvement or more long-standing neurologic dysfunction, may have an inherited peripheral neuropathy.

INHERITED PERIPHERAL NEUROPATHIES THAT MAY MIMIC GUILLAIN-BARRÉ SYNDROME

The variability and overlap in symptoms among the variants of GBS open the possibility of misdiagnosis, including diagnosing an inherited neuropathy as an acquired one. Some inherited neuropathies can mimic GBS, particularly in the initial presentation of neuropathic findings, although most show a chronically progressive course or involve multiple organ systems in a manner that ultimately suggests the underlying genetic nature of the disorder. Diagnosis becomes challenging when systemic manifestations are subtle, lacking, or temporally remote from the appearance of neuropathic findings, or when the disorder follows a relapsing-remitting or episodic course. In addition to evaluating for systemic signs and symptoms, key to determining whether an apparent case of atypical GBS may be caused by an inherited neuropathy is looking for subtle signs of long-standing motor, sensory, or autonomic neuropathy, such as weakness or gait abnormalities when asymptomatic, muscular atrophy in the affected limbs that is out of proportion to the duration of symptoms, or limb deformities secondary to neuromuscular weakness. Other features suggestive of inherited disorders include dysmorphic features or a family history of consanguinity.

Hereditary peripheral neuropathies are a heterogeneous group of disorders classified by type of neurons involved (sensory, motor, autonomic, or a combination), primary pattern of involvement (proximal or distal), and type of neuronal injury (demyelinating or axonal). Some have a relapsing-remitting or episodic course. An episodic nature to the disease or an apparent response to immunomodulation, often pursued when initial diagnostic impressions favor GBS, may suggest against an inherited disorder but does not adequately exclude a genetic mechanism, because intercurrent illnesses may unmask or worsen an underlying inherited disorder, particularly a mitochondrial disorder. Furthermore, positive sensory symptoms, such as paresthesia, may not be evident, and therefore the lack of such symptoms between episodes does not exclude the possibility of subtle but progressive sensory nerve dysfunction between episodes.

Similarly, some patients may show systemic manifestations long before or after the development of peripheral nerve disease, and this separation in time may make it challenging to recognize distinct findings as a part of the same underlying disease process. The authors evaluated a 19-year-old male patient who was admitted to our hospital for respiratory insufficiency secondary to severe neuromuscular weakness. His history before presenting to our institution was notable for an acute-onset and seemingly idiopathic restrictive cardiomyopathy at 8 years of age that required orthotopic heart transplant. At the time of transplant, he otherwise had no evidence of neuromuscular or systemic disease, and following transplant was stable on an antirejection medication regimen until age 12 years, when he developed a slowly progressive sensorimotor polyneuropathy heralded by episodes of severe lower extremity paresthesia and pain. EMG at that time showed a mixed axonal and demyelinating polyneuropathy. Over the next several years he developed signs of progressive neuromuscular disease, with foot deformities, scoliosis, and profound muscular atrophy. Whole-exome sequencing at 19 years of age revealed a mutation in *BAG3* consistent with myofibrillar myopathy, and review of preserved specimen slides from his diseased heart showed changes suggestive of myofibrillar myopathy as well.[23] Although the course of his neuropathy was more indolent and chronically progressive, some patients manifest with acute-onset peripheral neuropathy and either subtle or temporally remote systemic signs and symptoms that may make the recognition of an inherited disorder challenging.

Genetic disorders associated with pediatric-onset peripheral neuropathy are listed in **Table 2**.[24–43] These disorders can be broadly categorized as being part of the Charcot-Marie-Tooth or hereditary motor-sensory neuropathy spectrum and related disorders, as being secondary to mitochondrial disease, or as having a distinct genetically determined pathophysiology that interrupts peripheral nerve fiber function.

Charcot-Marie-Tooth Hereditary Neuropathies

The most commonly encountered inherited neuropathies are the hereditary motor-sensory neuropathies, or the Charcot-Marie-Tooth (CMT) neuropathies. There are multiple classification systems that group subtypes based on molecular genetics or clinical phenotype, with one such classification system delineating the following 9 clinical subtypes: demyelinating (CMT1), axonal (CMT2), Dejerine-Sottas (CMT3), spinal, pyramidal, optic atrophy, dominant intermediate type, recessive intermediate type, and X-linked. Of these, CMT1a is the most common and has the most frequent reported presentations with comorbid inflammatory neuropathies. Patients with CMT1a have presented with symptoms, physical findings, cerebrospinal fluid profiles, and EMG consistent with AIDP, Miller Fisher syndrome, or acute-onset CIDP, only to subsequently be revealed to have CMT1a when symptoms were treatment refractory or persistent, or when physical examination or family history revealed signs of chronic neuromuscular disease.[44] Patients with hereditary neuropathy with liability to pressure palsies have frequently been misdiagnosed as having recurrent AIDP. Symptoms typically develop following acute respiratory or gastrointestinal illnesses and consist of weakness and paresthesia. Distinguishing features allowing the appropriate diagnosis are the development of weakness in a mononeuropathy distribution, particularly at entrapment sites such as the peroneal nerve, ulnar nerve at the elbow, or the carpal tunnel, as well as a lack of response to immunomodulatory therapy.[44]

Mitochondrial Disorders

Mitochondrial dysfunction may also present with progressive weakness and peripheral neuropathy; these frequently have systemic manifestations including gastrointestinal, renal, ophthalmic, and cardiac. Infections can cause a worsening of existing symptoms, which may be mistaken for the infectious history commonly found in AIDP.

Mitochondrial neurogastrointestinal encephalomyopathy (MNGIE) is a rare autosomal recessive mitochondrial disorder presenting primarily with gastrointestinal symptoms as well as a variety of neurologic symptoms, in particular progressive external ophthalmoplegia, ptosis, leukoencephalopathy, and peripheral neuropathy. It is caused by mutations in the *TYMP* gene, which encodes thymidine phosphorylase, an enzyme involved in the salvage of pyrimidines after DNA and RNA degradation. Because mitochondrial DNA is more dependent on thymidine salvage than is nuclear DNA, inhibition of thymidine phosphorylase function causes accumulation of mitochondrial DNA errors and progressive mitochondrial dysfunction over time. The average age of presentation is approximately 18 years, although symptoms begin in childhood for most patients.[45] The most common initial symptoms are gastrointestinal (eg, dysmotility, pseudo-obstruction, diverticuli, failure to thrive), although up to 10% of patients present initially with peripheral neuropathy, foot drop, paresthesia, proximal muscle weakness, or gait instability. The presence of asymptomatic or symptomatic symmetric ill-defined white matter lesions on MRI, as well as the presence of gastrointestinal symptoms, may suggest that patients presenting with acute peripheral neuropathy may have MNGIE.[45]

POLG-spectrum disorders are mitochondrial disorders that may present as a seemingly acquired peripheral neuropathy. They are caused by mutations in the nuclear

Table 2
Genetic disorders associated with pediatric-onset peripheral neuropathy. Clinical features, diagnostic findings, and molecular genetics

Disorder	Age of Onset	Neuromuscular Findings	Systemic Findings	Diagnostic Evaluation	Course	Inheritance	Molecular Genetics
Monogenic Neuropathy Disorders							
Hereditary motor-sensory neuropathies (also referred to as CMT hereditary neuropathies)	Typically childhood or adolescence, although infantile hypotonia and developmental delays possible	• Chronic, progressive motor and sensory polyneuropathy • Wasting and weakness of distal extremities • Distal sensory loss • Decreased or absent tendon reflexes • Skeletal deformities (eg, pes cavus, hammer toes) • Hearing loss, dysphagia (*MPZ* mutations)	• Acrocyanosis • Optic atrophy (*MFN2* mutations) • Vocal cord and respiratory involvement (CMT2c subtype) • Early-onset glaucoma (*MTMR13* mutations) • Vocal cord paresis (*GDAP1* mutations)	• EMG/NCV: axonal or demyelinating sensorimotor polyneuropathy, depending on subtype • MRI: nerve roots on spinal MRI may show the onion-bulb sign, with T2 hyperintensity and bulbous tapering from the root to the nerve fiber • CSF: increased protein levels possible • Blood: neutropenia (*DNM2* mutations) • Other: sural nerve biopsy no longer routinely performed but may show onion-bulb formation	Chronic, progressive	Autosomal dominant, autosomal recessive, or X-linked, depending on subtype	Numerous genes are implicated in the pathogenesis of CMT. CMT1 accounts for up to 50% of all cases, and the most common form of CMT1, CMT1a, is caused by duplications in the *PMP22* gene. Duplications have also been identified in subtypes of CMT4. Deletions are implicated in subtypes of CMT2, CMT4, and CMTX. Pathogenic variants detected by sequence analysis detect most other subtypes

(continued on next page)

Table 2
(continued)

Disorder	Age of Onset	Neuromuscular Findings	Systemic Findings	Diagnostic Evaluation	Course	Inheritance	Molecular Genetics
HSAN	Early childhood to late adulthood. Symptoms of HSAN4 begin in infancy	• Severe, progressive peripheral sensory loss. Profound and early insensitivity to pain in HSAN4 • Severe, shooting pain in the extremities early in disease • Distal then proximal muscle weakness and atrophy. Strength may be preserved in HSAN5 • Decreased or absent tendon reflexes • Skeletal deformities (eg, pes cavus) • Dysautonomic crises with gastrointestinal and bladder symptoms, hypotension, temperature and sweating dysregulation (HSAN3, also known as familial dysautonomia or Riley-Day syndrome)	• Skin ulcerations and bone necrosis in affected extremities with possible spontaneous amputation • Fractures, infections, and unwitnessed injuries in the extremities secondary to decreased sensation (HSAN2, HSAN4) • Small stature, smooth tongue, cognitive delays, glomerulosclerosis (HSAN3) • Self-mutilating behaviors (HSAN4)	• EMG/NCV: axonal sensorimotor polyneuropathy with chronic denervation changes. Typically normal in HSAN5 • MRI: brain atrophy possible in HSAN3 • Urine: decreased vanillylmandelic acid excretion (HSAN3) • Other: sural nerve biopsy no longer routinely performed but may show loss of myelinated axons without demyelination; abnormal histamine and methacholine challenge responses (HSAN3)	Chronic, progressive	Autosomal dominant, autosomal recessive, depending on subtype	Numerous genes are implicated in the pathogenesis of HSAN. Subtypes of HSAN1 are associated with mutations in the *SPTLC1* and *SPTLC2* genes, as well as other genes. Subtypes of HSAN2 are caused by mutations in *WNK1*, *FAM134B*, and other genes. HSAN3 is caused by mutations in *IKBKAP*. HSAN4 is caused by mutations in *NTRK1*
Hereditary neuralgic amyotrophy	Second or third decade (median: 28 y)	• Sudden-onset severe pain in the arms or shoulders • Unilateral or bilateral brachial plexopathy developing within weeks of pain onset • Motor > sensory symptoms • Absent or diminished tendon reflexes in affected limbs • Paresthesia and hypoesthesia in affected limb • Atrophy of the upper extremity • Autonomic symptoms possible, primarily vasomotor changes	• Precipitants: infection, immunization, surgery, child birth, overuse of affected limb, cold exposure • Variable findings: bifid uvula, cleft palate, short stature, partial syndactyly, ocular hypotelorism	• EMG/NCV: chronic denervation changes • MRI: evidence of myelopathy or inflammatory plexopathy possible • CSF: increased protein levels possible • Blood: increased transaminase levels possible early in attacks • Other: sural nerve biopsy is rarely performed but may show reduction in number of myelinated fibers	Relapsing-remitting/episodic. Persistent and cumulative deficits possible	Autosomal dominant	*SEPT9*: up to 55% of affected patients have an abnormality in the *SEPT9* gene identified either by sequencing or deletion/duplication analysis

| Hereditary neuropathy with liability to pressure palsies | Second or third decade (range, 2–70 y; mean, 37 y) | None reported | • Acute-onset sensory and motor mononeuropathy in areas of compression (in decreasing order of frequency: peroneal nerve causing foot drop, ulnar nerve at the elbow, median nerve at the wrist causing carpal tunnel syndrome, brachial plexus and radial nerve)
• Paresthesia in affected distribution
• Reduced or absent tendon reflexes
• Mild polyneuropathy (focal weakness, atrophy, or sensory loss) possible
• Mild to moderate pes cavus deformity | • EMG/NCV: bilateral slowing of distal sensory and motor nerve conduction velocities at the carpal tunnel and at least 1 additional abnormal finding for motor conduction in 1 peroneal nerve; abnormal conduction across entrapment sites is supportive
• MRI: asymptomatic white matter lesions on brain MRI possible, decreased brain white matter volume possible
• Other: sural nerve biopsy shows tomaculous changes but is not specific | • Recurrent acute attacks
• Attacks last days to months
• Full recovery in approximately 50% of episodes
• Incomplete recovery with mild residual deficits is common
• Severe disability is rare | Autosomal dominant | PMP22: contiguous gene deletion of chromosome 17p11.2 in 80% of affected probands; pathogenic variant in 20% of affected probands |

(continued on next page)

Table 2
(continued)

Disorder	Age of Onset	Neuromuscular Findings	Systemic Findings	Diagnostic Evaluation	Course	Inheritance	Molecular Genetics
Mitochondrial Neuropathy Disorders							
Mitochondrial neurogastrointestinal encephalopathy disease	Between the first and fifth decades (60% of affected individuals present before age 20 y)	• Mixed demyelinating > axonal sensorimotor neuropathy • Paresthesia in a stocking-glove distribution • Symmetric distal muscle weakness • Unilateral or bilateral foot drop • Ptosis • External ophthalmoplegia • Asymptomatic leukoencephalopathy	• Severe gastrointestinal dysmotility and malabsorption • Cachexia	• EMG/NCV: decreased motor and sensory nerve conduction velocities, prolonged F-wave latency, partial conduction block • MRI: diffuse white matter abnormalities on T2 or FLAIR series • CSF: increased protein levels possible • Blood: markedly reduced levels of thymidine phosphorylase enzyme activity; increased plasma thymidine and deoxyuridine levels; lactic acidemia and hyperalaninemia possible • Urine: increased deoxyuridine and thymidine levels • Other: evidence of mitochondrial dysfunction in affected tissues	Chronic, progressive, degenerative	Autosomal recessive	*TYMP*: pathogenic variants on sequence analysis

Neurogenic muscle weakness, ataxia, and retinitis pigmentosa	Early childhood	• Proximal muscle weakness • Sensory or sensorimotor axonal polyneuropathy that can be clinically unapparent with episodic worsening in the setting of viral illnesses • Cerebellar ataxia • Seizures • Learning difficulties	• Variable retinitis pigmentosa • Short stature • Cardiac conduction defects	• EMG/NCV: axonal sensory or sensorimotor polyneuropathy • MRI: cerebral and cerebellar atrophy • CSF: increased lactate level • Blood: increased lactate level; increased alanine concentrations on plasma amino acid analysis • Urine: lactic aciduria • Other: isolated defects of mitochondrial complex I or IV enzymes	Chronic, progressive, degenerative	Mitochondrial	*MT-ATP6*: pathogenic variants in *MT-ATP6* are identified in approximately 50% of affected individuals
Ataxia-neuropathy spectrum (*POLG*-related disorders)	Infancy to adulthood	• Sensory ataxia • Cerebellar ataxia • Sensorimotor polyneuropathy • Most affected individuals have encephalopathy and seizures • Variable ophthalmoplegia and dysarthria	• Gastrointestinal dysmotility reported with some mutations • Liver disease: increased transaminase levels, mild liver synthetic dysfunction, or even liver failure possible	• EMG/NCV: axonal sensory, motor, or mixed polyneuropathy • MRI: hyperintense lesions in the thalami, cerebellar white matter, and inferior olivary nuclei on T2-weighted imaging • CSF: increased protein levels possible • Blood: increased transaminase levels, mild liver synthetic dysfunction, or even liver failure possible • Other: functional assays may show respiratory chain defects	Chronic, progressive	Autosomal recessive	*POLG*, which encodes DNA polymerase gamma, the only DNA polymerase found in mitochondria

(continued on next page)

Table 2
(continued)

Disorder	Age of Onset	Neuromuscular Findings	Systemic Findings	Diagnostic Evaluation	Course	Inheritance	Molecular Genetics
Metabolic and Other Neuropathy Disorders							
Refsum disease	Infancy to adulthood	• Asymmetric, waxing-waning but chronically progressive sensory and motor polyneuropathy • Distal weakness and paresthesia with muscular atrophy • Late-onset cerebellar ataxia • Sensorineural hearing loss	• Anosmia • Early-onset retinitis pigmentosa • Ichthyosis • Congenitally short metacarpals and metatarsals in ~35% of individuals • Cardiac arrhythmias and cardiomyopathy	• EMG/NCV: primarily demyelinating polyneuropathy with secondary axonal degeneration • MRI: progressive symmetric signal change in the corticospinal tracts, cerebellar dentate nuclei, and corpus callosum • CSF: increased protein levels possible • Blood: increased plasma phytanic acid concentration (typically >200 μmol/L; normal <10 μmol/L) • Other: deficiency of phytanoyl-CoA hydroxylase or PTS2 receptor • If molecular genetic testing is negative or ambiguous in patients with increased plasma phytanic acid levels and a consistent phenotype, enzyme analysis of phytanoyl-CoA hydroxylase should be performed	Chronic, progressive	Autosomal recessive	• >90% of identified affected individuals have pathogenic variants or deletions/duplications in *PHYH*, which encodes phytanoyl-CoA hydroxylase • <10% of identified affected individuals have pathogenic variants or deletions/duplications in *PEX7*, which encodes the PTS2 receptor

Disease	Presentation	Clinical features	Diagnostic findings	Course	Inheritance	Genetics
Krabbe disease (globoid cell leukodystrophy)	Infantile form presents before 6 mo. Late-onset forms present between 6 mo and adulthood	• Infantile form presents with irritability, stiffness, seizures, and developmental delays or regression. A subset of patients present with isolated peripheral neuropathy with absent tendon reflexes and weakness before appearance of other symptoms. Affected patients then develop spasticity and severe developmental regression that progresses to decerebrate posturing and blindness • Late-onset forms may present with distal weakness and paresthesia. Hypertonicity and developmental regression follow but may vary in severity	• Sterile pyrexias in infantile form • Fist clenching	• EMG/NCV: slow motor conduction velocities • MRI: diffuse severe demyelination • CSF: increased protein levels possible • Blood: decreased (0%–5% of normal) galactocerebrosidase enzyme activity • Other: EEG with diffuse slowing of background rhythm	Infantile form is severe and rapidly progressive, with death before 2 y. Late-onset forms are chronic, progressive, and variable in severity	Autosomal recessive	GALC: pathogenic variants and deletions
Acute intermittent porphyria	Adolescence to young adulthood	• Episodic neurovisceral attacks: sudden-onset severe abdominal pain, muscular weakness, autonomic changes (tachycardia, hypertension), mental status changes, possible seizures and hyponatremia • Progressive peripheral neuropathy, primarily motor, that can progress in an ascending fashion to include respiratory insufficiency or failure	• Hypertension • Chronic kidney disease • Risk of hepatocellular carcinoma • Attack triggers: numerous medications, alcohol intake, fluctuations in reproductive hormones, fasting, stress	• EMG: axonal motor neuropathy • MRI: findings consistent with posterior reversible encephalopathy syndrome possible • Urine: increased concentration of porphobilinogen during attacks	Recurrent attacks of variable length and recovery (days to months)	Autosomal dominant	HMBS: encodes hydroxymethylbilane synthase. Pathogenic variants and deletions/duplications, with variable penetrance

(continued on next page)

Table 2
(continued)

Disorder	Age of Onset	Neuromuscular Findings	Systemic Findings	Diagnostic Evaluation	Course	Inheritance	Molecular Genetics
Myofibrillar myopathies	Infancy through adulthood	• Proximal and distal muscle weakness (proximal > distal in up to a third of affected individuals, distal > proximal in up to a third) • Peripheral neuropathy with weakness and paresthesia	• Cardiomyopathy in up to 30% of affected individuals • Muscle aches and cramps • Restrictive lung disease	• EMG/NCV: fibrillation potentials, positive sharp waves, and other signs of electrical irritability. Mixed myopathic and neurogenic features • MRI: muscle inflammation possible • Blood: mild increases in serum creatine kinase level • Other: muscle histology with abnormal trichrome staining, decreased oxidative enzyme activity, and intense congophilia; muscle immunohistochemistry with ectopic expression of various proteins; muscle electron microscopy with myofibrillar degeneration commencing at the Z-disk	Chronic, progressive, resulting in severe disability or death	Autosomal dominant, with the exception of X-linked *FHL1* mutations and autosomal recessive *CRYAB* mutations	Sequence variants in the following genes have been identified. Deletions or duplications have not been reported: • *DES* • *CRYAB* • *MYOT* • *LDB3* • *FLNC* • *BAG3* • *FHL1* • *DNAJB6*
CD59 deficiency	Infancy through young adulthood	• Recurrent immune-mediated polyneuropathy following febrile illnesses • Risk for strokes	Coombs-negative hemolysis during episodes	• EMG/NCV: demyelinating, axonal, or mixed polyneuropathy • MRI: spinal root enhancement • CSF: increased protein levels during episodes • Blood: increased CRP level during episodes	Relapsing, chronic, progressive. Individual episodes respond to immunomodulatory therapy	Autosomal recessive	CD59: pathogenic variant CYS89TYR in the *CD59* gene on chromosome 11p13

Abbreviations: CMT, Charcot-Marie-Tooth; CoA, coenzyme A; CRP, C-reactive protein; CSF, cerebrospinal fluid; EEG, electroencephalogram; FLAIR, fluid-attenuated inversion recovery; HSAN, hereditary sensory and autonomic neuropathies; NCV, nerve conduction velocity.

gene *POLG*, encoding the gamma subunit of mitochondrial DNA polymerase, which replicates mitochondrial DNA. Children with *POLG*-spectrum disorders may present with a variety of symptoms that include ptosis, ophthalmoplegia, encephalopathy hepatic dysfunction, strokelike episodes, and myoclonic epilepsy. These clinical manifestations can vary significantly in severity, so the presence of subtle multisystem symptoms before onset of AIDP or between attacks of CIDP may be an indication of the presence of these disorders. The neuropathy seen in *POLG* mutations seems to be primarily axonal or mixed axonal-demyelinating.

Some patients with *POLG* mutations present distinctly with ataxia-neuropathy spectrum (ANS). Although ANS can be associated with encephalopathy and seizures, the findings can be mild in affected individuals. The ataxia tends to be a sensory ataxia related to a sensory or mixed sensory and motor neuropathy. Muscle cramps are present in up to 25% of affected individuals, although clinical myopathy is rare. Variable findings include myoclonus, blindness, liver dysfunction, headache, and depression. Genotype-phenotype correlation in this family of disorders is highly variable. A relapsing-remitting nature of illness may suggest against *POLG*-related disorders but does not entirely exclude them.[46]

Additional genetic disorders associated with pediatric-onset peripheral neuropathy are presented in **Table 2**.

THE DIAGNOSTIC EVALUATION OF INHERITED PERIPHERAL NEUROPATHIES

Patients presenting with the acute onset of symptoms suggestive of peripheral neuropathy should undergo a thorough evaluation focused on identifying the peripheral nerve as the cause of the patient's symptoms. The history and physical examination should delineate the acuity of onset and the presence or absence of systemic symptoms, as well as any exposures that would indicate exogenous causes of acquired peripheral neuropathy (see **Box 1**). Those whose presentation suggests GBS should undergo neuroimaging and neurophysiologic studies. Those whose presentation is indeterminate should have variant forms of GBS considered (see **Table 1**), as well as other causes of acquired peripheral neuropathy.

A positive family history, persistent symptoms, or indicators of systemic involvement or additional neurologic dysfunction may indicate an inherited peripheral neuropathy. Most patients with suspected inherited neuropathies have already had MRI studies of the brain and/or spine, lumbar puncture, and EMG, particularly if presenting with acute symptoms, and these investigations may provide valuable information regarding the type of inherited neuropathy (see **Table 2**). However, many require molecular genetic or functional investigations for confirmation.

Given the genetic heterogeneity of inherited neuropathies, targeted single-gene analysis is unlikely to yield a diagnosis, given that many disorders are associated with more than 1 gene. Multigene panels are available for numerous disorders, although whole-exome sequencing may be more cost-effective and have a higher yield than performing multiple multigene panels. However, exome sequencing is limited in its ability to detect genetic disorders secondary to copy number variations, tandem repeats, or mutations in mitochondrial genes. A tiered approach starting with whole-exome sequencing and deletion/duplication analysis is most appropriate. Although some mitochondrial disorders, such as *POLG*-spectrum disorders, are secondary to mutations in nuclear genes and may be detected via either sequencing or deletion/duplication analysis, others require assessment of mitochondrial DNA. Under these circumstances, when initial genetic studies are unrevealing and the suspicion for mitochondrial disease is high, mitochondrial DNA studies should be performed on the most accessible affected tissue, which is often muscle biopsy tissue.

Patients presenting with acute-onset peripheral neuropathy most often have an acquired cause for their disorder. However, the presence of systemic symptoms, a positive family history of neuromuscular disease, or the lack of a response to treatment may indicate an inherited neuropathy. A tiered investigative approach may lead to appropriate diagnosis and the avoidance of unnecessary immunomodulatory therapy.

REFERENCES

1. Yuki N, Hartung HP. Guillain-Barré syndrome. N Engl J Med 2012;366(24): 2294–304.
2. Kuitwaard K, van Koningsveld R, Ruts L, et al. Recurrent Guillain-Barré syndrome. J Neurol Neurosurg Psychiatry 2009;80:56–9.
3. Ruts L, Drenthen J, Jacobs BC, et al, The Dutch GBS Study Group. Distinguishing acute-onset CIDP from fluctuating Guillain-Barré syndrome. A prospective study. Neurology 2010;74(21):1680–6.
4. McGrogan A, Madle GC, Seaman HE, et al. The epidemiology of Guillain-Barré syndrome worldwide. Neuroepidemiology 2009;32:150–63.
5. Korinthenberg R, Schessl J, Kirschner J. Clinical presentation and course of childhood Guillain-Barré syndrome: a prospective multicentre study. Neuropediatrics 2007;38(1):10.
6. Dimachkie MM, Barohn RJ. Guillain-Barré syndrome and variants. Neurol Clin 2013;31(2):491–510.
7. Yikilmaz A, Doganay S, Gumus H, et al. Magnetic resonance imaging of childhood Guillain-Barre syndrome. Childs Nerv Syst 2010;26(8):1103.
8. Van den Bergh PY, Piéret F. Electrodiagnostic criteria for acute and chronic inflammatory demyelinating polyradiculoneuropathy. Muscle Nerve 2004;29(4): 565–74.
9. Evans OB, Vedanarayanan V. Guillain-Barré syndrome. Pediatr Rev 1997;18:10.
10. Genovese O, Ballario C, Storino R, et al. Clinical manifestations of peripheral nervous system involvement in human chronic Chagas disease. Arq Neuropsiquiatr 1996;54(2):190.
11. Pardo CA, McArthur JC, Griffin JW. HIV neuropathy: insights in the pathology of HIV peripheral nerve disease. J Peripher Nerv Syst 2001;6(1):21.
12. Wilder-Smith A, Wilder-Smith E. Electrophysiological evaluation of peripheral autonomic function in leprosy patients, leprosy contacts and controls. Int J Lepr Other Mycobact Dis 1996;64(4):433.
13. Bulun A, Topaloglu R, Duzova A, et al. Ataxia and peripheral neuropathy: rare manifestations in Henoch-Schönlein purpura. Pediatr Nephrol 2001;16(12):1139.
14. Lossos A, River Y, Eliakim A, et al. Neurologic aspects of inflammatory bowel disease. Neurology 1995;45(3 Pt 1):416.
15. Peyronnard JM, Charron L, Beaudet F, et al. Vasculitic neuropathy in rheumatoid disease and Sjögren syndrome. Neurology 1982;32(8):839.
16. Snavely SR, Hodges GR. The neurotoxicity of antibacterial agents. Ann Intern Med 1984;101(1):92–104.
17. Amato AA, Barohn RJ, Sahenk Z, et al. Polyneuropathy complicating bone marrow and solid organ transplantation. Neurology 1993;43(8):1513.
18. Kurczynski TW, Choudhury AA, Horwitz SJ, et al. Remote effect of malignancy on the nervous system in children. Dev Med Child Neurol 1980;22(2):205.

19. Yuki N. Guillain-Barré syndrome and anti-ganglioside antibodies: a clinician-scientist's journey. Proc Jpn Acad Ser B Phys Biol Sci 2012;88(7):299–326.
20. Wakerley BR, Yuki N. Mimics and chameleons in Guillain-Barré and Miller Fisher syndromes. Pract Neurol 2015;15:90–9.
21. Overell JR, Hsieh ST, Odaka M, et al. Treatment for Fisher syndrome, Bickerstaff's brainstem encephalitis and related disorders. Cochrane Database Syst Rev 2007;(1):CD004761.
22. Ito M, Kuwabara S, Odaka M, et al. Bickerstaff's brainstem encephalitis and Fisher syndrome form a continuous spectrum: clinical analysis of 581 cases. J Neurol 2008;255(5):674–82.
23. Konersman CG, Bordini BJ, Scharer G, et al. BAG3 myofibrillar myopathy presenting with cardiomyopathy. Neuromuscul Disord 2015;25(5):418–22.
24. Kuhlenbäumer G, Stogbauer F, Timmerman V, et al. Diagnostic guidelines for hereditary neuralgic amyotrophy or heredofamilial neuritis with brachial plexus predilection. On behalf of the European CMT consortium. Neuromuscul Disord 2000; 10:515–7.
25. Mouton P, Tardieu S, Gouider R, et al. Spectrum of clinical and electrophysiologic features in HNPP patients with the 17p11.2 deletion. Neurology 1999;52:1440–6.
26. Infante J, Garcia A, Combarros O, et al. Diagnostic strategy for familial and sporadic cases of neuropathy associated with 17p11.2 deletion. Muscle Nerve 2001; 24:1149–55.
27. Skjeldal OH, Stokke O, Refsum S, et al. Clinical and biochemical heterogeneity in conditions with phytanic acid accumulation. J Neurol Sci 1987;77:87–96.
28. van den Brink DM, Brites P, Haasjes J, et al. Identification of PEX7 as the second gene involved in Refsum disease. Am J Hum Genet 2003;72:471–7.
29. Ortiz RG, Newman NJ, Shoffner JM, et al. Variable retinal and neurologic manifestations in patients harboring the mitochondrial DNA 8993 mutation. Arch Ophthalmol 1993;111:1525–30.
30. Chowers I, Lerman-Sagie T, Elpeleg ON, et al. Cone and rod dysfunction in the NARP syndrome. Br J Ophthalmol 1999;83:190–3.
31. Holt IJ, Harding AE, Petty RK, et al. A new mitochondrial disease associated with mitochondrial DNA heteroplasmy. Am J Hum Genet 1990;46:428–33.
32. Verny C, Prundean A, Nicolas G, et al. Refsum's disease may mimic familial Guillain Barre syndrome. Neuromuscul Disord 2006;16(11):805–8.
33. Pareyson D, Scaioli V, Laura M. Clinical and electrophysiological aspects of Charcot-Marie-Tooth disease. Neuromolecular Med 2006;8:3–22.
34. van Alfen N, van Engelen BGM. The clinical spectrum of neuralgic amyotrophy in 246 cases. Brain 2006;129(2):438–50.
35. Sanahuja J, Franco E, Rojas-García R, et al. Central nervous system involvement in hereditary neuropathy with liability to pressure palsies: description of a large family with this association. Arch Neurol 2005;62(12):1911–4.
36. Husain AM, Altuwaijri M, Aldosari M. Krabbe disease: neurophysiologic studies and MRI correlations. Neurology 2004;63:617–20.
37. Nevo Y, Ben-Zeev B, Tabib A, et al. CD59 deficiency is associated with chronic hemolysis and childhood relapsing immune-mediated polyneuropathy. Blood 2013;121(1):129–35.
38. Rotthier A, Baets J, De Vriendt E, et al. Genes for hereditary sensory and autonomic neuropathies: a genotype-phenotype correlation. Brain 2009;132(Pt 10): 2699–711.
39. Henao AI, Pira S, Herrera DA, et al. Characteristic brain MRI findings in ataxia-neuropathy spectrum related to POLG mutation. Neuroradiol J 2016;29(1):46–8.

40. King PH, Petersen NE, Rakhra R, et al. Porphyria presenting with bilateral radial motor neuropathy: evidence of a novel gene mutation. Neurology 2002;58: 1118–21.

41. Pischik E, Kauppinen R. Neurological manifestations of acute intermittent porphyria. Cell Mol Biol (Noisy-le-grand) 2009;55:72–83.

42. Selcen D, Ohno K, Engel AG. Myofibrillar myopathy: clinical, morphological and genetic studies in 63 patients. Brain 2004;127:439–51.

43. Fischer D, Kley RA, Strach K, et al. Distinct muscle imaging patterns in myofibrillar myopathies. Neurology 2008;71(10):758–65.

44. Rajabally YA, Adams D, Latour P, et al. Hereditary and inflammatory neuropathies: a review of reported associations, mimics and misdiagnoses. J Neurol Neurosurg Psychiatry 2016. http://dx.doi.org/10.1136/jnnp-2015-310835.

45. Garone C, Tadesse S, Hirano M. Clinical and genetic spectrum of mitochondrial neurogastrointestinal encephalomyopathy. Brain 2011;134(11):3326–32.

46. Wong LJ, Naviaux RK, Brunetti-Pierri N, et al. Molecular and clinical genetics of mitochondrial diseases due to POLG mutations. Hum Mutat 2008;29:E150–72.

The Intersection of Medical Child Abuse and Medical Complexity

Hillary W. Petska, MD, MPH[a,]*, John B. Gordon, MD[a],
Debra Jablonski, RN[b], Lynn K. Sheets, MD[a]

KEYWORDS

- Medical complexity • Children and youth with special healthcare needs
- Medical child abuse • Munchausen syndrome by proxy
- Caregiver-fabricated illness • Child abuse • Child maltreatment

KEY POINTS

- Medical complexity and medical child abuse (MCA) may present similarly.
- Unusual and/or unfamiliar conditions or disease presentations may raise concerns about MCA when none is present.
- Recognizing MCA when a child presents with apparent medical complexity requires a high index of suspicion.
- In both conditions, clinical judgment, longitudinal observation, and consultation with appropriate specialists are often needed to arrive at a diagnosis while avoiding unnecessary medical diagnostic testing.

INTRODUCTION

Defining Children with Medical Complexity and Medical Child Abuse

Children with medical complexity (CMC) and children who are victims of MCA often have similar clinical presentations. This can lead to an erroneous diagnosis of MCA when not present or a missed diagnosis of MCA when it is an underlying or coexisting condition in a case of apparent medical complexity. Either of these outcomes results in harm to the child and family. The purpose of this article is to describe CMC and MCA, discuss factors that may complicate these diagnoses, and propose an approach to the assessment of CMC designed to avoid either an erroneous or missed diagnosis of MCA.

Financial Disclosure: The authors do not have any financial relationships relevant to this article to disclose.
Conflict of Interest: All authors confirm that there are no conflicts of interest.
[a] Children's Hospital of Wisconsin, Medical College of Wisconsin, Milwaukee, WI, USA; [b] Children's Hospital of Wisconsin, Milwaukee, WI, USA
* Corresponding author. Child Advocacy and Protection Services, Department of Pediatrics, Children's Hospital of Wisconsin, C615, PO Box 1997, Milwaukee, WI 53201.
E-mail address: hpetska@chw.org

Pediatr Clin N Am 64 (2017) 253–264
http://dx.doi.org/10.1016/j.pcl.2016.08.016
0031-3955/17/© 2016 Elsevier Inc. All rights reserved.

pediatric.theclinics.com

CMC are a heterogeneous subset of children and youth with special health care needs who typically have multiple chronic medical conditions.[1] Estimates of the prevalence of CMC are generally less than 1% of the US pediatric population but may be as high as 5%, depending on the number of chronic medical conditions and level of resource utilization used to define the population.[2] CMC often have neurologic impairment, functional limitations, and technology dependence and may have unusual diagnoses and treatments. Their care and treatment typically require multiple medications, multiple specialists, and significant home nursing or other specialized care. CMC also have high tertiary center resource use and very high health care costs, accounting for 30% to 40% of pediatric health care dollars.[1,3,4] Social determinants of health, such as language barriers, poverty, and poor access to care as well as mental or behavioral health problems, exacerbate the difficulties faced by CMC and their families in seeking care. Studies indicate there are multiple unmet needs for the children and considerable stress in the lives of families of CMC.[5,6]

MCA, often termed, *Munchausen syndrome by proxy*, is a form of child maltreatment in which a child receives unnecessary and harmful or potentially harmful medical care at the instigation of a caregiver.[7] Known by many names since it was first recognized (**Box 1**), MCA involves a caregiver who exaggerates or fabricates symptoms that cannot be independently verified or who intentionally induces symptoms or signs in a child. As in other types of child maltreatment, the abnormal caregiver-child relationship in MCA causes significant neurodevelopmental harm to the child that results in short-term and long-term negative health consequences of chronic toxic stress. In addition, MCA causes physical harm through unnecessary medical testing or procedures, including phlebotomy, repeated physical examinations, hospitalizations, surgeries, and medications with resulting pain, injury, and risk of complications. These unnecessary medical

---

Box 1
Evolution of terminology and definitions

Other Names for Medical Child Abuse	First Used by	Characteristics
Munchausen syndrome by proxy	Meadow,[8] 1977	Identified Munchausen syndrome by proxy as a form of child abuse, focused on caregiver motive
Factitious disorder by proxy	American Psychiatric Association, *Diagnostic and Statistical Manual of Mental Disorders* (Fourth Edition) (1994)	Psychiatric disorder in caregivers who falsify illness in a child for their own needs, focused on caregiver motive
Pediatric condition falsification	American Professional Society on the Abuse of Children (2002)	A child abused in this manner is a victim of pediatric condition falsification; focused on caregiver action
Child abuse in a medical setting	American Academy of Pediatrics Committee on Child Abuse and Neglect (2007)	Focused on the harm caused to the child
MCA	Roesler & Jenny,[7] 2009	Focused on the harm caused to the child
Caregiver-fabricated illness in a child	American Academy of Pediatrics Committee on Child Abuse and Neglect (2013)	Focused on caregiver action

Data from Refs.[7–11]

interventions result in a morbidity rate of 100% (eg, medical complications and disabilities) and mortality rate as high as 9%.[12] Regardless of a caregiver's underlying motivation, the child is harmed by the caregiver using the practitioner as the instrument of abuse.[13]

Factors Contributing to Erroneous or Missed Diagnosis of Medical Child Abuse

Although there are multiple situations that can result in unnecessary medical care, one of the more challenging is determining whether MCA contributes to or coexists with medical complexity. Delayed diagnosis of MCA has significant consequences and prolongs the suffering of a child (up to 21.8 months in cases of MCA).[14] Conversely, some CMC are suspected to be victims of MCA before they are eventually diagnosed with a medical condition explaining their symptoms and signs. The damage to the family and the caregiver-physician relationship arising from an erroneous suspicion of MCA can also have significant negative consequences on the child. There is also significant overlap between the 2 conditions in that up to 30% of children suffering from MCA do have an underlying medical condition.[12]

Patient, caregiver, and provider factors can singly or in combination contribute to an erroneous suspicion or a missed diagnosis of MCA. The former is demonstrated by the example of AB, a 6-year-old girl with failure to thrive, frequent infections, and abdominal pain who was repeatedly hospitalized at a tertiary center (case details throughout have been modified to protect patient confidentiality). The hospitalizations were often brief and she seemed to quickly return to baseline during admissions. Hospital personnel became concerned about possible MCA and consulted the hospital-based child protection team due to these concerns. Ultimately, further testing demonstrated a rare genetic disorder that fully explained her phenotype.

In contrast, CD was a 15-year-old boy with a diagnosis of intestinal pseudo-obstruction who was followed by his primary care physician and multiple specialists at a tertiary hospital. His mother had a mitochondrial disorder herself and reported that the child had feeding intolerance and pain with feeding. He had significant developmental delay, a seizure disorder, and other multisystem complaints consistent with a mitochondrial disorder. Over a period of several years, he underwent multiple procedures, became dependent on parenteral nutrition, and had multiple bouts of sepsis requiring intensive care. When MCA was eventually suspected, the parents' involvement in the child's care was suspended. Over the subsequent year, the child improved significantly to the point of no longer requiring parenteral or tube feeding. Although some features of medical complexity persisted, he rarely required hospital admission after MCA was diagnosed.

In these 2 cases, a common patient factor contributing to diagnostic uncertainty was a rare diagnosis: AB's diagnosis required novel testing and CD's was associated with multiple chronic conditions but never definitively diagnosed. The caregiver role also contributed to uncertainty. The parents of AB were confrontational and abrasive, and little rapport was established with the medical team. In contrast, CD's mother was medically sophisticated, interacted well with providers, and seemed to comply fully with medical team requests. These factors likely influenced the decision to consult the child protection team in the first case and the delay in consulting the child protection team in the second case.

Other factors that affect providers' suspicion of MCA include caregiver variability in reported symptomatology over time, perceptions of malingering, and discordance between objective and historical data. There are also several additional caregiver factors that may contribute to uncertainty about the contributing or coexisting diagnosis of MCA in CMC. First, health literacy limitations, such as those due to incomplete or erroneous understanding of medical terms or jargon, language barriers, and cultural barriers, may affect a caregiver's ability to accurately or consistently describe symptomatology. Other caregiver factors, such as fatigue, chronic stress, diminished cognition, mental illness, substance abuse, and inadequately met basic needs, can contribute to communication challenges. Caregiver misperceptions of medical information based on family lore or other unreliable sources, such as the Internet, can further contribute to inaccurate historical information. Secondly, caregiver requests for additional testing or treatment are common in both CMC and MCA. These may stem from dissatisfaction with the lack of a diagnosis, genuine fear or anxiety about the child's health, vulnerable child syndrome, or catastrophization.[15] Catastrophization is a common phenomenon in children with chronic illness and is characterized by the caregiver's perceptions and behaviors that reflect that each event in the medical journey is a disaster.[16] Although lack of understanding, hypersensitization to the medical environment, and secondary trauma from experiencing a child with complex medical needs may contribute to this phenomenon, when the behavior of a caregiver results in harm to a child, maltreatment has occurred regardless of the caregiver's motivation.[11] Finally, caregivers may seek out multiple specialists at multiple institutions because they are dissatisfied with services or a diagnosis or lack thereof, have heard that a particular physician is expert in the condition their child has or may have, or are using it as a subterfuge for MCA.

Provider factors also contribute to erroneous and missed diagnoses of MCA. CMC with multiple chronic conditions and uncertain diagnoses pose an enormous challenge to providers. The likelihood that any one provider has seen any given rare disease is unlikely and failure to recognize the disorder may lead to incorrectly branding it as factitious as in the case of AB. On the other hand, defensive medicine, the culture of medicine (pursuit of "zebras"), and acquiescence to caregiver demand for testing may identify a rare disease but may contribute to MCA.[17,18] In this era of rapidly advancing technology, increased information availability, and emphasis on family-centered care, navigation of appropriate diagnostic testing and what constitutes appropriate care-seeking behavior in CMC can be particularly challenging. Abnormalities of variable clinical significance are often discovered with extensive diagnostic testing, resulting in additional, and often unnecessary diagnostic studies. The pressure to make a diagnosis may cause both caregivers and providers to place a child at risk in search of a "cure."

The siloed nature of medical care in which specialists pursue diagnoses related to their specific body system coupled with limited communication among specialists can also contribute to delays in diagnosis.[17] Specialty provider input is often of significant value but is most beneficial when coupled with longitudinal observation and involvement of providers who know the child and caregivers well. For example, EF was a 3-year-old boy with mild developmental delay, a cheery demeanor, and an unremarkable examination. When the family began to repeatedly request a gastrostomy tube due to reported periods of difficulty eating, fatigue, and ataxic gait, providers began to suspect MCA since the child had been gaining weight appropriately and always seemed active and steady in clinic. However, a physiatrist was able to induce the fatigue and ataxia in clinic after prolonged physical exertion, and gastroenterology workup corroborated parental report of slow feeding and neurologic dysphagia. The child was ultimately diagnosed with a mitochondrial disorder and, after a gastrostomy tube was placed, his overall development and endurance was markedly improved.

Provider bias can create diagnostic challenges as well. Unconscious or not, biases, especially those involving perception of the caregiver, can affect the objectivity of the diagnostic process. For example, 2 children, GH and IJ, were referred to a program for

CMC at a tertiary care children's hospital. Both had multiple similar medical problems that could be objectively identified (seizure disorder, mild hypothyroidism, intermittent hypoxia, and intestinal pseudo-obstruction) as well as multiple complaints identified by their mothers (abdominal pain and fatigue) that were not consistently associated with objective findings. The parents of both children had been previously suspected of MCA at other institutions. In the case of GH, the family was very engaged and cooperated actively with medical providers, and ongoing work-up led the medical team to conclude that she had a mitochondrial disorder despite failing to identify a specific genetic cause. In contrast, the family of IJ had difficulty engaging with providers and was perceived as confrontational. Unlike GH, many providers initially suspected that IJ was a victim of MCA despite the fact that the 2 children had virtually identical phenotypes. Both children had a history of multiple procedures, parent-reported pain out of proportion to appearance, dependence on parenteral nutrition, and multiple medications, and in both cases, parental responses to physician-perceived minor problems was often as vociferous as those to major problems. The key difference in these 2 cases was the relationship the mothers had with the health care team, which highlights the importance of awareness of biases in cases involving contentious caregivers.

Although a contentious caregiver may increase the level of suspicion for malicious intent, this does not necessarily suggest MCA and should prompt further exploration of the caregiver's understanding, motivations, fears, and concerns. Although secondary gain (eg, attention/sympathy, resources/benefits, status, or money/donations) is often a motive for MCA, a caregiver seeking or publicly soliciting secondary gain in isolation does not meet criteria for MCA. For example, the parents of a CMC with modest heart and kidney disease told his school that he required heart and kidney transplant and the parents of a child who was relatively stable despite multiple chronic conditions told the school he was in hospice. In both cases, the history given to the school was false and raised concerns about potential MCA. On further discussion with the hospital-based child protection team, however, the cases did not rise to the level of MCA because the children were not receiving unnecessary medical care. Both cases, however, raise a concern for emotional harm to the child who may be forced to play a sick role that is out of proportion to reality. Finally, providers must guard against making assumptions based on the perception that the family or caregiver is "nice" as this may lead to missed diagnosis of MCA. Perpetrators of all types of child maltreatment can appear to be "nice" or "good" caregivers in their brief interactions with medical professionals.

APPROACH

CMC are cared for by a wide range of practitioners in a variety of settings, including primary care practices and tertiary hospitals. Over the past decade, there has been a growing recognition of the needs of CMC and their families with a concomitant growth in the new field of complex care. Complex care programs provide medical management and care coordination for CMC often in collaboration with primary care physicians, thus ensuring an "enhanced" medical home for these children and their families.[1,3,4] Practitioners in the field come from various disciplines within pediatric medicine, nursing, social work, and so forth. Whether care is provided by a primary care or complex care program, a comprehensive patient/family-centered approach to assessing a child with medical complexity resulting in a detailed plan of care is essential (**Box 2**).

As with any medical evaluation, assessment of a child with medical complexity begins with a history and physical. This generally includes a detailed interview with the

---

Box 2
Example of elements of a plan of care for children with medical complexity

Initial assessment and care plan

Medical history
  Chief complaint
  History of present illness (a narrative of the issues identified by child and caregiver)
  Code status/health care goals
  Primary diagnosis
  Current problem list (a comprehensive review of systems using informants and chart review)
  Past history (medical and surgical)
  Medication list
  Nutrition
  Growth
  Allergies
  Immunizations
  Family history

Care coordination (essentially a very detailed social history)
  Family structure, including siblings and caregiver occupations
  Immediate goals of care
  Child likes/dislikes
  Coping/support systems
  Ongoing patient care team
    Primary care provider
    Specialists
    Home services
  Transportation
  Nursing needs
  Technologies and equipment (including suppliers)
  Insurance
  Community resources
    School/early childhood program/therapies
  Unmet needs/immediate concerns

Physical examination (eg, vital signs, general description, and complete examination)

Relevant laboratory tests (eg, recent or critical values that support the assessment and plan)

Assessment and suggestions/plans (consists of both a narrative overview of the child and families care coordination and medical status and needs as well as a tabular summary)

---

caregiver that focuses on the child's medical history, child and caregiver goals, social supports, barriers to care, and home and other services. The physical examination often focuses not only on the child's medical issues but also on functionality, comfort, and capabilities. After the initial visit, considerable time is spent reviewing the medical records and speaking with other providers both at the hospital and in the community, with a focus on objective findings rather than just past diagnoses. Synthesis of multiple symptoms described by the caregiver, physical findings, information gleaned from chart review, and information from other providers is then attempted to best treat the child and meet the caregiver's goals of care enunciated in the initial visit. Subsequent visits and ongoing communication with the caregivers and multiple hospital-based and community providers are standard practice for most complex care programs.

After the initial visit, there is often a period of searching for a diagnosis, during which considerable testing and referral to subspecialists may occur. Many caregivers of CMC are cure-seeking and would like to know what is wrong with their child and what can be done to improve their health and/or quality of life.[19] Commonly, children in a complex care program lack a definite unifying diagnosis that explains all of their chronic conditions. With longitudinal observation, results of testing and specialists' opinions, and care conferences designed to promote communication, working diagnoses and a plan of care can often be developed even in the absence of a definite diagnosis, although the search for answers is often ongoing.

MCA should not be viewed as a diagnosis of exclusion but rather considered concurrently with other possible medical explanations for the illness. Certain risk factors have been identified as common features in cases of MCA but should not be considered in isolation. For example, although perpetrators are often female caregivers with a health care background, this is nonspecific as other caregivers with varied backgrounds also can be perpetrators.[11,13] In addition, there is significant overlap between characteristics of caregivers who have children with organic disease and those who perpetrate MCA. Although providers should be aware of the more common presentations of MCA (ie, bleeding, seizures, central nervous system depression, apnea, feeding problems, diarrhea, vomiting, fever, and rash), the range of illness often involves multiple organ systems and is limited only by the imagination.[12,14,20]

There are several features of the history, physical, and follow-up period that should prompt consideration of MCA (**Box 3**). A history that is inconsistent with objective findings or that does not make sense should lead to further questioning, exploration of caregiver factors as previously discussed, and/or consideration of alternative diagnoses. Periodic checking for comprehension by encouraging the caregiver to express their understanding in their own words can be helpful in clarifying the situation. Suggested questions could include

- "Tell me what you think is going on."
- "What is your understanding of your child's illness/symptoms?"
- "To make sure I explained this well, can you tell me why your child is on this medication; what does it do and how and when do you give it?"

Longitudinal observation is essential in identifying symptoms that wax and wane and objectively describing a symptom. Failure to objectively identify a key symptom

---

Box 3
Red flags for medical child abuse

- History discordant with objective findings over multiple visits

- Unexplained, unexpected signs and symptoms, which may only be observed by a single caregiver

- Atypical response of child's illness to its standard treatments

- Incongruent caregiver affect
  - Persistent negative affect in the face of reassurance
  - Behavior inconsistent with expressed distress

- Caregiver insistence that excessive or invasive interventions are needed

- Caregiver resistance to release of records when care is sought from multiple providers/institutions

- Caregiver or sibling(s) with history of unusual, unexplained illness

- Disclosure of abuse by child

Adapted from Flaherty EG, Macmillan HL, Committee on Child Abuse and Neglect. Caregiver-fabricated illness in a child: a manifestation of child maltreatment. Pediatrics 2013;132:590–7.

over a prolonged period is a red flag, particularly when unexplained signs or symptoms occur only in the presence of a certain caregiver and cannot be independently verified. Repeated treatment failures and/or request for interventions that are inconsistent with stated goals for care (eg, cure or quality of life) should also prompt re-evaluation of provider/caregiver expectations and consideration of MCA. If the child is verbal, a medical history from the child separate from the caregiver should be conducted if possible. Lack of disclosure, however, from a verbal child does not rule out the possibility of MCA. Children who are being abused or neglected may collude with the perpetrator in maintaining secrecy about or be unware of the true etiology of signs and symptoms.[21] Finally, a caregiver who resists reassurance that a child is healthy, focuses on normal or minimally abnormal results without clinical significance, and/or does not adhere to medical recommendations should also raise concerns for MCA.[11,20]

The review of the chart may also suggest MCA when multiple providers or health institutions have been involved in a child's care. CMC, particularly those with unusual diagnoses, often seek care at multiple institutions when the caregiver is not satisfied with the expertise available, diagnostic answers, or care provided at one institution. Similarly, a caregiver who perpetrates MCA may seek care at multiple sites to obtain desired testing or to evade detection of the true nature of the child's health problems. Such doctor shopping prevents a unified team approach and limits the ability of providers to share information that might suggest a diagnosis of MCA. Doctor shopping, however, may also inadvertently raise the possibility of MCA in CMC with unusual diagnoses requiring input from additional subspecialists. The motivation for seeking care from multiple providers or institutions should be sought, and, whenever possible, previous medical records should be obtained and discussion with providers familiar with the child should be attempted. Most caregivers are cooperative with providing medical records. Refusal by a caregiver to allow sharing of health information between institutions should prompt consideration of MCA, although such reluctance may be due to many reasons, such as embarrassment about prior behavior or fear that providers at the first institution will refuse to see the child because the family sought another opinion. Other possible indicators of MCA are previous concern of MCA by medical personnel and siblings with similar unexplained illness or death, both of which also may be found in CMC.

MANAGEMENT

Once a concern about MCA has been raised, consultation with a child protection team, child abuse pediatrician, or other provider with advanced training or expertise in child maltreatment should be considered since few complex care team members have experience with diagnosing MCA. This consultant may recommend commonly used strategies to clarify red flags, which can help differentiate between CMC and MCA (**Table 1**). If red flags remain or these strategies have already been tried, the child protection team likely will perform a record review of the medical care the child has received. This consultation typically includes a compilation of known problems and diagnoses, problems without clear diagnoses, and testing and procedures completed (**Table 2**). In the process of review, the consulting team/provider may invite input from others involved in the child's care and/or experts in rare diseases and their mimics, including members of the complex care team, the child's primary care physician, and subspecialists with expertise in the conditions in question.[10] The goal of this review is to determine the appropriateness of diagnostic testing and whether the caregiver appropriately advocated for their child. These consultations are resource

Table 1
Examples of strategies to address and clarify concerns for medical child abuse

Basis of Concern for Medical Child Abuse	Strategies
Objective information is discordant with history.	• Define with precision what was known and what was reported by the caregiver. • Encourage the health care team to document verbatim when the caregiver discusses the history.
Symptom only occurs when caregiver is present.	• Encourage respite time with close monitoring in caregiver absence (eg, sitter). • Consider talking with the child alone if verbal.
Caregiver request for procedures seems incongruent with previously stated goals.	• Assess caregiver understanding (eg, teach back) and whether goals have changed. • Consider social work consult to better understand psychosocial factors. • Involve other caregiver supports (eg, health psychologists) if struggling with grief or other issues. • Consider ethics consult.
Caregiver obstructs release of outside records.	• Plan a family meeting to explain rationale and to develop a contract about expectations of the caregiver and health care team. • Ask whether there are specific people at other institutions with whom one can speak.
Caregiver obtains secondary gain from child's condition.	Unless causing the caregiver to seek additional procedures to maintain the sick role or causing other harm to the patient, no specific interventions are needed.
Health care team is being triangulated by the caregiver.	Schedule a care conference to ensure consistent message from and to the caregiver.
Members of the team make negative assumptions about the caregiver's behavior.	• Consider social work consult to better understand psychosocial factors. • Involve other caregiver supports (eg, health psychologists) if struggling with grief or other issues.

intensive because all available medical records are obtained and documentation is reviewed for inconsistencies, contradictions, and/or exaggerations.[22] Nursing notes in particular can provide rich detail about a caregiver's behavior.

Most cases of MCA can be diagnosed through record review and longitudinal medical care. If lethality risk is high, however, or if there is suspicion that a caregiver is actually inducing illness, covert video surveillance as an additional diagnostic tool may be considered. This should serve as a last resort given the ethical implications of potentially placing the child back into harm's way.[7] If covert video surveillance is used, it should be done with guidelines that are consistent with best practice. When used, covert video surveillance may assist in making a diagnosis of MCA and, in some cases, may demonstrate a genuine medical problem.[11,23] Diagnosis also may require a trial separation between the child and caregiver; rare conditions would not be expected to resolve when the caregiver is removed from the child's environment.

After completion of the investigation by the consulting team/provider, the results should be presented to the multidisciplinary team involved in the child's care, potentially leading to re-evaluation of the care plan. The threshold for mandated reporting—reasonable suspicion— is even more challenging in these cases, resulting in many cases going unreported.[11] This is particularly true when a child also has elements of

Table 2
Sample template for record review

Date, Type of Visit	Provider and Facility Name	Reason/Chief Complaint	Final Diagnosis	Diagnostic Testing Performed Including Blood Draws	Discrepancy Between Caregiver Report and Objective Data (Observed Behavior, Examination, Laboratory Tests, Test Data)			Specific Location in the Medical Record	Other Comments
					Caregiver Report	Objective Data	Reason for Concern		

Adapted from Flaherty EG, Macmillan HL, Committee on Child Abuse and Neglect. Caregiver-fabricated illness in a child: a manifestation of child maltreatment. Pediatrics 2013;132:594.

true medical complexity. Although not necessary for diagnosis, a caregiver's motivation may become clearer during the investigation by child protective services and law enforcement.

In cases of medical complexity, including those with concerns for MCA, providers should remain vigilant for evidence of neglect (medical noncompliance, emotional, physical, or educational), physical abuse, sexual abuse, and psychological abuse since disabled children are at a heightened risk of all forms of child maltreatment.[24] If reasonable suspicions for child maltreatment arise, a mandated report to authorities should be made in accordance with state laws. For example, KL was a 5-year-old boy with a known chromosomal abnormality, developmental delay, seizures, and chronic lung disease who was nonverbal/nonmobile and presented on several occasions with long bone fractures. Due to his degree of osteopenia and plausible explanations for the fractures (physical therapy), child physical abuse was not initially considered. At the age of 7 years, he was admitted with evidence of facial trauma and the presence of an abuser in the home was identified. Although the long bone fractures were ultimately indeterminate for abuse, the child's medical complexity may have led to a delay in reporting suspected maltreatment.

MCA has significant effects on the child.[9,25] After a diagnosis of MCA, every attempt should be made to repair the physical and psychological damage a child has suffered in the least restrictive manner that still ensures the child's safety.[13] Recovery may involve reversal of medical procedures and intensive mental health therapy, although some children will suffer long-term or permanent injury.

SUMMARY

Differentiation of medical complexity and MCA may be difficult in the clinical setting. A thoughtful, multidisciplinary approach to these conditions can prevent adverse consequences for children and families.

REFERENCES

1. Cohen E, Kuo DZ, Agrawal R, et al. Children with medical complexity: an emerging population for clinical and research initiatives. Pediatrics 2011; 127(3):529–38.
2. Berry JG, Agrawal R, Kuo DZ, et al. Characteristics of hospitalizations for patients who use a structured clinical care program for children with medical complexity. J Pediatr 2011;159(2):284–90.
3. Berry JG, Hall M, Neff J, et al. Children with medical complexity and Medicaid: spending And cost savings. Health Aff (Millwood) 2014;33(12):2199–206.
4. Gordon JB, Colby HH, Bartelt T, et al. A tertiary care–primary care partnership model for medically complex and fragile children and youth with special health care needs. Arch Pediatr Adolesc Med 2007;161(10):937–44.
5. Kuo DZ, Berry JG, Glader L, et al. Health services and health care needs fulfilled by structured clinical programs for children with medical complexity. J Pediatr 2016;169:291–6.e1.
6. Mandic C, Johaningsmeir S, Corden TE, et al. Impact of caring for children with medical complexity on parents' employment and time. Community Work Fam 2016;1–15.
7. Roesler TA, Jenny C. Medical child abuse: beyond Munchausen syndrome by proxy. Elk Grove (IL): American Academy of Pediatrics; 2009.
8. Meadow R. Munchausen syndrome by proxy. The hinterland of child abuse. Lancet 1977;2(8033):343–5.

9. Ayoub CC, Alexander R, Beck D, et al. Position paper: definitional issues in Munchausen by proxy. Child Maltreat 2002;7(2):105–11.

10. Stirling J Jr, American Academy of Pediatrics Committee on Child Abuse and Neglect. Beyond Munchausen syndrome by proxy: identification and treatment of child abuse in a medical setting. Pediatrics 2007;119(5):1026–30.

11. Flaherty EG, Macmillan HL, Committee on Child Abuse and Neglect. Caregiver-fabricated illness in a child: a manifestation of child maltreatment. Pediatrics 2013;132(3):590–7.

12. Rosenberg DA. Web of deceit: a literature review of Munchausen syndrome by proxy. Child Abuse Negl 1987;11(4):547–63.

13. Jenny C, editor. Child abuse and neglect: diagnosis, treatment and evidence. St Louis (MO): Saunders; 2011.

14. Sheridan MS. The deceit continues: an updated literature review of Munchausen Syndrome by Proxy. Child Abuse Negl 2003;27(4):431–51.

15. Thomasgard M, Metz WP. The vulnerable child syndrome revisited. J Dev Behav Pediatr 1995;16:47–53.

16. Quartana PJ, Campbell CM, Edwards RR. Pain catastrophizing: a critical review. Expert Rev Neurother 2009;9(5):745–58.

17. Bass C, Glaser D. Early recognition and management of fabricated or induced illness in children. Lancet 2014;383(9926):1412–21.

18. Emanuel EJ, Fuchs VR. The perfect storm of overutilization. JAMA 2008;299(23):2789–91.

19. Feudtner C, Blinman TA. The pediatric surgeon and palliative care. Semin Pediatr Surg 2013;22(3):154–60.

20. Mash C, Frazier T, Nowacki A, et al. Development of a risk-stratification tool for medical child abuse in failure to thrive. Pediatrics 2011;128(6):e1467–73.

21. Awadallah N, Vaughan A, Franco K, et al. Munchausen by proxy: a case, chart series, and literature review of older victims. Child Abuse Negl 2005;29(8):931–41.

22. Doughty K, Rood C, Patel A, et al. Neurological Manifestations of Medical Child Abuse. Pediatr Neurol 2016;54:22–8.

23. Hall DE, Eubanks L, Meyyazhagan LS, et al. Evaluation of covert video surveillance in the diagnosis of Munchausen syndrome by proxy: lessons from 41 cases. Pediatrics 2000;105(6):1305–12.

24. Nowak CB. Recognition and prevention of child abuse in the child with disability. Am J Med Genet C Semin Med Genet 2015;169(4):293–301.

25. Bryk M, Siegel PT. My mother caused my illness: the story of a survivor of Münchausen by proxy syndrome. Pediatrics 1997;100(1):1–7.

Ending a Diagnostic Odyssey
Family Education, Counseling, and Response to Eventual Diagnosis

Donald Basel, MBBCh, Julie McCarrier, MS, CGC

KEYWORDS

- Diagnostic odyssey • Whole exome sequencing • Genetic counseling
- Variant calling • Categorical model for WES results disclosure
- Patient experiences-Case series

KEY POINTS

- Genomic sequencing is the diagnostic test of choice for families with undiagnosed or rare diseases seeking an explanation for their child's complex medical concerns.
- The concept of sequencing all of the known genes and grasping the enormity of the data generated within this process is challenging to comprehend for most physicians, let alone patients and families who have been struggling with a life-altering disease.
- The desire to find answers can easily bias interpretation of sequencing results, and thus the counseling process is designated to facilitate informed decision making and clearly set realistic expectations for possible outcomes.
- The patient case examples serve to highlight the various challenges and complexities encountered with the clinical application of genomic sequencing and to reflect some of the data that have been accrued during the past 5 years of clinical experience.

THE ODYSSEY

To end the odyssey, one must first understand the journey. This term diagnostic odyssey is used freely in the lay press and has been the subject of several recent publications in the scientific literature. Is the odyssey the legions of investigations undertaken by the health care providers in an attempt to define and diagnose the cause of the symptoms that brought the patient to medical attention? Is it the frustration of the person impacted and his or her family with the seeming futility of modern medicine, or the doctor shopping in an attempt to identify a provider who is able to listen and compute that the myriad of seemingly disparate symptoms are connected in some way? These encompass any individual odyssey that ends, not necessarily in

Department of Pediatrics, Medical College of Wisconsin, Children's Hospital of Wisconsin, 9000 West Wisconsin Avenue, MS 716, Milwaukee, WI 53226, USA
E-mail address: dbasel@mcw.edu

Pediatr Clin N Am 64 (2017) 265–272
http://dx.doi.org/10.1016/j.pcl.2016.08.017
0031-3955/17/© 2016 Elsevier Inc. All rights reserved.
pediatric.theclinics.com

treatment, but in defining the underlying cause. The average time taken to reach a diagnosis in a rare disease (typically defined as a disorder affecting <1 person in 2000) is 6 years, requiring multiple visits to health care providers.

The advent of massively parallel sequencing has enabled genomic sequencing technologies to be used to identify rare and previously undiagnosed diseases and is a real game changer for modern diagnostics. This article explores the process of how patients initially engage with this technology and how the outcomes impact their ongoing ability to cope with illness and disease and explore the range of feelings and reactions that may arise.

GENETIC COUNSELING

Genetic counseling is the process of helping people understand and adapt to the medical, psychological, and familial implications of genetic contributions to disease".[1] Families with undiagnosed or rare diseases are often on a diagnostic odyssey seeking an explanation for their child's illness. For these patients, genomic sequencing, either whole-exome sequencing (WES) or whole-genome sequencing (WGS), is the diagnostic test of choice. Currently the majority of genomic sequencing relates to WES, and further discussion will focus on this technology. Genetic counseling is warranted in these cases to facilitate informed consent, discuss key parental concerns, and explore the patient/family experience surrounding the consent process and results disclosure for WES.

Identifying realistic expectations of WES is a critical part of obtaining informed consent. There is often a misunderstanding that if all the genes are sequenced, the answer to the ailments will be revealed. However, WES may only provide such an answer in a quarter to a third of analyses despite most all participants hoping that it is the final step in their diagnostic journey.[2] Genetic counseling for WES requires educating the patient or family about the test and implications, as well as working with families to facilitate informed decision making. This process can be cognitively and emotionally taxing. Families are presented with complex possibilities, predictions, and uncertainty and asked to make sophisticated comparisons between the benefits and limitations of testing.

Uncertainty or limitations of medical and scientific information, the clinical utility of treatment or preventative care, and even consideration of trade-off between risk and benefit are key elements of discussion during the counseling for consideration of clinical WES testing. Given that all individuals interpret and react to uncertainty differently, how the individual patient/family deals with stress and coping must be taken into consideration. Uncertainty may differ for each family. For many families, this may include clinical symptoms the patient experienced, the treatment decisions at hand, and concern for the health of additional family members. It also includes the potential of a molecular diagnosis, lack of a molecular diagnosis, and the likelihood of finding an undesired or uncertain molecular result.

There are some common questions and concerns that may arise during informed consent for WES, including the chance of the test providing a diagnosis, privacy and confidentiality of the test result(s) and data, impact on other family members, the anticipated response to results, insurance discrimination, and the impact of results on the patient's medical management. Common misperceptions include that a negative result excludes a genetic diagnosis, that the laboratory report will include numerous secondary or incidental findings, and that the test will provide a diagnosis.[3] Patients and families who have elected to know incidental findings from WES often express disappointment when the report is negative.

Results from WES are classified into 2 main categories: primary results and secondary results or incidental findings. Testing can yield positive or negative results, or variants of uncertain significance. Primary results are likely pathogenic changes felt to be responsible for the phenotype investigated. Secondary results are likely unrelated to the phenotype under investigation, felt to cause disease/risk, or greatly modify risk for disease.

A categorical model for results disclosure (**Figs. 1** and **2**) is used to establish a cognitive framework for patients/parents, who have the option to choose the results that they would like to receive based on category:

- Primary result: likely pathogenic DNA variants felt to be responsible for the phenotype investigated
- Secondary result: DNA variants likely unrelated to the phenotype under investigation
- Medically actionable: variant in a gene where knowledge of the particular variant will affect medical decision making such as initiation of a treatment
- Not medically actionable: variant(s) that increase an individual's risk for disease where no treatment is proven to significantly change medical decision making

From a population of 139 WES cases, 37 patients (26.6%) declined to know any incidental findings; 70 patients (50.4%) elected to know untreatable childhood onset conditions, and 78 patients (56.1%) elected to know treatable adult onset conditions. Fifty-eight patients (41.7%) elected to know untreatable adult onset conditions, and 79 patients (56.8%) elected to know carrier statuses (**Table 1.**).

The categorical model for results disclosure is unique from the laboratory standard used for molecular variant calling, which was established in 2015 for the determination of the relevance of a specific variation detected on sequencing.

This classification system is based on the likelihood that a variant is (or is not) associated with the phenotype in question. The specific variant modifiers used are as follows: (i) pathogenic, (ii) likely pathogenic, (iii) uncertain significance, (iv) likely benign, or (v) benign. The details for deriving these designations is beyond the scope of this discussion but is clearly defined by Richards and colleagues.[4] The highest level of patient misunderstanding and frustration centers around the subgroup (iii): variants of unknown significance (VUS). These are neither clearly disease associated nor more likely to be benign and thus insignificant in the context of the ongoing quest. There is often a desire for these to be causative, and they are frequently misinterpreted as such when relaying the medical history to other providers. This can also be challenging for providers who are not familiar with genomic medicine; thus the role of the genomics team is to ensure clear communication of these results with both the patient and his or her providers.

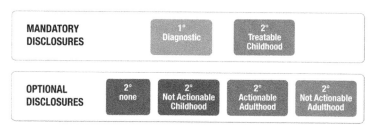

Fig. 1. WES results categories. Mandatory primary results and optional secondary results categories.

Patient Choices for Incidental Findings

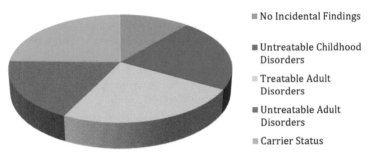

- ■ No Incidental Findings
- ■ Untreatable Childhood Disorders
- ■ Treatable Adult Disorders
- ■ Untreatable Adult Disorders
- ■ Carrier Status

Fig. 2. Secondary/incidental findings choices by percentage. Graphic representation of choices for incidental findings during WES counseling.

Patient Experiences—Case Series

The following quote is taken from the public blog of Yoni Maisel (http://www.primary-immunodeficiency.com/blog/genomics-the-psychology-of-the-rare-disease-diagnostic-odyssey):

> I wept openly in the offices of two physicians - the occasions being when each of my Rare Disease diagnoses were presented to me. The first occasion was in 2006 when told I had CVID, a 1 in 25 to 50,000 genetic disorder of the immune-system, the second, when diagnosed with the even more rare Sweet's Syndrome in 2011, making me only the second case in medical literature of having the two disorders at the same time.

These stories, filled with raw emotion, are becoming more abundant in the public media and are the key driver for patients, parents, and their health care providers for seeking out the availability of this newer diagnostic tool.

Known Diagnosis

Patient A presented to the hospital with fever, urinary incontinence, and cold extremities, with onset of symptoms the week prior to admission. The child had a long history of complex neurologic disease of unknown etiology with onset of symptoms at age 2 years, and was followed by multiple specialty clinics. The child had a history of paresis predominantly of the upper extremities, truncal muscles, and diaphragm, and had a slow decline over almost a decade. The child was initially thought to

Table 1
Secondary/incidental findings decision making

Secondary/Incidental Findings Choices	Percent of Patients
No incidental findings	26.6
Untreatable childhood disorders	50.4
Treatable adult disorders	56.1
Untreatable adult disorders	41.7
Carrier status	56.8

Data reflecting individual choices for WES outcomes.

have a transverse myelitis and then thought to have a chronic dysimmune neuropathy. The progression from upper to lower extremities appeared to be halted by steroids and intravenous immune globulin, and then stabilized over several years, with gradual decline in functionality and sudden worsening of symptoms. The current episode of acute or chronic weakness was thought to represent natural progression of disease versus relapse of disease versus worsening due to acute illness. Extensive genetic testing was nondiagnostic; metabolic workup was negative, and neurologic testing did not yield a definitive diagnosis. Family history was uninformative. WES was undertaken, and results confirmed a diagnosis of an autosomal-recessive riboflavin transporter deficiency neuronopathy. Riboflavin treatment was initiated, and Patient A made some improvement. Parents were extremely appreciative that their diagnostic odyssey had come to an end and that a treatment existed. They expressed concern for Patient A's siblings, as onset of symptoms can vary from infancy to young adulthood, and they expressed sadness that a diagnosis had not been made sooner.

Variants of Uncertain Significance

Patient B has a complex medical history compatible with a diffuse small fiber neuropathy including postural orthostatic tachycardia syndrome, daily migraines, epigastric pain without esophagitis and with lactose intolerance, increased acid exposure on pH impedance, retrograde duodeno-gastric peristalsis of bile on esophagogastroduodenoscopy, postprandial nausea, CARP (confluent and reticulated papillomatosis of the skin), hypermobility syndrome, back pain, mild von Willebrand disease and platelet function defect, anxiety, and depression, with onset of symptoms at 12 years of age. Chronic constipation was diagnosed at age 2 years. Family history is significant for mother with joint pain, anxiety, and erythema nodosa. Because of chronic health concerns, Patient B was no longer able to compete at a high level in sports. The patient followed in numerous specialty clinics, and comprehensive workup was not diagnostic. The patient did not meet clinical criteria for a diagnosis of Ehlers Danlos syndrome (Beighton score of 3/9). WES – duo analysis was undertaken, and results showed 3 heterozygous variants of uncertain significance in RYR1, RYR2 (maternal), and SCN2A (maternal). Results of muscle biopsy, performed to evaluate for pathologic findings associated with the RYR1 VUS, and mitochondrial DNA analysis were nondiagnostic. Evaluation by an electrophysiology cardiologist to assess for catecholaminergic polymorphic ventricular tachycardia (CPVT) in regard to the RYR2 VUS was normal.

Although the family received appropriate pre and post-test genetic counseling and was informed of the approximately 32.5% diagnostic rate from WES, Patient B's parent has expressed extreme frustration at the lack of a diagnosis and has had great difficulty accepting that the variants identified on testing are inconclusive. Annual reanalysis of WES data was recommended.

Multiple Diagnoses

Patient C is a grade school student who was initially evaluated because of a history of CFTR-related metabolic syndrome (CRMS) and concern for a connective tissue disorder. Family history was concerning for a parent, grandparent, and sibling who all have similar symptoms suggestive of a connective tissue disorder. Previous testing of the CFTR gene revealed a pathogenic variant and a 5T variant. Patient C followed in multiple specialty clinics and had a history of weight gain, lack of increase of stature in a year, delayed bone age, body pains, hypermobility, gastrointestinal dysmotility, and fatigue, leading to concerns for a connective tissue disorder. A previous bone age study revealed Patient C was 4.2 standard deviations below the mean. The patient did not fit criteria for classical growth hormone (GH) deficiency, although a trial of

GH treatment was recommended since Patient C's sibling, who was thought to have the same genetic condition and had a history of adrenal insufficiency, GH deficiency, and central hypothyroidism, along with CRMS, had shown improvement on GH. Patient C's copper and ceruloplasmin levels were normal, and the periodontal type of Ehlers-Danlos syndrome or short stature, hyperextensibility, hernia, ocular depression, Rieger anomaly, and teething delay syndrome was considered. A specific underlying condition was thought to be causative of Patient C's symptoms and as directed connective tissue disorder testing was unlikely to be helpful, WES quad analysis was pursued in the hope of yielding a diagnosis for which other interventions could be proactively implemented.

Results of WES revealed 2 pathogenic variants in trans (1 variant from each parent), confirming a diagnosis of odontoonychodermal dysplasia (OODD) in the patient and sibling. The current associated features of OODD do not completely explain Patient C's history/presentation but do explain a significant portion of symptoms.

Patient C was also found to be heterozygous for a likely pathogenic POMC variant that was inherited from a parent, and was thought to be contributing to the adrenocorticotrohic hormone (ACTH) deficiency. The POMC gene is associated with autosomal-recessive adrenal insufficiency and obesity (proopiomelanocortin deficiency), which occurs at an early age. Affected individuals have low levels of ACTH and tend to have fair complexions and red hair. As WES can miss some types of pathogenic variants, it is possible Patient C and sibling have a second variant that was not detected through WES. Interestingly, both the POMC and WNT10A genes reside on chromosome 2, and it is thought that both children share the same parental alleles.

This case shows multiple layers of medical and diagnostic complexity. WES analysis did not identify a cause for the underlying connective tissue disorder but did identify that Patient C has a compound, multigenic phenotype, which in combination can explain many of the individual clinical concerns. This family struggles with the uncertainty of the variant for proopiomelanocortin deficiency, which remains a finding of interest. A second variant has yet to be identified.

Significant Secondary Results

Patient D was a preschooler with a history of unusual facial features, spasticity, developmental delay, and autism. An extensive genetic and metabolic work up was nondiagnostic, and therefore WES was performed in the hope of revealing a unifying diagnosis. Results of WES revealed that Patient D had a heterozygous likely pathogenic variant in the KAT6B gene that is associated with autosomal-dominant/recessive genitopatellar syndrome, Say-Barber-Biesecker variant of Ohdo syndrome. This variant was inherited from a parent. Additionally, a likely pathogenic variant was also identified in SHANK3, which is associated with autosomal-dominant Phelan-McDermid syndrome and other neurodevelopmental disorders/autism. The SHANK3 variant was not confirmed via Sanger sequencing, and as it was unconfirmed, the significance of this finding was unknown. The presence of a rare or novel variant in a dominant gene alone is insufficient to determine pathogenicity. The SHANK3 variant appeared to be de novo in Patient D. Confirmatory analysis of the SHANK3 variant at an outside laboratory was recommended (and results were negative).

At the time of informed consent for WES, Patient D's parents elected to know secondary results/incidental findings, including treatable adult-onset conditions. The patient was found to be heterozygous for a pathogenic variant in BRCA1, which was both surprising and concerning to the parents, although family history was significant for Patient D having a great aunt who passed away at a young age from breast cancer. Subsequently and unbeknownst to Patient D's parents, the great aunt's sibling (grandparent of Patient D) underwent genetic testing for BRCA1/2, and a pathogenic variant was identified. After the WES results disclosure appointment, Patient D's parent spoke to the grandparent who was a sibling of the patient's great aunt. The grandparent disclosed that genetic testing following the death of the aunt was positive for a pathogenic BRCA1 variant and s/he had elected at that time not to disclose test results to the family to avoid worrying or alarming relatives.

Because this information was now out in the open given Patient D's WES results, the patient's parent was now forced not only to comprehend this information, but also to consider the significant implications for personal health and medical management. It was recommended that the at-risk parent undergo single-site BRCA1 analysis to confirm the finding so that the result could become part of his or her own medical record. This case is an example of WES being nondiagnostic for the patient, but "Pandora's box" being opened, and the family having to address and deal with an unexpected secondary result that could have significant implications for family members. It also brings to light the complexities of intrafamilial communication and the risks associated with withholding of medical information due to the potential uncomfortable nature of addressing heritable information, as well as the presumption that the information will be negatively received, or cause fear, alarm, and anxiety within the family unit. Genetic counseling is crucial to assist families with navigating the complex issues that may arise with genetic testing.

The examples provided represent an insight into the complexities encountered with the clinical application of genomic sequencing in the practice of medicine. The uncovering of multiple diagnoses, modifiers of disease, and frequent lack of additional actionable data are commonplace, but regardless of the outcome, patients and parents generally express a deep sense of gratitude knowing that they have explored the diagnostic possibilities to the fullest capacity. The authors' experience has additionally demonstrated that there always needs to be some form of forward planning, either initiation of appropriate treatment recommendations or formulating next steps clearly so that the families are not left wondering what should or could happen next. The clinical utility of this testing has been demonstrated previously,[5–7] and given the rapid advancement of technology, whole-genome sequencing is anticipated to be the new standard of care in the near future. To accommodate this, the rules for variant calling and assignment will need to be robust in order to minimize unnecessary anxiety to patients and their families.

REFERENCES

1. Resta R, Biesecker BB, Bennett RL, et al. A new definition of genetic counseling: National Society of Genetic Counselors' task force report. J Genet Couns 2006;15: 77–83.
2. Tomlinson AN, Skinner D, Perry D, et al. "Not tied up neatly with a bow": professionals' challenging cases in informed consent for genomic sequencing. J Genet Couns 2016;25:62–72.
3. Bernhardt BA, Roche MI, Perry DL, et al. Experiences with obtaining informed consent for genomic sequencing. Am J Med Genet A 2015;167A:2635–46.
4. Richards S, Aziz N, Bale S, et al. Standards and guidelines for the interpretation of sequence variants: a joint consensus recommendation of the American College of Medical Genetics and Genomics and the Association for Molecular Pathology. Genet Med 2015;17:405–23.
5. Manolio TA, Chisholm RL, Ozenberger B, et al. Implementing genomic medicine in the clinic: the future is here. Genet Med 2013;15:258–67.

6. Valencia CA, Husami A, Holle J, et al. Clinical impact and cost-effectiveness of whole exome sequencing as a diagnostic tool: a pediatric center's experience. Front Pediatr 2015;3:67.
7. O'Donnell-Luria AH, Miller DT. A clinician's perspective on clinical exome sequencing [review]. Hum Genet 2016;135:643–54.

Index

Note: Page numbers of article titles are in **boldface** type.

A

Abatacept, for VEO-IBD, 154
Abdominal pain
    fever in, 220
    in Henoch-Schönlein purpura, 188–190
    in polyarteritis nodosa, 199
Abductive reasoning, 8–9
Abuse, child. *See* Medical child abuse and/or medical complexity.
Access center, 24–25
Acetretin, for interleukin-36 receptor antagonist deficiency, 116
Acne, in PAPA syndrome, 114–115
Acrodermatitis enteropathica, 47–48
Acute disseminated encephalomyelitis, 74–75
Acute inflammatory demyelinating polyradiculoneuropathy, 231–234
    differential diagnosis of, 237
    versus acquired peripheral neuropathy, 233–234
Acute intermittent porphyria, 247
Acute motor axonal neuropathy, 237
Acute motor-sensory axonal neuropathy, 238
ADAM gene, in VEO-IBD, 147, 149
Adaptive dysfunction, in intellectual disability, 132–133
Adenosine deaminase 2 deficiency, 119, 200–201
Adopted children, fever in, 211
Affective errors, 5–6
Agammaglobulinemia, X-linked, 150, 152
Aicardi-Goutières syndrome, 59–60, 83
Airway inflammation
    in granulomatosis with polyangiitis, 195–196
    in polyangiitis, 197–198
Albinism, oculocutaneous, 95–96
Alemtuzumab, for FHLH, 98
Alpers syndrome, 163
American College of Rheumatology classification of vasculitis, 186
Amino acids, in mitochondrial disease, 165
Amyloidosis
    in cryopyrinopathies, 52–53
    in tumor necrosis factor receptor-associated periodic syndrome, 117–118
Anakinra, 116, 154
Anemia, dyserythropoietic, in Majeed syndrome, 118
Angiitis, primary, 63–64, 82
    angiography-negative, 78

Pediatr Clin N Am 64 (2017) 273–290
http://dx.doi.org/10.1016/S0031-3955(16)41136-3
0031-3955/17

pediatric.theclinics.com

Moving?

Make sure your subscription moves with you!

To notify us of your new address, find your **Clinics Account Number** (located on your mailing label above your name), and contact customer service at:

Email: **journalscustomerservice-usa@elsevier.com**

800-654-2452 (subscribers in the U.S. & Canada)
314-447-8871 (subscribers outside of the U.S. & Canada)

Fax number: **314-447-8029**

Elsevier Health Sciences Division
Subscription Customer Service
3251 Riverport Lane
Maryland Heights, MO 63043

*To ensure uninterrupted delivery of your subscription, please notify us at least 4 weeks in advance of move.

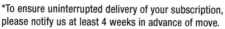

Printed and bound by CPI Group (UK) Ltd, Croydon, CR0 4YY

03/10/2024

01040398-0012